Atlanta's Living Legacy
A History of Grady Memorial Hospital and Its People

Martin Moran, M.D.

KIMBARK PUBLISHING, LLC
Atlanta, Georgia
2012

Published by
KIMBARK PUBLISHING, LLC
3180 West Paces Ferry Road
Atlanta, GA 30327
kimbarkpublishing.com

Copyright © 2012

All rights reserved. No part of this
publication may be reproduced, or
stored in a data base or retrieval
system, or transmitted, in any form
or by any means, without the prior
written permission of the Publisher.

Printed in the United States of America
on acid free paper

First Printing: September 2012
9 8 7 6 5 4 3 2 1

ISBN: 978-0-615-53009-3
LCCN: 2011940250

Designed by Esther Patrick

www.gradyhistory.com

To Harriet
and the memories of our parents

Introduction

Opened in 1892, Grady Memorial Hospital is one of the largest public hospitals in the United States. Located in the heart of Atlanta, Georgia, its campus is dominated by an imposing 23-story structure that holds nearly 1,000 beds and contains dozens of outpatient clinics. Snuggled tight against the Interstate 75-85 Connector that runs through the middle of the city, Grady has the only Level One Trauma Center in the sixth largest urban center in the United States.

The story of Grady hospital is complicated, made more so by its financial health depending for years on property taxes paid by the residents of Fulton and DeKalb counties—most of whom would never use the hospital. It has been a teaching hospital for medical students and a research institution from the start. Both have had a major impact on the practice of medicine in Georgia and around the world. Most importantly, Grady has been a safe haven for the unfortunate sick or injured who had no other place to receive care.

Because of its care for the indigent and the uninsured, Grady is often called Atlanta's safety net hospital. Significantly, however, it also has been a vital safety net for private hospitals throughout Atlanta, relieving them of many of the costs associated with caring for the indigent and the uninsured. But Grady has been much more than a safety net for individuals and institutions. Grady Hospital has trained approximately twenty-five percent of the physicians practicing in the state of Georgia and trained hundreds of others that practice in all 50 states and many that serve across the world.

It is a hospital that has impacted the lives of millions of individuals since its founding in 1892 and continues to do so. No hospital can be successful without dedicated staff and volunteers. Grady Memorial Hospital has been blessed with both. This is their story.

Contents

Introduction	iv
The Setting	3
Henry Woodfin Grady	21
A Living Monument	29
Building Patterns, 1892-1917	40
Building Dreams, 1918-1941	86
Expansions, 1942-1965	137
Desegregating the Gradys After World War II	169
Pioneers in Children's and Maternal Health	194
Expanding Grady as Georgia Grows, 1965 - 1989	199
The Whirlwind, 1990-2008	238
Into the Twenty-First Century	268
Acknowledgments	269
Selected Sources and Suggested Reading	270
Photo/Illustration Credits	273
Endnotes	274
Index	299

"I consider the Grady hospital the grandest institution that was ever founded in Atlanta. It will nurse the poor and rich alike and will be an asylum for the black and the white. ... Without money, the trustees can do nothing."

Captain James English,
Trustee, Grady Memorial Hospital, May 25, 1892.

"The Grady Hospital is the grandest and noblest institution in the city, and we should be proud of such an institution, maintain and support it. Hundreds of lives will be saved each year by this noble institution, for the fact, many wounds and diseases cannot be treated successfully unless we observe strict hygiene, cleanliness and proper nursing of the patient. It is impossible for hundreds of poor to afford this, [who] therefore die of septic wounds [when] their lives could have been saved in a properly kept hospital."

Report of the Relief Committee
Atlanta City Council, January 2, 1893

"What concerns me most, is my inability to take care of the City's sick as I should like to. Every day I am compelled to reject cases applying for admission, for the reason, that I have no beds, - [sic] a deplorable situation indeed."

Steve Johnston
Superintendent, Grady Memorial Hospital, February 3, 1920

"We don't neglect a single patient. ... We work to our utmost to save the life of every patient and we work to our utmost to get the full value out of every dollar. But, we never neglect one for the other."

Joseph Hines, M.D.
Medical Director, Grady Memorial Hospital, March 21, 1936

"Grady comes in close contact with every home in Atlanta through the public schools and domestic service in the home. Therefore, Grady's problems are your problems."

J. Moss Beeler, M.D.
Superintendent, Grady Memorial Hospital, November 9, 1939

"If politicians run the hospital, the quality of care will go to hell."

Manuel J. Maloof
Chairman, DeKalb County Board of Commissioners, April 21, 1988

"We took the patients no one else would take. And we were happy to have them."

J. W. "Bill" Pinkston
Chief Executive Officer, Grady Memorial Hospital, 1964 -1989, April 28, 2009

Atlanta's Living Legacy

Atlanta Medical College 1857-1906

Chapter 1

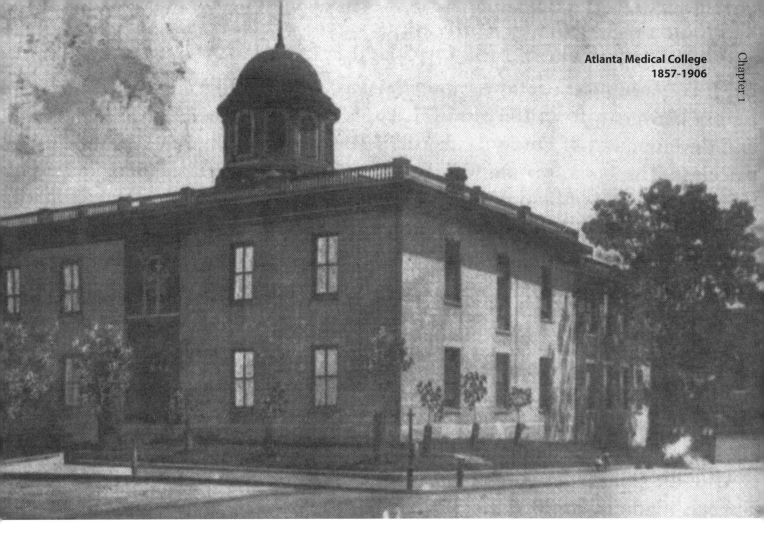

The Setting

It was an age when hospitals belonged in cities and the United States had relatively few of either. With 7,303 residents in 1830, Savannah, Georgia, was the 37th largest city in the nation. It also was home to one of the few hospitals in the country. Organized in 1804 to treat sick sailors, the Savannah Poor House and Hospital Society ran the only hospital in the state until 1818 when one was formed in Augusta to house that city's "sick poor." The two hospitals in Georgia, like those elsewhere in the United States, served people with nowhere else to turn. Usually these were sailors and other sojourners to a city, or residents without friends or family to care for them.

Upon entering the hospital, a new patient met a collection of cots in a large room called a ward. The people resting there were likely to be very poor and very ill. Linked in misery, patients of that era went to the hospital to convalesce or die rather than to receive a diagnosis or a cure. In short, most American hospitals amounted to little more than warehouses for the poor, hopeless cases in the city.[1]

In the 1830s, people living in central and western Georgia had little direct access to medical care. For them to reach a physician in a city or town often required a difficult and tedious journey by horseback. For the most part, people in the countryside relied on folk remedies until a circuit-riding doctor or midwife showed up. Even then, the ability to get competent medical help was mostly a matter of luck. A good physician or midwife was hard to find, even as the number of medical practitioners became more abundant.

> ### Medical Pioneers
>
>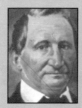
>
> Dr. Joshua Gilbert (1815-1889) is considered the first physician in Atlanta. He was a member of the city's first Board of Health. Dr. Gilbert is buried with his wife in the Utoy Church Cemetery in southwest Atlanta.
>
>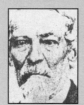
>
> Dr. Noel D'Alvigny (1800-1877) was born in France and arrived in Atlanta in 1848. The character of Dr. Mead in Margaret Mitchell's novel, *Gone with the Wind*, is rumored to have been based on Dr. D'Alvigny. He is buried in Atlanta's Oakland Cemetery.
>
>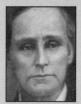
>
> Dr. John Westmoreland (1816-1887) was born in Monticello, Georgia, graduated from Augusta Medical College in 1843, and was elected to the state legislature in 1857. He also founded the Atlanta Medical College. Dr. Westmoreland is buried in Oakland Cemetery.

Concerned about the prevalence of "quacks" and a lack of professional standards, medical school graduates in Georgia, like many across the United States, wanted the government to regulate the practice of medicine. Until the states determined who could practice medicine (there were no national standards for defining either medical competency or acceptable levels of health care) the relatively few physicians who graduated from medical schools competed with midwives and doctors trained in an apprenticeship. Far from enjoying a lucrative career, the medical school graduates on Georgia's plains and hill country worked hard to eke out a living.[2] Eager to see as many people as possible, doctors roaming the countryside in the late 1830s would stay only briefly in small, start-up towns like Terminus, Georgia.

Set along a ridge where Appalachian foothills intersect with the Piedmont in the forest of northwest Georgia, little distinguished Terminus from other small communities in the area—except for its origins. Some towns in the Georgia countryside formed where ancient crossroads or the lay of the land offered an agreeable place for farmers, merchants, and others to socialize and trade. Other settlements grew up near rivers and streams where someone built a mill or set up a ferry. In the 1830s, a few towns sprang into being because Georgia's first railroads were being planned and built. Stretching from the Atlantic coast to developing farmlands in the center of the state, the railways spurred speculators to build up towns that would serve the roads and their customers. Terminus, however, was different. Instead of rising from the speculative dreams of entrepreneurs, it was established to satisfy Georgia's legislature.

Representatives from the Monroe and Georgia railroads led a convention in Macon, Georgia, in November 1836 to plan the creation of a publicly owned railroad. Running between the Tennessee River and DeKalb County, Georgia, the railway would connect Augusta and Savannah with the American West. A month later, William W. Gordon, who in addition to serving as president of the Central Rail Road and Banking Company also was a state representative from Savannah, sponsored a bill in Georgia's legislature to adopt the Macon convention's plan. Following the passage of Gordon's bill, the State of Georgia formed The Western & Atlantic Railroad of the State of Georgia.[3] Few of the forward-looking statesmen who legislated the railroad into being might have cared that the State of Georgia would continue to own the line into the 21st Century. They were focused on giving a huge boost to the state's economy (and its privately-owned railroads). Georgia's legislators, like other advocates of internal improvements in the United States—from the Cumberland Road to the Erie Canal—were bent on using public money to stimulate economic expansion.[4]

There were few railroads in the United States when the legislature gambled on building a rail line running to the Tennessee

River and past the headwaters of the Coosa River (which flows into the Gulf of Mexico).[5] The Western & Atlantic was an ambitious venture that depended on public financing; it would be one of only a handful of railroads in America to be owned and operated by a state government.[6] In 1837, Georgia's state legislature mapped out an endpoint for the railway. With creative energy apparently exhausted by laying out the Western & Atlantic, the railway workers simply referred to the end of the line as Terminus. It would take another five years for the railway to decide exactly where to place the terminal within the new village. By the time it did, the settlement, which consisted of a few buildings and about thirty residents, had been renamed Marthasville.[7] Even later that year when the first train ran between Marthasville and Marietta (fifteen miles to the northwest), the town was mostly a promise. Little had changed when the state legislature officially incorporated the hamlet in 1843.

Two years later, in 1845, regular rail service began between the town and Marietta. By then Marthasville had grown to 200 residents and was getting ready to welcome a second rail line. That summer, as Marthasville's promise of growth was being set in iron, Henry David Thoreau went homesteading along Walden Pond, President Polk saw to the annexation of the Republic of Texas, and the entire United States had a little more than 4,000 miles of railroad track. Late into a muggy September night, as summer turned toward autumn, for the first time the train cars of Marthasville's second rail line, the Georgia Railroad, steamed into town.[8] Amazingly, at that moment nearly four percent of the train track laid in the United States ended in tiny Marthasville, Georgia.[9]

Renamed Atlanta in December 1845, the village was flourishing. Perhaps railroads would turn the town into a great city; and why not? Trains were beginning to bring the world to Atlanta. While it would be another six years before the 137 miles of road to Chattanooga were completed, the arrival of the Georgia Railroad and improving financial conditions in 1845 helped brighten the area's prospects.[10]

Given the promise of a growing population, it made sense to believe that the end of the line would be a good place to start a practice of medicine. Undoubtedly the town's prospects for development (combined with the likelihood of a high number of accidents among railroad employees) attracted Dr. Joshua Gilbert to Atlanta. How else could the recent graduate of Augusta Medical College (which later became the Medical College of Georgia) have seen a village of two hundred people as a place of promise? (It may have helped that his brother, also a physician, lived fairly close by.)

The town's first physician, Dr. Gilbert hung out his shingle in the summer of 1845; by the end of the year a second physician, Dr. Stephen Terry Biggers, a graduate of a medical school in Macon, opened an office in Atlanta.[11] Within two years, the town's population quintupled to over one thousand residents. As Atlanta swelled from hundreds to thousands of residents, more doctors came. Considering the town's growth and the rising number of physicians, it seems reasonable to expect that someone would start thinking about building a hospital in the area. After all, Atlanta was beginning to look like a city.

Necessity rather than civic ambition or foresight sired Atlanta's first hospital. In July 1853, eight years after Dr. Gilbert established his practice, a smallpox epidemic hit the area. To limit the outbreak, the town isolated the afflicted at a special facility located at the fairgrounds on Fair Street, slightly southwest of Oakland Cemetery. When the smallpox outbreak ended, so did the community's first sickbay.[12]

Even with its rapid growth, Atlanta was still far from reaching the size or significance of Cincinnati or Memphis, much less St. Louis. With 2,572 residents in 1850, Atlanta barely qualified as a city. (It topped the census bureau's definition of a city by 72 residents.) Four years after the census, and one year after the smallpox outbreak, physicians in Atlanta launched a venture common to communities with grand ambitions—an institution of higher learning.[13]

The city's first medical school, Atlanta Medical College was organized in 1854. Originally the college faculty borrowed space at city hall (when it was available) to give their lectures. The school first held classes in its own building in May 1857.[14] A short stroll down the hill from Peachtree Street, the college's new facilities featured a short-term residence for ill patients. This infirmary made it easy for the school's faculty members to treat patients in a ward near their offices. A convenience for physicians and their patients, the small infirmary was a crucial part of the business of medical education since medical schools needed access to patients in order for professors to teach and students to learn. At a time of intense competition between medical schools, when students actively sought institutions that had an ample supply of patients, Atlanta Medical College's success was closely tied to that of its infirmary.[15]

Unlike hospitals, infirmaries were part of an enterprise that was supposed to be financially profitable—the proprietary medical school. Patients at the Atlanta Medical College's infirmary were charged for room and board (15 cents per day) in addition to fees for treatment. While satisfaction was not guaranteed, sometimes the infirmary's physicians waived their consultation charges. For example, the Atlanta Medical College promised slave-owners that treatment for a slave would be free if the patient was not cured.[16] In addition to being a source of income, patients were used in teaching demonstrations.[17] In contrast to the medical college's infirmary, up until the Civil War most American hospitals treated charity patients; they were rarely available for teaching. Simply put, at the time infirmaries and hospitals served different constituencies and had different ambitions.

For most of the nineteenth century Americans saw hospitals as little more than temporary housing for the impoverished who were ill. Often owned by religious groups or voluntary societies, and sometimes by a city government, hospitals generally were non-profit institutions with civic and philanthropic aims. They improved public welfare by offering a place of healing to those who could not help themselves. In doing so, hospitals helped establish access to care for all as a defining virtue of American city culture.[18]

To provide the poor with care, nineteenth-century American hospitals depended on volunteerism. Countless guilds of civic-minded women raised money, furnished buildings, visited the sick, brought flowers,

Atlanta Medical College

The state granted a charter to the city's first medical school, the Atlanta Medical College, in 1854. A year later, on June 21, 1855, the school's officials laid the cornerstone for their own building at Butler Street and Jenkins Street (now Armstrong Street). Elected to the legislature two years later, the school's founder, Dr. John Westmoreland, used his political seat to obtain funding from the State of Georgia for the private institution. The school closed during the Civil War but its facilities remained open to allow physicians and nurses to treat casualties from the battlefield.

In 1864, as intense fighting neared Atlanta, the hospital was overwhelmed with wounded and dying men (a scene dramatically depicted in the film version of *Gone With the Wind*). Medical school faculty member Dr. Noel D'Alvigny, a 64-year-old surgeon, remained in the city during the Battle of Atlanta. When General Sherman's federal troops captured Atlanta in September 1864, all of the city's physicians were ordered to leave except Dr. D'Alvigny. He soon became a prisoner of the Union Army but continued with his practice, caring for both Northern and Southern soldiers. When Union troops began burning the city, D'Alvigny misled them in order to spare Atlanta Medical College from the torch. (The building survived until it was demolished by the wrecking ball in 1906.)

and spread cheer. At the urging of clergy and colleagues, leading businessmen made crucial financial gifts to keep the buildings together and pay for supplies. Charity hospitals also depended on the good graces of volunteer medical staff to treat patients at no charge, a crucially important philanthropy that helped both patients and doctors.

Physicians began seeking appointment to non-paying positions on a hospital's staff as a way to gain professional status. In the absence of other official recognition, being associated with a hospital could help a doctor's reputation. This was because the philanthropists who funded hospitals tended to guard their institutions from incompetent physicians—not only for the common good but also to protect their own reputations. Because the self-appointed doctor peddling various quack tonics and cures was unlikely to be associated with a hospital, being named to a hospital's staff quickly became a mark of public confidence in a physician. Significantly, the doctors' efforts, like those of American hospitals, reflected a charitable commitment to the common good. While the poor in the nineteenth century turned to hospitals for help, the middle class had a different story.

Through the nineteenth century, middle class Americans preferred to be treated in the comfort of their own home. Settled in familiar surroundings, they hired private caretakers to attend to daily needs and relied on their physician for house calls. Being at home offered a quieter, more restful space in which to heal. Convalescing in one's own castle also offered greater privacy than being in a crowded hospital ward with a dozen or more patients in an open room. Lack of privacy may have been worth the sacrifice if hospitals had provided diagnostic equipment or medical remedies that one could not get at home—but hospitals offered no such benefit.[19] With nothing to gain and much to lose, the middle class stayed away.

The Civil War helped alter popular attitudes toward hospitals, primarily by changing their character. Until then, hospitals were filthy, smelly, and chaotic. In the war, hospitals were cleaner and better managed.

Support for a "Free Hospital"

Among the earliest evidence for an effort to start a charity hospital in Atlanta is a notice published in the *New York Times* late in 1866. Seven prominent New Yorkers including Henry Ward Beecher, the most renowned preacher in the United States, and the prominent journalist Horace Greeley signed a letter supporting the effort of Dr. J. W. Wood to raise money for a "Free Hospital" in Atlanta. They intended to help the people of Georgia recuperate from their suffering during "the late war." The proposed institution would attend to "all residents and strangers, irrespective of color or condition." The article noted that contributions could be sent to Robert W. Lowry of the National Bank of the Republic located at the corner of Wall Street and Broadway. The funds deposited there would be forwarded to Mr. John Rice, president of the Georgia National Bank in Atlanta.

To treat the many casualties (and, more often, soldiers suffering fever or dysentery), hospitals were forced to be better organized and more efficient. The massive influx of patients led military hospitals to order, store, and dispense enormous quantities of medicine, bandages, bedding, food, and other supplies as no single hospital had earlier. The war brought other big changes to hospitals. By adopting the sanitary reforms that Florence Nightingale popularized after the Crimean War ended in 1856, Civil War military hospitals reduced the spread of infections between patients. Improved ventilation and more effective waste removal helped push military hospital mortality rates drastically downward; they fell to below ten percent.[20]

The war affected popular attitudes toward hospitals in a second way: it led a large number of middle class women, most of them for the first time, to volunteer in hospitals.[21] During the war they cared for people from a broad range of backgrounds—rich and poor, urban and rural, laborers and gentlemen. It was the first time American hospitals treated citizens from all social ranks.

The Civil War forced people in the North and South to face injury, illness, and death on a scale they had never known before.[22] With the arrival of wounded soldiers, Atlantans turned almost any space they could find into a hospital. Schools, churches, and other large buildings became makeshift hospitals for injured and ill soldiers.[23] The sheer number of people requiring medical attention, and the enormous number of recently created hospitals calling for sanitary supplies and other necessities, pushed the community to organize and cooperate in distributing medical care.

At the onset of the Civil War almost 10,000 people called Atlanta home. Less than half as large as Savannah, Atlanta was only one-sixteenth the size of St. Louis, the largest American city west of Pittsburgh. Although smaller than the nation's biggest cities, the railroad junction was a bona fide boomtown when the unpleasantness between North and South broke into open hostilities. During the war the city became a magnet for refugees from the hinterlands, an arms-maker to the Confederacy, and an important center for shipping goods.

Decimated by General Sherman on his destructive march to the sea, Atlanta rebuilt quickly after the war; its population mushroomed from several thousand residents when Robert E. Lee laid down his sword at Appomattox to 20,288 inhabitants two years later.[24] As Atlanta grew during Reconstruction, the city began a few public works projects. By the early 1870s it was building a municipally owned waterworks and a sewer system to serve the central business district and adjoining white upper class and middle class neighborhoods.[25]

In 1873, the city council appointed a committee "to make arrangements for establishing immediately a temporary or permanent hospital in the city."[27] The effort was soon stymied as the Panic of 1873 upended city finances.

Because it shared the low-tax consensus common to American cities, and because the municipal government was deeply in debt for a decade after the Panic of 1873, Atlanta had little money to spend on a hospital much less on sanitary improvements, clean water, or waste disposal during the 1870s. Reform of the city charter in 1874 was designed to keep public spending low by forcing the city to pay for its debt and public works from current income. It also required that residents approve the issue of public bonds through a referendum. With limited resources and an ideology favoring low taxes, the city chose to focus its public improvements on the central business district area.[26] This meant that water service and sewers would be denied to most of the city's neighborhoods. While municipal programs that would have improved public health stalled, medical care for Atlanta's indigent began to evolve.

In 1874, as the city charter was being rewritten, a group of prominent women led by Mrs. William Tuller organized the Atlanta Benevolent Home. Neither an almshouse nor a hospital, the benevolent home was designed to provide a place for indigent white women and children.[28]

Started on a shoestring, the benevolent home suffered financial trouble from the start. Relying on fairs, rummage sales, donations from churches, and on pledges paid out in monthly installments of 25 cents, the home raised much of its original funding by gathering nickels and dimes. While most of the financial support came from private sources, the city contributed the final $700 of the $4,500 needed to purchase a facility for the home. Even with the city's help, the home was seriously underfunded.

Two years after the founding of the benevolent home, the city council created a new committee to analyze Atlanta's need for a hospital.[29] In short order the Atlanta Benevolent Home and the Atlanta Medical College, whose infirmary had grown to thirty beds, issued competing proposals.[30] To analyze them, the council's hospital committee dutifully surveyed what was being done in cities of similar size, including Mobile, Nashville, Charleston, Memphis, and Worcester, Massachusetts.[31] While the council was working on its study, the women who ran the benevolent home and the men who owned

Atlanta Medical College joined forces to create a unified proposal.³² Still, the council kept investigating.

Presenting its report early in May, the council's committee acknowledged that a hospital would "prevent and arrest the spread of disease." In that way, a hospital would aid everyone in the city. While it believed a hospital would "indirectly benefit all classes," the committee felt it would be "by far the greatest blessing to the poor and indigent." In its report, the city council's committee indicated that Atlanta needed a hospital to provide for "victims of disease and accident" with "scanty means" who otherwise would not receive "the care and comfort to which they are entitled by the ordinary dictates of humanity." Although in favor of creating a hospital, the council committee was wary of putting politicians in charge; it preferred that a private group operate a charity hospital "free from the manipulations of politicians."³³

The distinction between private and public, however, was somewhat blurry since the committee claimed that city taxes could be used to acquire land and buildings for the "private" institution. To be governed by seven trustees, the envisioned hospital would do more than make the prosperous feel good about attending to the poor. The hospital and its benefactors would benefit every citizen since having a hospital was expected to lessen spending on private doctors. Terming hospitals "an expression of Christian philanthropy," the committee emphasized that the institution would help patients and their families without robbing them of "self-respect, or self-reliance." While arguing for the need, the committee believed acquiring a site, erecting buildings, and forming a "model institution" required more money than the cash-strapped city could afford. This provided another reason to leave the creation of a charity hospital in private hands.

While there was strong support for organizing a hospital, opposition to the movement carried the day. The *Daily Constitution* explained a few weeks later, "the fact that Atlanta is subject to no epidemic, except small pox, partially accounts for the singular want of a public hospital." Having a salubrious city, however, was only one argument against the hospital. The fears of attracting paupers to Atlanta and of increasing city expenditures seemed to be more powerful reasons for resistance. The *Daily Constitution,* which supported creating a charity hospital, claimed those who feared the hospital would attract paupers failed to understand the difference between a hospital and a poorhouse. The *Daily Constitution* saw no "reason why Atlanta should continue to be the only city of 30,000 inhabitants in the country that has no hospital." It also rejected predictions of added expense and, by implication, higher taxes. Indeed, the *Daily Constitution* argued that having a hospital would be more cost-effective (and humane) than existing forms of care.³⁴

Although the city did not fund a hospital in 1876, the council committee, Atlanta Benevolent Home, and Atlanta Medical College all saw the need, if not the means, to create a city hospital. In the context of financial stringency, Atlanta's leaders continued to struggle with how to provide charity care. Two years after the city council rejected a public hospital, an event beyond anyone's control seemed to provide ammunition to people who claimed Atlanta didn't need a hospital.

As it became a leading city of the South after the Civil War, Atlanta cultivated the unusual status of being a healthy city. In the nineteenth century, Americans usually considered cities to be unhealthy—which they were. Crowded and filthy, cities like New York, New Orleans, and Chicago were associated with high rates of disease and early death. By the 1870s, however, Atlanta was developing a reputation for being a healthy city.³⁵ Its standing would be enhanced when the biggest medical scourge to hit the South in years bypassed Atlanta.

The Great Mississippi River Basin Yellow Fever Epidemic of 1878 hit the region hard. The best estimates indicate the fever infected 120,000 people in the Mississippi River Basin; approximately 20,000 people died in the epidemic. The fever struck cities with special force. Five thousand, one hundred-fifty people died from the fever in Memphis. Nearly 4,000 died in New Orleans. Many smaller towns also suffered enormous loss of life.[36]

Fearing for their health and safety, many people across the area fled to escape the storm of illness. By some strange fate, the scourge barely touched Atlanta; six cases entered the city and only one death occurred. Although the *Daily Constitution* and others had pushed for sanitary reform well before the yellow fever first appeared that summer in New Orleans (by way of Cuba and Brazil), it took the epidemic's threat to prompt Atlanta to implement precautionary sanitary reforms—which it did with vigor.[37] Frantic once the epidemic became known, Atlanta's civic leaders became obsessed with keeping the city clean. Anticipating that ill refugees would descend on the city, Atlanta built a special hospital on the outskirts of town to greet them. Opened in September, it was barely needed and soon closed. Civic leaders took the city's freedom from the epidemic as proof of its immunity to such illnesses. The *Daily Constitution* interpreted the city's good fortune as simply natural: "the atmosphere of Atlanta is not only a preventive [for yellow fever], but a cure for the disease."[38]

In addition to missing the epidemic, Atlanta escaped the economic hardships that the contagion inflicted elsewhere. The city's boosters grasped the situation with alacrity. It was easy to notice the sharp contrast between Atlanta's commercial prosperity and the economic doldrums that infected areas where the epidemic raged.[39] Seeing a close link between prosperity and public health, civic leaders hoped to begin protecting their city from potential outbreaks of disease.[40] This makes it easy to understand why important public health and sanitary reforms began attracting interest from Atlanta's business and civic leaders.[41]

Although the city had developed a few municipal services earlier in the 1870s, the yellow fever epidemic prompted business leaders to ask the municipal government for more. They hoped the city would extend access to clean water, fix drainage problems, begin regulating garbage disposal, and provide privy maintenance. When first implemented, the reforms were limited to the central business district and adjacent white neighborhoods. Within this limited sanitary district, which mirrored the fire district, four night soil wagons made rounds twice a week. In 1880, the first year that the sanitary service in the center of the city got underway, only one-fifth of the privies in the city were cleaned. Because the city lacked an official disposal site, workers were free to empty the carts wherever it was convenient outside of the sanitary district.[42]

The desire for sanitary improvements led the city to look for more money to spend on infrastructure and public services. At the same time, however, the lingering economic depression, the city's debt, and the restrictions that the city charter imposed all helped limit spending on sanitary improvements. With more than half of the city's tax revenue—which stayed flat during the latter 1870s despite a growing population—devoted to debt repayment, paying for sanitary improvements seemed to require imaginative solutions.[43] As it turned out, Atlanta's future would be financed by a system long used in other American cities.

The effort of Mayor James W. English to modernize Atlanta's infrastructure and services during his term in 1881 and 1882 required him to find more money. Hamstrung by the city charter, Mayor English moved the city toward financing public improvements with a fee-for-services model. In Atlanta, public improvements had long been paid for out of general funds and by floating public bonds that all of the taxpayers subsidized. Under Mayor English's model, the adjoining property owners would pay for two-thirds of the cost for street and sewer improvements. While special assessments had been common in American cities for decades, a large number of affected residents in Atlanta, encouraged by newspapers like the *Atlanta Journal*, sued the city to stop it from levying new taxes for public works.[44]

The broad public support for improving public health that emerged with the Yellow Fever epidemic seemed to wane within a few years. Certainly the business community's anxiety about potential outbreaks did little to turn public health into the city's highest priority. Civic leaders kept boasting that Atlanta was a naturally healthy city. Despite some reform efforts during the 1880s, in Atlanta during those years, as the historian John H. Ellis concluded, "health matters never occupied the place in public consciousness that they achieved in New Orleans and Memphis, so ingrained was the myth of local vitality."[45]

The business district and wealthier adjoining neighborhoods gained more (and sooner) from public sanitary improvements than did other parts of the city.[46] White neighborhoods closer to the core of the city benefited from better sewage and drainage. The white working class tended to live farther from the center of the city, and, as a result, was slower to benefit from municipal improvements like paved streets and a sewage system. Black communities, usually occupying low-lying areas, received very little except the run-off from white neighborhoods. Black areas lacked a sewer system and access to clean drinking water; their drinking wells were polluted by fecal runoff that swept through the neighborhoods during heavy rainstorms. Most of the streets in the city's overcrowded and filthy black neighborhoods were as dreary as the living quarters were squalid.[47]

While sanitary improvements remained limited in the first years after the epidemic, Atlanta's medical institutions began to grow up alongside its commercial interests.

In the first twelve years after the Great Mississippi Basin Yellow Fever Epidemic, from 1878 to 1890, three major hospitals, three specialized infirmaries, three medical schools, and several smaller medical institutions opened in the city.[48] A pair of physicians opened The Taliaferro and Noble Infirmary, dedicated to "diseases of women," in 1883. The same year the National Surgical Institute opened on East Alabama Street. Led by Drs. Kells Boland and Charles Wilson, the facility responded to the need to treat diseases and deformities not usually seen or treated by physicians. The institute included a workshop for making body braces and other appliances needed in the treatment of patients.[49] Two years later, in 1885, another group of surgeons began the Atlanta Surgical Infirmary on Marietta Street. Nearly all of these were proprietary, for-profit institutions. While these began to take off as the city regained prosperity in the 1880s, non-profit charity institutions seemed to struggle.

The Atlanta Benevolent Home continued to have trouble finding solid financial footing. Finally, at the end of 1880, the women who ran the home, and whose husbands were part of Atlanta's civic leadership—including Mrs. Henry Holcombe Tucker, Mrs. C. C. Rhodes, Mrs. A. O. Adair, and Mrs. John Milledge—gave their charity baby over to an all-male board of trustees. In doing so, they explicitly provided that the home would be nonsectarian and its board of trustees religiously diverse, consisting of a representative from each of several Protestant denominations plus a Roman Catholic and a Jew.[50] The new board of trustees included two former mayors and one of the city's leading businessmen, Samuel Inman. They were among Atlanta's most prosperous citizens and at the heart of the city's social leadership. Despite their guidance, the Atlanta Benevolent Home continued to have difficulty raising enough money.

Led by the Reverend Doctor Henry Holcombe Tucker, a former chancellor of the University of Georgia and one of the most influential Baptist preachers in the South, the new board of trustees extended the institution's service to the "sick and destitute and all who need a home." The women who had run the home remained ambitious. Even as they gave up control, they continued to believe that the home's purpose would "be reached when it is managed only as a hospital for the benefit of the city."[51] A few days after the new board took over, the city agreed that the benevolent home could run a hospital out of a house on Alabama Street.[52] Paid $75 per month by the city, the benevolent home would treat all of the white patients that the city's ward physicians sent for hospitalization. In order to provide this service, the benevolent home relied on volunteer medical service from physicians. This was a form of charity expected of reputable physicians; the public assumed it to be part of the doctor's vocation. To pay a physician for treating charity patients would never have crossed anyone's mind. Yet even with this free care, the benevolent home continued to struggle financially.

Their view of humanity may help explain why the city's white commercial and civic leaders left the benevolent home to run on a shoestring budget. Atlanta's white business leadership was made up of men who began coming of age at the same time that the Old South yelled its first battle cry. In the Civil War's wake, these sons of farmers rued the apparent loss of the region's economic system. They looked down their noses at blacks as inferior and viewed the region's poor whites as lazy, hopeless cases. If the city's civic leaders had believed in Darwinian evolution, they would have seen poor whites as having little capacity to adopt the skills and habits needed for long-term survival. Respecting neither poor whites nor most blacks, the city's white civic leaders seemed to reject any democratic dogma that would have required them to believe in the essential dignity of every human being. They would have viewed such an idea as being at odds with human reality. More than that, the democratic idea conflicted with the society they were building. Despite their parsimony, these prominent people saw the support they gave to the home as a sign of their concern for their fellow man.

Atlanta's local government practiced charity with similarly measured generosity. For example, in 1886, the city reimbursed the Atlanta Benevolent Home at the miniscule rate of a fraction over 16 cents per patient per day.[53] Even as the benevolent home struggled, new houses of healing were being planned for the growing city.

Some of Atlanta's new medical facilities were started because religiously devoted people wanted to live out their faith by bringing comfort and healing to the sick. In the same year that the women from the Atlanta

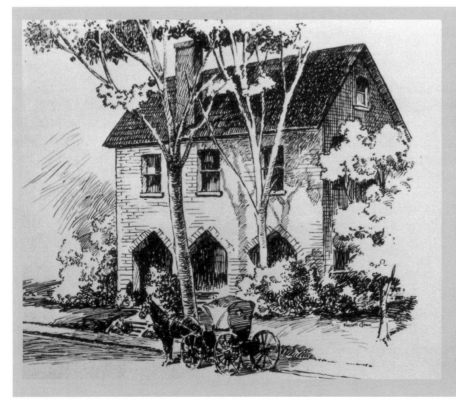

St. Joseph's Infirmary was started in 1880 by four Sisters of Mercy from Savannah, Georgia, in a ten-room house at 210 North Collins Street. The community immediately embraced the institution.

Benevolent Home gave its institutional reins to a group of men, four nuns from Savannah who belonged to the Sisters of Mercy came to Atlanta to care for the city's sick. Arriving in 1880 with very little money and few earthly goods, they made up for their sorry finances with an abundance of compassion and determination. None of the sisters had formal medical training; they were teachers. It may not have mattered greatly if any of the sisters understood medicine; they moved to Atlanta to establish a sanitarium, not a medical practice.

Led by the indomitable Sister Cecilia, the nuns purchased a two-story brick house (at the corner of Baker and North Collins Streets) and quickly adapted the space for their needs. Local physicians including Drs. Abner W. Calhoun, James J. Knott, and Charles R. Upton provided medical service. Other distinguished physicians, including Drs. Joseph P. Logan, James F. Alexander, and Charles Pinckney served on the medical advisory board for the hospital. Dedicating the facility (it had ten beds) on April 21, 1880, the nuns from Savannah named it for the city they would serve. A year later the sisters changed its name from Atlanta Hospital to St. Joseph's Infirmary. Started when there were few other medical facilities in the city, it offered an especially bright beacon of hope.[54]

In 1883, the leaders of Atlanta's second medical school, the Southern Medical College (formed in 1878), helped spur a group of philanthropic white women to create Central Ivy Street Hospital. A pioneer institution in Atlanta, Ivy Street became the first hospital in the city to accept black patients and to treat emergency cases. More than that, Ivy Street set an important precedent in making emergent care available to the poorest people. The women who organized the hospital soon turned it over to an all-male board of trustees. Their transfer agreement mandated that Southern Medical College control Ivy Street's medical services and that the college's faculty be allowed to use the facility for private patients. In addition, the college's physicians were to treat the indigent at no cost to the patients. To cover the cost of treating them,

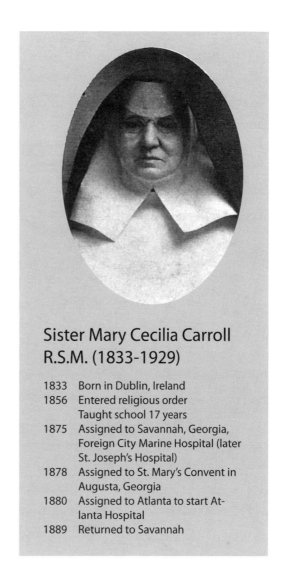

Sister Mary Cecilia Carroll R.S.M. (1833-1929)

1833	Born in Dublin, Ireland
1856	Entered religious order Taught school 17 years
1875	Assigned to Savannah, Georgia, Foreign City Marine Hospital (later St. Joseph's Hospital)
1878	Assigned to St. Mary's Convent in Augusta, Georgia
1880	Assigned to Atlanta to start Atlanta Hospital
1889	Returned to Savannah

Ivy Street hospital soon arranged a contract whereby Atlanta's city government would pay the hospital for treating the poor. Without reimbursement from the city and without volunteers, Ivy Street hospital would have been unable to pay its bills.[55] In this regard it had much in common with hospitals far and near. None of Atlanta's houses of healing had yet developed a business model that freed it from the need for assistance from taxpayers or philanthropists.

As a result, the rates medical institutions charged and received for treatment gained greater financial significance. In the 1880s, some wealthier Americans began being admitted to hospitals. Charging a fixed rate based on accommodations or length of stay was relatively unusual. Instead of a flat rate, patients typically negotiated the price of boarding at sanatoriums on an individual basis. The amount that they were charged often depended as much on the physician's diagnosis as on the hospital's opinion of the patient's pocketbook. In the end, few patients paid for the full cost of their hospitalization.

The system of negotiated fees made it nearly impossible for hospitals to accurately predict income. More importantly, the financial set-up prevented hospitals from being able to count on revenue from paying patients to subsidize charity care—an idea that was starting to spread across the United States but had yet to take hold in Atlanta. Even without charging wealthy patients slightly higher fees to subsidize care for the poor, during the 1880s each of Atlanta's major hospitals provided general care to the city's poorest residents. None of them turned away people who were unable to pay for treatment. Yet, in order to stay open, Atlanta's hospitals needed more income to cover the cost of providing room and board to the poor.

Recognizing the financial problem that charity patients posed to private institutions, Atlanta's city government promised to reimburse hospitals for the expenses incurred in caring for the indigent. Unfortunately, the city failed to adequately follow through on its pledge; it paid only a small percentage of the cost connected to charity care. Physicians and hospital administrators soon became frustrated with the city's tight-fisted approach. With little hope of seeing their true costs covered by the municipal government, physicians and hospitals—along with many of Atlanta's leading citizens—looked for a new way to provide health care to the poor.

In April 1886, a group of Atlantans and prominent people from other cities, including the architect Daniel H. Burnham of Chicago and John D. Rockefeller, the oil magnate from Ohio, took the first steps toward organizing a charity hospital for blacks in Atlanta. Leading physicians like Drs. Willis F. Westmoreland and Joseph P. Logan, businessmen including Samuel Inman, public servants like Levi B. Nelson, and clergy including the Reverend W. J. Gaines were among the organizers. The projected Franklin Hospital hoped to limit operating expenses by using "donated" labor. For nurses they would rely on students from a local training school for black women, Spelman Seminary.[56]

At about the same time that the businessmen looked into starting a hospital for black residents, city officials began investigating Ivy Street Hospital's treatment of African Americans. Led by Levi B. Nelson, a city council member and an officer of Fourth National Bank, the council spent more than a year looking into what was happening at Ivy Street. At the end of 1887, after extensively reviewing the hospital's practices, the city council refused to renew its annual contract with the hospital for the treatment of indigent blacks. Instead, the council continued its arrangement with Ivy Street on a month-to-month basis pending improvements by the hospital.

In the fall of 1887, as the city council continued to examine practices at the Ivy Street hospital, Miss L. J. Bothwell arrived from Boston to lead Spelman's nursing school. Within several weeks the Franklin Hospital Association acquired two acres of land near Spelman Seminary.[57] The movement for the new black hospital picked up more steam shortly after the start of the next year when eighteen nursing students from Spelman Seminary demonstrated their skills to an audience that included at least one organizer of Franklin Hospital, Samuel Inman. The journalist Henry Grady and several other prominent Atlantans in attendance were impressed by the ability of the student nurses and with their knowledge of medical conditions including typhoid fever and seizures.[58] The organizers of Franklin Hospital who were there that night must have been pleased with their prospective laborers. Satisfied they could rely on the free labor of black nursing students, Franklin Hospital's founders hoped they could rely on white physicians to provide medical treatment—also for free.

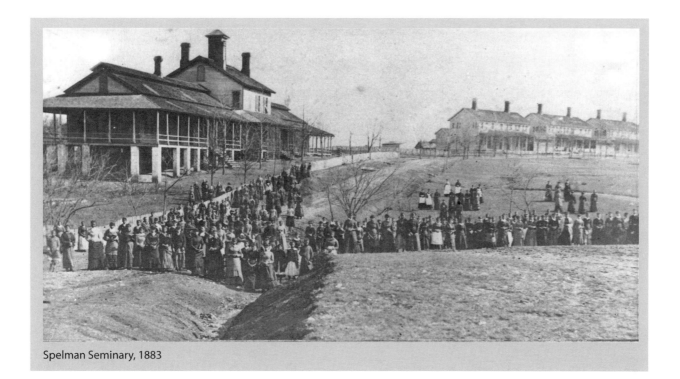
Spelman Seminary, 1883

For reasons that are unclear, Franklin Hospital went little further than winning a charter from the superior court and acquiring land. Nevertheless, the effort to create the institution stands out. Organized by physicians, businessmen, and clergy, the hospital was intended to provide charity care to African Americans in Atlanta. The anticipated association with Spelman Seminary, befriended by John D. Rockefeller, hints at the relationship that would emerge between medical care and northern philanthropy after the turn of the century.

Seven months into 1888 the city council decided to stop paying Ivy Street for treating charity cases. In ending the month-to-month extensions of its expired contract the city council declared that "our dependent sick do not receive the care and attention the amount paid by the city entitles them to."[59] While initially concerned about "the care of the colored sick," the collapse of the relationship between the city and Ivy Street was more complete.

The city council's relief committee ended its connection with the hospital in clear terms: "hereafter no city patients, white or black, shall be sent to the Ivy St [sic] Hospital by any branch of the city government."[60] The ill could be treated elsewhere. In short, Ivy Street wasn't the only hospital in town. In light of the city government's decision, Ivy Street Hospital—facing significant debt and an end to its steadiest source of revenue—changed management. At nearly the same time, the King's Daughters Hospital, organized only weeks earlier by a group of women associated with St. Luke's Episcopal Church, announced that it would treat the poor of Atlanta.[61]

Founded by a small group of Episcopal women in New York City in 1886, the King's Daughters rapidly expanded across the United States. With dozens of chapters formed in Episcopal congregations throughout the nation, the King's Daughters quickly became an umbrella organization for Episcopal women interested in charitable work. In many cities, existing Episcopal women's groups signed up with the new organization. Particularly effective in attracting young women to the church's social mission, the King's Daughters led many new groups to form. Their membership engaged in a wide range of charitable activity, ranging from direct assistance to needy families to visiting the sick in hospitals.

In Atlanta they went further, organizing a hospital.[62]

Although it had Episcopalian roots, the King's Daughters Hospital in Atlanta would admit patients of any religious faith. Indeed, the Daughters were self-consciously nonsectarian in their approach. Guided by Mrs. Nellie Peters Black, a doer and leader among the city's philanthropic women, the King's Daughters originally wanted to create a children's ward. Within days their mission expanded to cover adults too. Even before the women put together their project, however, two Episcopal physicians—Dr. A. J. Woodward, a pediatrician, and Dr. F. O. Stockton, a nose and throat specialist—began making their own push for an Episcopalian hospital in Atlanta. By the time the King's Daughters developed their plans, the physicians already had quietly gained support for a church-sponsored hospital from rectors in the diocese and its bishop, John Beckwith.

With the church's blessing, the two groups met to see if they could combine forces. The main stumbling block appears to have been the men's insistence on having an Episcopal hospital while the women were resolute about creating a nonsectarian institution. The men compromised, agreeing the hospital's religious identification would not prevent people of other faiths or no faith from being admitted. Within weeks, at the start of August 1888, the nascent hospital opened in a small house at 180 South Pryor Street near the new St. Luke's Cathedral.[63]

The organizing group assembled a solid board of trustees for the hospital, including Bishop Beckwith, Samuel Inman, Drs. Woodward and Logan, and Henry W. Grady. Quickly accepting the King's Daughters offer to help, the trustees created a woman's auxiliary for the hospital board. In addition, the trustees turned over internal management of the hospital to a group of hard-charging women led by Mrs. Nellie Peters Black, Mrs. John C. Olmsted, and Mrs. Levi B. Nelson. Some of Atlanta's most esteemed physicians were on the hospital staff at its opening, including Drs. Olmsted, Westmoreland, Noble, Crawford, Woodward, and Stockton. Other notable physicians, including Drs. Abner Calhoun, William P. Nicolson, J. S. Todd, A. G. Hobbs, and T. D. Longino, a future city council member, joined the hospital's consulting medical board.[64]

Several months before the King's Daughters Hospital first became a gleam in Bishop Beckwith's eye, at a time when the city council was scuttling its contract with Ivy Street Hospital, city leaders stimulated public discussion about providing medical care to the poor. In mid-February 1888, at the urging of the city council's relief committee, Drs. J. S. Todd, K. C. Divine, and W. M. Durham called for a mass meeting of citizens interested in improving how Atlanta cared for its ill and injured.[65]

On the night of February 16, as the temperature outside hovered slightly above forty degrees and cloudy skies threatened rain, dozens of physicians, businessmen, and clergy gathered in the basement of the courthouse in downtown Atlanta. The more than sixty physicians present dominated the debate about improving medical care for Atlanta's indigent. The discussion that night produced two significant results. The first involved recommendations for reforming Atlanta's system of delivering medical care to the needy, the ward physician system.

At the time, medical care for the poor revolved around six physicians in private practice that the city employed on a part-time basis. Each was assigned to one of Atlanta's six aldermanic wards and received a small annual stipend for their public service. The ward physicians, however, soon found that their busy private practices left them with little time to attend the destitute. As the city's population grew during the 1880s, physicians regularly handled a dozen or more calls per day from their private patients. With almost all of those requiring a visit to the patient's home, the doctors had little time to treat the poor—a situation that horrified the ward physicians themselves. Clearly the existing program was ineffective for physicians and indigent residents alike.[66] Frustrated with a system it recognized as unworkable, the medical profession eagerly addressed the issue of indigent care. There is little doubt that leading physicians in the city had been bending the ear of their representatives in city hall.

The group that gathered in the courthouse proposed a simple reform: replace the part-time ward physicians with two doctors devoted full time to caring for the city's indigent. One physician would serve residents in the north section of the city while the other physician would care for people living on Atlanta's south side. Under their plan, the city would pay these physicians a salary large enough for them to devote their entire practice to the poor. The meeting's other major recommendation that night concerned how to provide hospital care for Atlanta's indigent.[67]

With Dr. J. S. Todd serving as chairman of the meeting, the assembled men debated the city's need for a public hospital. Dr. T. S. Powell, the founder of Southern Medical College and head of Central Ivy Street Hospital, objected to creating a competing institution. He claimed Ivy Street and St. Joseph's hospitals had more beds than patients and therefore, in his view, Atlanta had no need for a public hospital. (His fellow faculty members later boasted that Ivy Street Hospital alone could handle three times as many white charity patients as it did "without interfering with our private patients received from the railroads and other sources.")[68] Besides claiming there were too few patients to support a city hospital, Dr. Powell argued that a public hospital would force unnecessary tax increases for Atlanta's already overburdened taxpayers. In addition, Dr. Powell warned that a public charity hospital would draw "an influx of hundreds of paupers" from outside the city.[69]

Having restated the arguments against a public hospital that had been given in the 1870s, Dr. Powell also appealed to the booster's pride in Atlanta. Defending the city's reputation, he claimed the absence of a general city hospital proved that Atlanta was the healthiest city in the world. He argued that by building a public charity hospital, Atlanta would simply signal that it was becoming "unhealthy like Mobile or New Orleans or Birmingham." (Moments after Dr. Powell finished his speech, a wag in the audience suggested Atlanta abolish graveyards lest the city develop a reputation for being a place where people died.)[70]

Despite his arguments against the proposed charity hospital based on lack of need, the likelihood of tax hikes, the prospect of attracting undesirable slackers, and his concern about the city's reputation, Dr. Powell suggested one circumstance under which he would support a city hospital: if Atlanta built a "large and magnificent" hospital that would be available for teaching purposes to all of the medical schools in the city and accessible to "all classes of patients." If this happened, he expected that Atlanta would become "the great medical center of the south"—one of his dearest ambitions.[71] As he acknowledged, however, turning Atlanta into a great medical center—a dream that would live on for generations—was not on the agenda that night. The more limited nature of the discussion allowed Dr. Powell to stick with his arguments against creating a public hospital. The rest of the crowd of physicians and other citizens easily dismissed Dr. Powell's claims, especially his characterization of Atlanta as the city too healthy to have a public hospital.

Supporters of the public charity hospital offered a broad mandate. They favored having a general city hospital available to all (white) physicians. It would not be the province of a single medical school in the manner of Ivy Street Hospital. In addition, they hoped the general hospital would attract medical students from "all over Georgia, and the south, to learn from it."[72] Physicians at the meeting also wanted the hospital to be owned and controlled (directly or indirectly) by the city. A publicly-owned hospital would accept any citizen as a patient without considering race or religious affiliation; more importantly, they dreamed, it would never deny a physician the right to treat patients there. In their view, a public hospital would be open to the patients of every white physician practicing in the city, and they emphasized its accessiblity to physicians.

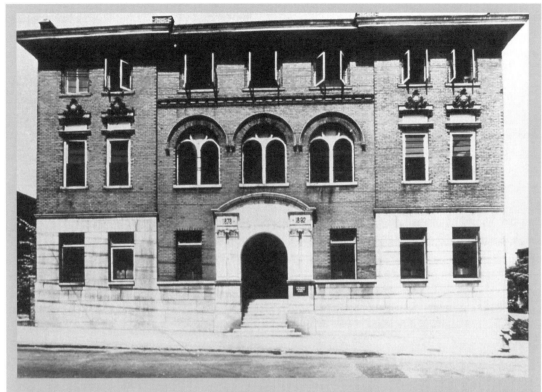

Southern Medical College opened in 1878 under the leadership of Dr. Thomas Powell. The school was located on Porters Alley (changed to Equitable Place in 1913). Dr. Powell was behind the creation of the Ivy Street Hospital and, in 1892, the Southern Dental College.

The physicians at the meeting were less concerned about politicians in city hall controlling the hospital than about a small group of doctors hijacking the institution for themselves and their patients. They also hoped for democratic governance, allowing physicians from a broad range of medical philosophies to participate in management and have access to the hospital. By keeping the hospital "free from sectarianism," they hoped to prevent a few physicians from controlling its internal affairs. Even more importantly, they aimed to build a place where everyone could find medical care.

The physicians and laymen gathered in the courthouse basement agreed that everyone in Atlanta, regardless of race or income, had a right to basic health care. They also knew that, even as they met, people in the city were dying from medical neglect. All but a few physicians present on that winter's night in 1888 believed that a new hospital was essential for the city of 70,000 people.

Although they were aware of the need, they recognized that creating and operating a comprehensive public hospital was too large of a project for a few individuals to finance. The failed effort to adequately support a small hospital associated with the Atlanta Benevolent Home showed that building and sustaining a suitable charity hospital required more resources than a few rich men could muster. A charity hospital in Atlanta would demand public ownership for financial reasons as much as for professional ones. With all that in mind, that night the citizens passed resolutions supporting both a new hospital and its public ownership.

Even with public control and funding, they knew that money would continue to be a problem for the venture. But they seemed to believe that public control and accountability would foster the trust needed to gain solid financial support from the city council. Frustrated by the way things were, and driven by practical concerns about how to properly care for their fellow man, they looked for a public solution. Without one, many of their fellow citizens would continue to die from neglect. And so that night a group of Atlanta's physicians, businessmen, clergy, and other citizens organized a committee to plan and promote a publicly owned charity hospital for Atlanta.*[73]

The citizens' hospital committee began by researching charity hospitals in other American cities. Drawing on what was being done elsewhere, the committee developed broad ideas for Atlanta's circumstance. Although its work was completed by mid-summer, the committee waited until that autumn to deliver its report to the city council. It hoped that by then the city's coffers would be replenished—they had become depleted thanks to appropriations for paving streets with bricks. In July, as he announced the delay in presenting the report, Dr. Cooper, the committee's chairman, promised his group would keep pushing for a city hospital to be run "solely for the good of the sick and helpless in our midst."[74]

Several months passed before the committee provided its substantial report to the city council. Having studied public hospitals in American cities of comparable size, including Memphis, Louisville, and Hartford, the committee determined Atlanta should start with a relatively small hospital. It proposed building one with a capacity for treating 50 inpatients, making it one-third the size of the charity hospital in Memphis and about one-fifth as large as Louisville's city hospital.

Expecting the hospital to be enlarged over time, the committee proposed building it in a way that would allow additions to be made easily. The committee offered ideas about the future hospital's design, construction and operating costs, funding, management, and racial accommodations that it believed the city should consider in planning the institution. The committee also suggested several sources for financing. These included endowment funds of from $500 to $1,000 to support individual beds, income from private-pay patients, bequests from estates, and an annual fund-raising fair. In addition, it proposed that on one weekend each year the hospital request financial support at houses of worship.[75] As 1888 ended, the city had a reasonable, well thought-out plan for organizing a public hospital. Although relatively small at the outset, over time it would grow in pace with the population to meet the needs of what civic leaders assumed would be the foremost city of the region.

As a new city council was about to take office at the start of 1889, leading physicians, clergy, businessmen, and politicians had come to a consensus about Atlanta's need for a general hospital. Although the city government was ready to start building a new hospital early that year, its efforts would be blocked by legal questions about proper title to the land the city hoped to use. For most of 1889, Atlanta's push to create a publicly owned and operated charity hospital stalled. By that December, eighteen months after the city announced it would stop paying for the care of indigent patients at Ivy Street Hospital and seventeen months after the tiny King's Daughters Hospital opened, Atlanta's city council reported still having "no definite arrangement for the building of a city hospital."[76]

Ironically, the final impetus for the life-giving services of a hospital dedicated to caring for the poor emerged from the death of a wealthy man. Two days before Christmas 1889, the city's most prominent citizen, Henry Woodfin Grady, died. The journalist and after-dinner speaker had earned a national reputation during the 1880s. Together with other southern journalists like Henry Watterson of Louisville and Richard H. Edmonds of Baltimore, Grady boosted a big cause: making a New South. Grady took

---

*Chaired by Dr. Hunter P. Cooper, the hospital's organizing committee included Drs. Joseph P. Logan, Frances H. Orme, W. M. Durham, William Perrin Nicolson, Judge William L. Calhoun, the Reverend Dr. Henry Holcombe Tucker, and Samuel Inman.

the lead in claiming that America's South could create itself anew; Atlanta's civic and commercial leaders followed in his promotional footsteps.

Atlanta's most prominent citizens believed that increasing the area's wealth depended on having a healthy population. Although this tenet was not part of the New South gospel, Atlanta's leaders increasingly came to see provisions for public health as a sign of civic significance. Of course, the leaders who held that view also had other beliefs. Most were native southerners who were born before the Civil War.[77] Prospering in Atlanta's post-war economy, these men shared a faith in capitalism.

Several of the city's most important civic leaders, however, had different roots. No less loyal to a capitalist creed, these men were Jewish immigrants from Germany. Moving across the ocean as young men, most briefly settled in the north before establishing themselves in Atlanta shortly after the Civil War. An important part of the city's civic leadership by the 1880s, they played major roles in expanding health care in Atlanta. They included Joseph Hirsch, the person who would become most responsible for creating Atlanta's public hospital. For him, the desire to provide a public hospital was more moral than mercenary, rooted largely in a humanitarian impulse that led to the creation of what a perceptive historian in the 1970s described as "perhaps the greatest monument to Jewish philanthropy" in Atlanta.[78] He would be his brother's keeper.

In the end, the city's civic leaders joined in a view that was both moralist and practical. While perhaps only a few stood for the democratic belief in the essential dignity of every human being, all concluded that every citizen should have access to adequate health care. Those men—who had become especially attuned to the link between prosperity and good public health after the Mississippi River Basin Yellow Fever Epidemic of 1878—believed civic betterment went hand in hand with the making of a prosperous New South. If one person was the spokesman for this class of men, it was Henry Woodfin Grady.

Henry Woodfin Grady

"Few American journalists have been better loved than Henry W. Grady."
Frank Luther Mott, *American Journalism, A History, 1690-1960*

As much as he was a forward-thinking man eager to remake the American South, Henry Grady was in full a man of his own era. Born in Athens, Georgia, a little more than a decade before the onset of America's Civil War, Grady was the oldest child in his family. He learned at an early age to work hard and persevere through adversity; he shared in many of the hardships afflicting people across the South during the Civil War. A child of the Old South, Grady matured toward manhood during that devastating conflict and would finish his formal education a few years after the Confederacy surrendered. Growing into a young man with ideas, Grady freely expressed his opinions during the years of post-war reconstruction. Indeed, he first articulated his central theme three years before the last federal troops ended their patrol of the South in 1877.[1]

Grady was twenty-four years old when he issued his signature cry—the creation of a "New South." While he did not originate the phrase—historians have traced it back earlier—Grady popularized the phrase. He soon developed a stump sermon urging southern entrepreneurs to attract capital from northern investors to finance new factories. The resulting industry would bring jobs and help make the region rich. At bottom, his "New South Creed" was designed to turn the region into a land of milk, honey, and money.[2] More than that, enriching the region would change relations with the North. The South, Grady expected, would gain greater influence in national politics if the region became more prosperous. His main idea, in the end, concerned enhancing the region's political power as much it did improving the welfare of southerners.[3]

Grady's prophetic call for a New South of greater wealth, political influence, and national impact may have seemed audacious to his readers. Perhaps it was. For him and his comrades, however, the effort to make America over seemed anything but absurd. Perhaps this was because his call was quite cautious. He wanted to create wealth in the region, but under a system that rewarded investors far more than laborers. He was far from aiming to create a region that provided equal opportunity for all. Neither would the riches be evenly distributed. The southern residents most likely to gain from his idea were the urban elites whom Grady represented.

Perhaps Grady thought his long-standing hope to build a New South was on the cusp of reality when he died in December 1889. It is hard to tell; perhaps the growing discontent of farmers and others who would become part of the Populist movement made him less sanguine about the prospects for erecting a New South. In either case, by the time he died the hope for creating the South anew had become an important theme for the region. Its significance would only grow in the decades that followed. Invoking the phrase

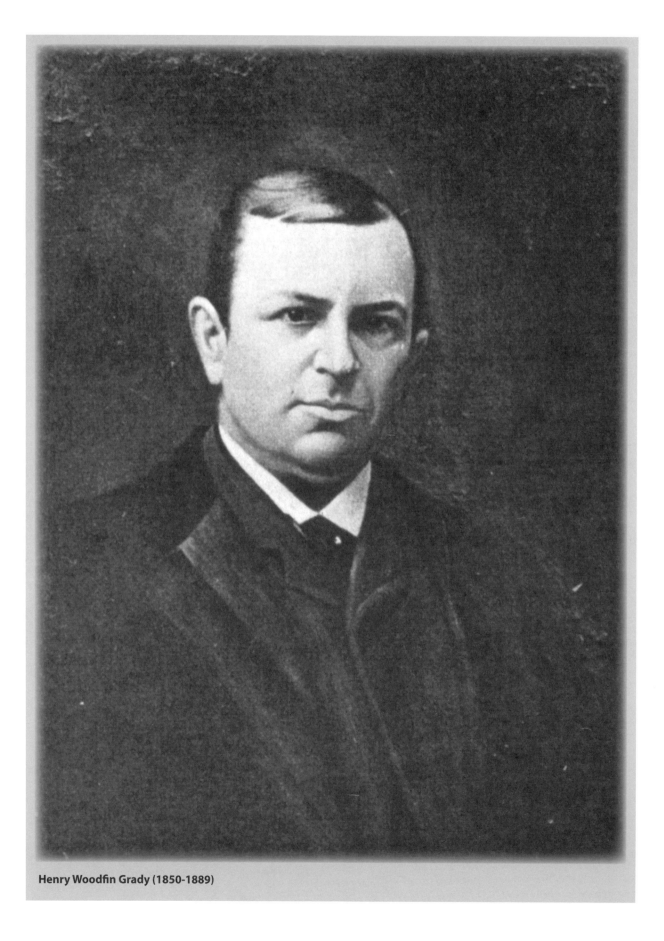
Henry Woodfin Grady (1850-1889)

for more than a century after Grady's death, generations of southern leaders reworked the idea of a "New South" to suit their own needs. In that way the region continued to benefit from Henry Grady's effort. It is helpful to understand, however, that his bequest to the South and the nation was rooted in Henry Grady's own inheritance.

In the late eighteenth century, during a time of terrible turmoil in Ireland, William O'Grady moved to North America from County Donegal. Like many Irish immigrants then, O'Grady settled in North Carolina. It is likely that his reasons for coming to North America were similar to those of others who left the old sod for new woods. Many eighteenth-century Irish emigrants left to escape economic hardship, political unrest, and religious intolerance. They also came to North America in order to build something for themselves and their heirs. Pushed out of Ireland and attracted to North America, O'Grady's choice of northeastern North Carolina allowed him to build his life in the company not of strangers, but of kinsmen. The first generations of his heirs would share William O'Grady's ability to establish fresh roots in new land.

His descendant Jonathan Grady would move north from Bertie County, North Carolina, to Halifax County, Virginia. The generation of Gradys after Jonathan headed south and west. Jonathan's son Henry (born in 1788) and daughter-in-law, Leah King Grady, started their own family in Virginia. Leah gave birth to William Sammons Grady, their fourth child, in 1821. William Sammons Grady, the son of Henry and Leah and great-grandson of the immigrant William O'Grady, was only eight years old when his mother died in 1829. His father, Henry, who was then forty-one years old, soon left for Cherokee County, Georgia, together with his sons John and William.

The three Gradys arrived in the hills of northern Georgia in 1830, two years after gold was discovered in the area. Prospectors soon unearthed so much of the precious metal that the United States Mint set up an operation in the boomtown of Dahlonega.[4] Although Henry joined the land rush that the find fueled, he was a farmer rather than a miner. Grady rapidly went to work helping create the settlement of Mountaintown in the county's Dyer Gap. (The community was about six and a half miles northwest of present-day Ellijay, Georgia—which itself sits on the site of an ancient Indian village).

About ten years later—after the forcible removal of the Cherokee—the two sons of Henry and Leah Grady did what the Grady men had done for the past few generations: move away from home. John W. Grady moved thirty miles east of the family's home to the gold mining town of Dahlonega. His brother, William, left Gilmer County for Athens, Georgia, where he became a successful

Cherokee Nation

Approximately 17,000 members of the Cherokee Nation lived in northern Georgia when the Gold Rush started in 1829. The Cherokee were farmers and cattle ranchers who had built Christian churches, laid down roads, and adopted European clothing styles. In 1827 they formed an independent Cherokee Nation. Even before the discovery of gold, however, the Cherokee confronted a rapid increase of Anglo-Saxon settlers in Georgia. The United States Congress offered the Cherokee no relief. Indeed, "The Indian Removal Act" of 1830 served the opposite effect.

The state of Georgia, which had been eager to remove the Cherokee for years, used the new law to acquire the Native Americans' land. The Cherokee sued to block Georgia's action. Despite winning their case in the United States Supreme Court, the Cherokee could not make the state of Georgia abide by the court's ruling. The state allowed The Land Lottery of 1832 to move forward, dividing the Cherokee land among whites.[5] In 1835, a renegade group of Cherokee signed a removal treaty with the United States on behalf of the Cherokee Nation. Ratified by the United States Senate, The Treaty of New Echota gave the federal government a pretext to remove the Cherokee from Georgia. Under the leadership of General Winfield Scott, the United States Army began moving the Cherokee Nation along their "trail of tears" to Oklahoma in 1838—the forced march that cost nearly 8,000 Cherokee lives.[6]

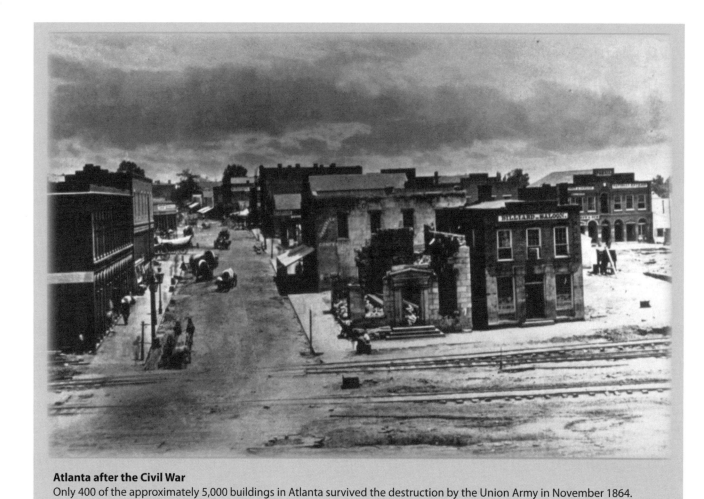

Atlanta after the Civil War
Only 400 of the approximately 5,000 buildings in Atlanta survived the destruction by the Union Army in November 1864.

businessman. William Grady married Ann Elizabeth Gartrell in 1848. Henry Woodfin Grady, the future journalist and evangelist of the New South gospel (and first of the couple's four children), was born on May 24, 1850. (Annie, their youngest, would die in infancy in 1857.) William S. Grady joined the Confederate Army shortly after the outbreak of the Civil War. While home on leave he purchased a large house on Athens' fashionable Prince Street. After returning to duty, Major Grady died in combat during the Battle of Petersburg, Virginia, on October 21, 1864. His family continued to live in Athens after the war ended.

Henry Woodfin Grady, who was fourteen years old when his father died, attended the nearby University of Georgia. After graduating in 1868, young Henry Grady continued his education at the University of Virginia. While there, he developed a reputation for being a skilled orator and refined his writing skills as a reporter for the university's newspaper. When Grady finished his formal education at Virginia, he—like his father, grandfather, and great-grandfather before him—moved to a new town to start his career.

Seeking to become a journalist, Grady, then nineteen years old, went to work as an associate editor for the *Courier* in Rome, Georgia. Grady left the newspaper after the editor blocked him from investigating local political corruption. Without missing a beat Grady purchased two competing papers, combined them into the *Rome Commercial*, and proceeded to go after public corruption. The *Rome Commercial* earned much respect but very little money; indeed, it was a financial flop. Hardly deterred by losing money in his first newspaper business, Grady soon invested in Atlanta's *The Daily Herald*. This venture collapsed after four glorious years of offering the city "the newsiest and liveliest paper Atlanta had ever seen."[7] Grady found a different sort of success in the midst of these disappointments. He met, courted, and—in 1871—married Julia King. (Their union produced two sons and one daughter.) After *The Daily Herald* failed in 1876, Grady joined Robert Alston in founding *The Atlanta Courier*. That newspaper lasted three weeks. Grady's next venture, the *Sunday Telegram*, survived longer: it endured for five weeks.

Even in the midst of business losses, Henry Grady continued to build his reputation as a skilled journalist. His reporting captured the attention of Captain Evan P. Howell who had become editor of the *Atlanta Constitution* in 1876. Howell, who was a lawyer and an industrialist, had a keen eye for good writing and he saw it in Grady's reporting for the *New York Herald* on the contested presidential election of 1876. Grady soon accepted Howell's offer to become an editorial writer for the *Constitution*. A short time later Grady made a find of his own when he hired Joel Chandler Harris to be an editorial paragrapher. (Harris spent the next twenty-four years with the *Constitution*, writing colorful articles on daily life and spinning memorable tales of "Uncle Remus.") Four years later Grady borrowed $20,000 in order to acquire a one-quarter interest in the *Constitution*'s ownership. The enterprise's new part owner also became its managing editor.

Grady wielded political influence in Georgia nearly from the start of his career and his stature only grew as he refined his persuasiveness in print and in person. His skill in articulating the state's (and region's) trials in rebuilding after the Civil War enhanced Grady's authority as a public spokesman. In 1873, he endorsed former Confederate General John B. Gordon for the U.S. Senate. While Grady's action certainly was not the only reason, the state legislature subsequently elected Gordon.[8] Grady's political influence grew in the following years as candidates for local and state political office regularly sought his support, hoping his endorsement might help them win election. The historian C. Vann Woodward elegantly summarized Grady's political power: "As a practical politician with the wires of a powerful machine in his hands, he helped see to it that Georgia was governed by the new industrialists."[9]

Grady's political participation meshed with his increasing involvement in commercial affairs across Georgia. He consistently urged business leaders to try new ventures. (He seemed to think they needed his prompting to keep their eyes open.) Grady saw southern businessmen regularly overlooking chances to attract financial investment and create jobs. To emphasize his point, he often told a story about what happened after a certain Georgia farmer died. Manufacturers in the north made the farmer's burial clothes and coffin. The shovel used to dig his grave came from Pittsburgh. The marble marker for the grave came from a firm in Vermont. In the end, Georgia provided only two things for the funeral: the man's body and the hole in the ground. This happened even though all of the raw materials the farmer's family needed for the man's burial existed in Georgia. The moral of Grady's funeral tale was simple: People in Georgia and across the South failed to exploit the economic opportunities that their surroundings provided. If southerners would take advantage of the area's natural bounty, then the region would prosper.

Grady's words reached a broad national audience. During the 1880s, the weekly edition of the *Constitution* had the largest circulation of any weekly newspaper in the United States—140,000 copies by the end of the decade.[10] The *Constitution* had subscribers in every state of the union, sent out 20,000 sample copies each week, and saw its editorials reprinted in newspapers published elsewhere. Grady's editorials appealed to businessmen, politicians, and commercial boosters on both sides of the Mason-Dixon Line. His reporting also garnered praise from across the nation; his coverage of the Charleston earthquake of 1886 captured enormous public attention.

His already rising reputation would make a quantum leap later that year.

A speech he delivered to the New England Society of New York on December 21, 1886, dramatically enhanced Grady's national prominence. Standing before northern civic and business leaders in the banquet hall of Delmonico's restaurant, Grady presented a rosy picture of the "The New South." In that speech, as in his editorials, Grady leaned on the pulpit of a prophet rather than the lectern of a scholar. Advertising his region, he claimed more changes had taken place in Southern politics, race relations, and economic growth than an honest appraisal should have allowed. His audiences would not have cared—neither those attending his lecture on the winter solstice of that year nor whites at home who later read his words. Grady's message reassured his audiences that the Old South died at Appomattox. In its place a New South was rising.

That news, if it was news to him, probably thrilled one of the other men at the dais that night—J. Pierpont Morgan, America's greatest financier. Morgan's vast wealth had hardly quenched his appetite for making money. You can practically see Morgan's ears perk up at hearing that the South was rising for investment. Several years later, in 1894, he would form the Southern Railway from the ruins of railroads that fell apart during the financial panic of 1893. Combining dozens of corporations, Morgan's Southern Railway soon controlled 7,500 miles of rail, giving Morgan control over the transportation of a large percentage of southern goods, raw materials, and agricultural products. Less than ten years later J. P. Morgan and Company would gain control over the Louisville and Nashville Railroad before profitably financing the sale of the company to the Southern Railway's largest rival—the Atlantic Coast Line.[11] It seems that when Henry Grady spoke, J. P. Morgan listened.

That night at Delmonicos, Henry Grady opened his optimistic address with words Georgia's former Senator Benjamin H. Hill spoke at Tammany Hall in New York in 1866. In the Civil War's aftermath, Hill proclaimed the South had reached the end of an era. He said, "there was a South of slavery and secession—that South is dead. There is a South of Union and freedom—that South, thank God, is living, breathing, growing every hour."[12] Apparently, Grady wanted his audience to know that the South "of Union and freedom" had expanded in the two decades since Hill's rhetorical surrender. Grady continued his oration with a tribute to President Lincoln—a standard procedure in the North that was somewhat less familiar in the states of the former Confederacy. Grady also paid respects to General Sherman (who was present and preceded Grady on the program). He described Sherman as "one who is considered an able man in our parts, though some people think he is a kind of careless man about fire."[13]

Having tipped his hat to the general who burned Atlanta, Grady moved to his theme: the South was establishing a new era. His meaning was clear. Without apologizing for the past, the New South was creating itself most honorably. Grady assured his audience that the South "of Union and freedom" would continue to gain by the hour. To his listeners he came across as a safe man with whom to do business. More significantly, Grady made the South seem like a place where Yankee capitalists could invest with confidence. J. Pierpont Morgan might have wanted to raise his glass and toast the prospective profits to be had in the southern states.

Henry Grady's well-heeled audience received the speech very well, to say the least. Northern politicians and businessmen saw Grady as someone with whom they could work. If he believed the time had come for the South to deal with regional issues by itself, then they would be more than willing, nearly a decade after the end of Reconstruction, to have the South handle the "race problem" on its own. Certainly Grady believed racial peace and economic development depended on each other. A political moderate by the standards of his time and place, Grady's conservative speech reassured northern investors about the prospect for racial harmony in the sunny southland. In addition to indicating that racial peace was within sight, he essentially promised that the region teemed with an untapped workforce ready for industrial jobs. His audience must have salivated over their dessert as they pondered Grady's invitation to come south and hire low-wage industrial labor.

The speech significantly enhanced Grady's professional and personal reputation and opened new opportunities for him. Over the next three years Grady traveled widely as lecturer, toastmaster, and after-dinner speaker. His appeal was so broad that in 1888 some political observers suggested he would make a good running mate for Grover Cleveland, the Democratic Party's nominee for President. One northern newspaper even suggested Grady should be a presidential candidate.

The pride of Atlanta gave what turned out to be his final prepared speech at the annual banquet of the Boston Merchants Association on December 12, 1889. Speaking on "The Race Problem in the South," the ever-optimistic salesman of the New South assured his audience that justice was at hand for southern blacks. He told the Bostonians, as he did so many others, that southerners could handle race relations on their own; they didn't need Yankee help to create an equitable racial climate. Yet, even as he spoke Jim Crow laws were taking hold across the South.

While Grady may have liked the applause that greeted his address, he was barely able to enjoy the accolades that followed. Although apparently exhausted, the next morning Grady visited Plymouth Rock. That afternoon he gave an impromptu speech to the Bay State Club.[14] As he headed home that night, something more immediate than the audience's response captured his attention—something that had been nagging at him for a few days before he arrived in Massachusetts.

Shortly before leaving Atlanta, Grady had decided to see his physician, Dr. Frances H. Orme. A distinguished physician and founder of the Southern Homeopathic Medical Association, Dr. Orme determined that Grady was too ill to travel.[15] He advised the orator to cancel the trip, but Grady declined to follow his doctor's suggestion. Thus, neither Grady nor his journey to Boston started out well. Perhaps Grady expected that resting aboard the train would help him feel better; unfortunately, his condition worsened as he traveled. Stopping off to see a physician in New York City, Grady again heard a doctor tell him to cancel his engagement in Boston. Prescribed a dose of rest, Grady instead decided to push farther north.

Following his demanding journey, the tired and ill Grady endured a long evening in Boston. The program lasted eight hours. It included a formal dinner and speeches by former President Grover Cleveland and Andrew Carnegie, the steel baron turned philanthropist. Taking his turn at the podium, Grady summoned the strength to speak for more than an hour. It could not have helped his health. His illness became progressively worse on the journey home. Grady suffered from a debilitating fever and cough when he returned to Atlanta on December 17. His doctor saw him immediately and quickly diagnosed pneumonia. Despite valiant efforts to treat his illness during the next few days, Grady died at 3:40 on the morning of December 23, 1889.

People from across the United States sent telegrams and letters bringing condolences to his family, city, and region. Two days after he died thousands of people from all walks of life gathered at Atlanta's First Methodist Church for Grady's funeral. The service marking his passing held that Christmas Day cast a somber mood across the city. (His remains were temporarily interred in a friend's tomb at Oakland Cemetery while his crypt was being prepared in Westview Cemetery.) The eulogies his friends gave proved to be only the start of the city's recognition of Grady's impact on his friends, readers, and fellow citizens.

Henry W. Grady achieved a great deal beyond writing influential editorials at the *Atlanta Constitution* and giving noteworthy lectures. The once financially plagued journalist had enjoyed substantial political influence in Georgia and wielded significant social authority in Atlanta. He helped organize institutions that became important for the city, including its first Young Men's Christian Association (YMCA), first public library, the Georgia Institute of Technology, and the city's Confederate Soldiers Home. In addition, Grady helped plan and develop major events in Atlanta. The International Cotton Exposition of 1881 and the Piedmont Expositions of 1887 and 1889, each of which attracted tens of thousands of visitors, were the largest among these. Finally, Grady is also known for having helped bring organized professional baseball to Atlanta. (In addition, he served as president of the Southern League, an association of professional baseball teams). With his death, Atlanta lost an influential editor and businessman, the South lost an eloquent advocate, and the nation lost a man who dedicated his short life—brief even by late nineteenth century standards—to enhancing southern wealth, increasing the region's political power, and healing the rift between North and South, albeit on terms suitable to American business interests.

A Living Monument

Let [our children] see that the living monument of Henry Grady is far grander and more glorious than the dead monument of stone, erected to perpetuate his memory.
—Belle K. Abbott, *Atlanta Constitution*, February 9, 1890.

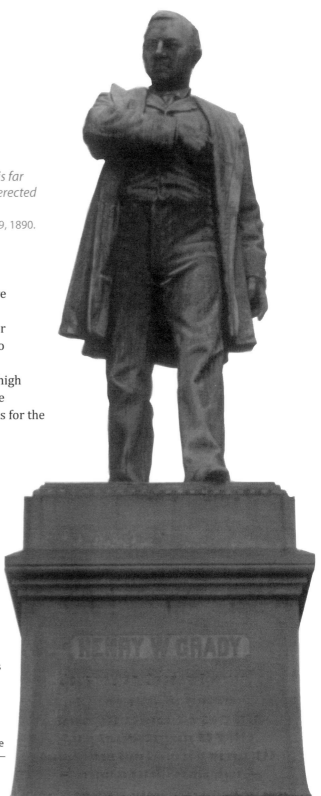

Henry Grady's death stunned and saddened friends and admirers. It hardly surprises that on the day after he died more than one hundred shocked friends and colleagues gathered in the *Atlanta Constitution* building to consider how to best honor Grady's life.[1] To firmly establish his memory for generations to come, the assemblage decided to erect a bronze statue of his likeness in the heart of downtown Atlanta. The gesture was a high honor reserved for only the most significant public men. Those gathered that day quickly formed a committee to oversee plans for the monument.*

Soon after the mourners decided to erect a statue to help preserve the memory of Henry Grady, a letter published in the *Atlanta Constitution* indicated that some of Atlanta's most respected citizens found a full-size bronze too small of a memorial. No matter how tall or imposing or magnificently rendered, a bronze statue would never convey adequately Henry Grady's achievements or his vision for what the New South might become. Mr. William A. Moore, the senior partner of the Moore

---

* After reviewing proposals from fifteen artists, the committee chose a plan submitted by one of the most famous (and expensive) sculptors in the United States, Alexander Doyle. His work was familiar to Georgia's civic leaders who only five years earlier had unveiled his bronze sculpture of former United States Senator Benjamin H. Hill. Following a series of revisions to Doyle's proposal and more than a year of his labor, Atlanta's civic leaders presented the bronze Henry Grady to the public on October 21, 1891. Now an Atlanta landmark, Grady's statue commands the middle of Marietta Street, one of the busiest thoroughfares in downtown Atlanta. At the time it was dedicated near the intersection with Forsyth Street, the statue stood directly across from the ornate United States Customs House and near where the *Atlanta Journal-Constitution*—the successor to Grady's newspaper—would build its offices.

and Marsh Company—a large wholesale dry goods company formed in 1864—refused to contribute funds for the statue. His hesitancy had nothing to do with the committee and everything to do with his belief that Grady deserved a greater tribute. Moore sought a civic gesture that would better fit and recognize Grady's life.[2] The late journalist and New South booster had consistently suggested ways to make life in the New South not only more bearable, but significantly better. A living monument that improved people's lives, bringing them the kind of hope Grady had inspired, seemed to Moore to be a more appropriate way to extend the booster's legacy. A breathing tribute could continually infuse Atlanta's civic life with Henry W. Grady's ethos, his vision of serving the city and bettering the lives of its people.

The way that Moore proposed his idea for an active memorial is noteworthy. Although Atlanta's civic leaders regularly conducted public business in private, Moore stated his opinion in a letter to the *Constitution*. Perhaps he chose to make his case public out of a sense of urgency. In any case, the *Constitution* published Moore's suggestion that the city do more to honor Grady. Moore promised to give $5,000 in cash and designate another $5,000 in his will to help fund a specific proposal: have the city honor Henry W. Grady's life and vision with a hospital that would serve all of Atlanta.[3]

The city's civic boosters, Moore's fellow members of Atlanta's business and social establishment, must have smiled as they took notice. You can almost hear them approving of Moore taking advantage of Grady's death to attract attention to an old cause. Many civic leaders had been pressing for a city hospital since the middle of the 1870s. For more than a decade, ever since the Yellow Fever Epidemic of 1878, Atlanta's leading businessmen had looked for ways to provide better public health in their city. Nearly a year before Henry Grady died, the city council's Relief Committee recommended Atlanta set aside $10,000 per year for a new city hospital in each of the next three years. With their plan, the city would accumulate $30,000 for a charity hospital by 1892.[4]

Although there is little direct evidence suggesting that Henry W. Grady had sought a city hospital for very long, he too showed interest in Atlanta's hospital movement in the two years before he died. As noted in Chapter 1, Grady accompanied Samuel Inman and other civic leaders to see students from Spelman Seminary demonstrate their nursing skills in January of 1888. That summer, shortly after the King's Daughters Hospital was founded, Grady joined Inman as a member of the hospital's board of trustees. Editorials published in the *Constitution* in 1888 and 1889 that expressed support for a city hospital probably reflected Grady's views.[5] While Grady may not have been the first or greatest booster of Atlanta's city hospital movement, those who knew him well decided that a forward-looking institution designed to improve the welfare of his city and its people was a fitting tribute to the spokesman for a New South.

On January 6, 1890, within days of Moore's suggestion being printed in the *Constitution*, Mayor John Thomas Glenn stood before Atlanta's Board of Aldermen and Councilmen. Looking out over his friends, Mayor Glenn asked them to create a hospital in honor of Henry W. Grady. Taking his cue from the mayor, Joseph Hirsch, a remarkably successful businessman with philanthropic instincts, introduced a formal resolution to the body: the city would create a public hospital. Following a favorable report from a special committee of the council, the people's representatives approved the measure at their next meeting.[6] Atlanta would solve two problems efficiently—honor its most famous citizen appropriately and fill the need for a charity hospital.[7]

Joseph Hirsch, together with Colonel Robert J. Lowry—each had been a close friend of Henry Grady—organized the effort to turn the plan for a memorial hospital into reality. Their first step was to create a blue-ribbon committee made up of some of Atlanta's most prominent citizens. At the city council's request, this group would form the

A Leading Philanthropist Behind Grady Hospital

Jacob Elsas was born on October 6, 1842, in Württemberg, Germany. Orphaned as a child, he was raised by an uncle. As a teenager, Elsas worked in a factory and sold goods until, faced with being drafted into the army when he was eighteen, he headed to the United States. Practically destitute when he left Germany, Elsas is reported to have borrowed a dollar from a fellow passenger in order to complete his journey to Cincinnati.[38] After arriving in that heavily German-accented city, Elsas went to work for another uncle, a very successful merchant-manufacturer who ran a department store and was part of Cincinnati's growing garment industry.[39] Jacob's labors in Cincinnati, however, would not last long.

Having come to the U.S. shortly before the start of the Civil War, Elsas soon struck out on his own. He began as a traveling salesman, selling merchandise in Ohio and Tennessee. Shortly after ending a business venture in Nashville, Elsas met the fate he avoided in Germany. Drafted into the Union Army, he was posted in Cartersville, Georgia. He settled there after the war and opened a store. Three years later, in 1868, the restless and ambitious immigrant moved south to Atlanta

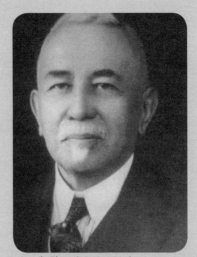

Jacob Elsas (1842-1931)

where he quickly started different ventures—including a general store and a used goods store. Together with two partners, he also started a business making "paper and cotton bags for flour, grain, and other commodities."[40]

The firm prospered greatly after another German immigrant, Isaac May, joined the team and helped it secure a $9,000 loan from a banker in Cincinnati. By 1879, Elsas, May and Company reached $400,000 in annual sales. Two years later, in 1881, they restructured their firm as the Fulton Cotton Spinning Company. With access to capital, they built a new complex of buildings east of downtown Atlanta, near the city's Oakland Cemetery.

In 1889, a year after Isaac Mays' death, Jacob Elsas formed the Fulton Bag and Cotton Mill Company. It soon became the largest industrial enterprise in the city. Elsas added an astonishing 40,000 spindles when he started a second factory in Atlanta in 1895. Twelve years later he added another 50,000 spindles in a third mill he erected in the city. The company expanded across the United States, eventually acquiring and opening plants in New Orleans, Dallas, Kansas City, St. Louis, Brooklyn, and Minneapolis. Although his firm had a national presence, Elsas remained devoted to Atlanta and continued to play a major role in the city's civic establishment.

A disciple of Grady's New South creed, Elsas strongly supported projects he hoped would boost Georgia's prosperity. For example, Elsas was an early supporter of having the State of Georgia charter a school of technology. During a meeting (that Henry Grady chaired) to discuss the idea in 1885, Elsas echoed a familiar New South theme. In short, he believed Georgia needed to attract factories in order to prosper. Starting a school of technology might help stimulate industrial production. It certainly would help relieve Georgia of a shortage of engineers. Sounding a little bit like Henry Grady, he told the group, "we are selling our raw materials for 5 dollars a ton to states that have trained engineers who fabricate it and sell it back to us at 75 to 100 dollars a ton."[41] He also told the group he was prepared to send his son (then attending Boston Latin School) to the Massachusetts Institute of Technology. The businessmen at the meeting each pledged $1,000 for the new school.

To the relief of Elsas and many other civic leaders, the state provided a charter for the new Georgia School of Technology that same year. (The school was renamed the Georgia Institute of Technology in 1948.) Along with many other businessmen in Atlanta, Elsas contributed to the fund-raising campaign for what became Georgia Tech's first building. Over time, Elsas would have his hand in a wide range of civic activities, including a major role in building the Hebrew Orphans Home, establishing Capital City Bank, and planning a modern water works system for the city.

new institution.* Since a planning committee had laid the groundwork for a city hospital only months earlier (see Chapter 1) much of the new committee's work would center on raising money.

Several sources provided the first gifts for the project. Individual contributors donated a total of $5,600 to the cause at the first meeting of the citizens' committee.[8] Atlanta's city council soon appropriated $30,000 for the project. By February 5, barely a month after W. A. Moore made his proposal, citizens and businesses had pledged over $11,000, with Moore himself donating $5,000.[9] The sale of property belonging to the city's defunct benevolent home generated another $20,000 for the Grady hospital fund.[10] Additional contributions lifted the building fund to nearly $68,000 by the first anniversary of Grady's death (December 23, 1890).

In addition to raising money, Hirsch and Lowry organized two subcommittees to oversee the hospital's construction. Captain James W. English, an established entrepreneur and former mayor of the city, chaired the group looking at potential sites for the hospital. His support for the hospital was evident in an initial pledge of $500 at the first meeting of the citizens' committee. Within a month his Chattahoochee Brick Company would pledge $1,000 to the hospital fund.[11] Jacob Elsas, whose firm had already given $1,000, would lead the building subcommittee.

In his role as chief of the embryonic hospital's building subcommittee, Elsas went on an inspection tour of recently built hospitals in the northeastern United States. Finding a new hospital in Providence, Rhode Island, especially impressive, Elsas enthusiastically supported hiring its architectural firm. Following his advice, the Grady Memorial Hospital planning committee soon signed a contract with the firm of Gardner, Payne, and Gardner. Ironically, given Henry Grady's view that hiring homegrown talent would help the New South prosper, the hospital hired an architectural firm based in New England. As it turned out, however, the head of the firm, Mr. Eugene Clarence Gardner, recently had moved to Atlanta for health reasons. A nationally renowned architect and pioneer in American domestic architecture, Eugene Gardner designed a wide range of buildings. In addition to the hospital in Providence, Gardner planned the hospital for his hometown of Springfield, Massachusetts, wrote a book about church design, laid out residential subdivisions, crafted industrial space, and even planned a cemetery.

The building subcommittee and the hospital's board of trustees enthusiastically adopted Gardner's concept for the hospital. Although Jacob Elsas had been impressed by the hospital in Providence, Gardner's work in Springfield provided the template for Grady hospital. Perhaps oblivious to the irony of it all, the building subcommittee awarded the general contract for constructing the hospital to another company from New England, Darling Brothers of Worcester, Massachusetts. (The firm submitted the lowest of the three bids offered.)[12] The architect and contractor expected to complete the new hospital within twelve months. Before building could commence, however, Captain English's subcommittee had to select a building site.

The location committee settled on a three-acre tract east of Atlanta's main South-North thoroughfare, Peachtree Street. The property, set between Edgewood Avenue and Decatur Street, occupied relatively high ground. This was important because the architect insisted that hospitals needed to be on land with good drainage. It was also rare to find such a spot near the center of the city. Many available areas near downtown Atlanta were relatively low-lying and regularly flooded during the 1880s. The location had another important

---

* Committee members included Joseph Hirsch, Samuel M. Inman, Robert J. Lowry, Dr. Abner Calhoun, Jacob Elsas, Albert Howell, Hugh T. Inman, William A. Moore, Dr. Hunter Cooper, Julius Brown, Captain John Milledge, Mayor John Glenn, and Governor Rufus B. B. Bullock.

advantage: Atlanta's streetcar line* ran only one block from the property, making the site easily accessible to potential patients and employees. The hospital also would front Butler and College Streets, placing the facility near Atlanta Medical College—one of the medical schools that would play a major role in Grady Memorial Hospital's story.

The planning committee bought the property for $13,500.[13] With an eye to the future, it purchased more land than it immediately needed. (Having the land in hand helped when Grady later expanded its facilities—at a time when the price of land near downtown had risen dramatically.) The total price was reduced when Colonel Lemuel P. Grant returned $1,000 of the purchase price after hearing that the land he was selling would be used for the charity hospital. (Such generosity was hardly out of character for Colonel Grant, a well-respected engineer who during the Civil War laid out Confederate lines of defense for the city. Eight years before selling the land for Grady, Colonel Grant donated 100 acres to the city for what became Atlanta's Grant Park.)

With the land acquired, the architect and hospital committee could begin to move from idea to plan. For Grady, as for his hospital in Springfield, Massachusetts, Gardner suggested using the pavilion plan made famous in the United States thirty years earlier by Philadelphia's Presbyterian Hospital. In this scheme, wards were set apart from each other and placed perpendicular to a central hallway. The idea was to allow for air to flow as freely as possible through the wards—and to provide as much daylight as possible. Of course, the way the idea was implemented varied from one institution to the next. The Johns Hopkins University Hospital in Baltimore was a somewhat more direct antecedent for Grady than Philadelphia's Presbyterian. Gardner had used Hopkins as the model for the hospital in Springfield and he would recycle the central concepts in Atlanta. Because of a difference in institutional size, he also would make some adjustments. Springfield, a town with 40,000 residents, erected a hospital that could hold fifty patients; Grady was supposed to open with twice as many beds.[14]

The vision of the planning group from 1888—presented more than a year before Henry Grady died—was for Atlanta's public hospital to start small and grow over time. The building subcommittee for Grady hospital followed the same idea. Compared to the hospitals in cities of comparable size—like Memphis, Louisville, and Hartford—Grady would be quite modest. The plans Grady's founders pushed (and could afford) were more in keeping with those of Springfield, whose hospital had one bed for every 800 residents. Following the guidelines from the building committee, Gardner planned on the same ratio of patient beds to population for Grady.

At first glance, the arrangement for Grady appears remarkably shortsighted. Even Gardner realized that Atlanta's rapid growth would quickly bring the ratio of beds to patients to an unacceptably low level. By his calculations in 1890, Grady hospital would have to double its original size within a decade just to keep pace with the expected population increase.[15] Gardner believed Atlanta's status as a railroad town only exaggerated the need for more beds at Grady.[16] Instead of designing a hospital that would serve the city for the next ten years, Gardner and the hospital committee were creating a hospital that would need to grow continually alongside the city. Perhaps their caution resulted from the city's experience with the benevolent home—a constant shortage of operating funds.

Maybe the plans for Grady hospital were so conservative because the boosters proclaiming the city's inevitable growth did not fully believe their own rhetoric. The choice

---

*The Atlanta and Edgewood Line was the first electric street car in Georgia. It was built by Joel Hurt, the President of East Atlanta Land Company, and was designed to connect downtown Atlanta with the residential Inman Park neighborhood to the east. It began operating on August 22, 1889, four months prior to the death of Henry Grady.

to start small would have made sense if civic leaders expected Atlanta to stagnate.

A relatively large and growing city, optimistic about its future, Atlanta nevertheless was already behind other cities by the time it decided to build a public hospital. Atlanta was not only playing catch-up to Memphis and Louisville, but also to smaller cities like Springfield, Massachusetts. Following the strategy of smaller cities—to begin small and add beds as the population grew—would doom Grady hospital to decades of difficulties. Another element in the planning for the hospital would provide its own set of challenges for generations to come.

In April 1890, as Gardner was moving from conceptual design to building plans, he pointed to a temporary aspect of the hospital. Gardner's original plan called for three wards for black patients to be built facing Jenkins Street, at the opposite end of the lot from the main administration building. A kitchen and a laundry separated the ward buildings for blacks from those for white patients. The wards to be built for black patients, however, would not last long. In the original plans, the wards for blacks were merely a temporary convenience.[17] Gardner told the *Constitution* in April 1890, "The idea is that a separate hospital will be provided for colored people in a few years, and the whole lot will be covered with wards for white people so as to give accommodations for two hundred, besides rooms for fifteen pay patients on the second floor of the administrative building."[18] Perhaps Atlanta's civic leaders still hoped that the proposed Franklin Hospital would be built near Spelman Seminary. In any case, the committee originally planned to turn Grady into an all-white hospital within a few years of its founding. With that configuration, Grady's growth would, for the next decade, easily keep pace with a growing white population. This meant that from the outset there was supposed to be a single Grady for whites only. Just as there were two Atlantas—one white and one black—there would be two racially separate charity hospitals.[19]

While the hospital in Springfield cost a little under $60,000, Atlanta's would be more expensive because it would be larger. Neither hospital, however, had the financial resources to duplicate the campus at Johns Hopkins; both, however, could borrow its principles. First among these was having plenty of air and sunlight in the wards. To achieve this the wards would be detached from each other—although connected by airy corridors. The other standards Johns Hopkins set and Gardner followed were equally simple: good "lighting, ventilation, drainage, and all sanitary conditions."[20] The administration building would house the operating room, and, on the top floor, have private rooms for patients who paid their own way. Gardner's preliminary drawings featured a brick "Tuscan" design that Gardner described as the only architectural style "adapted to brick." He found it advantageous because "it is simple and free from the elaborate detail."[21]

Gardner's main worry about Grady in April 1890 was that the $55,000 in hand would not go very far in erecting the first six ward buildings and the administration building. Joseph Hirsch, who had taken the lead in raising money for the hospital, shared Gardner's worries. Fortunately, the county chain gang performed the extensive grading the building site needed—which saved the hospital $3,000.[22] Cutting costs with free labor, however, would not be enough. When the construction contract was signed in November, the committee still needed another $25,000 to complete the project. This was in part because the initial cost estimate had risen to $90,000. It was also because enthusiasm for the public subscription campaign seemed to have declined despite Joseph Hirsch's monumental efforts.

Hirsch repeatedly appealed to the public, and the city's newspapers supported the cause. An editorial in the *Constitution* put the need in graphic terms: "[The people of Atlanta] have seen men ground up on the railroads, or mangled in machinery, and they have wondered why there was no suitable place to care for the sufferers. There is a simple answer to this: it was the lack of funds to build a hospital." Invoking the biblical parable of the Good Samaritan, the editorial urged Atlanta to care for the afflicted. It asked, "shall we let them die for lack of attention because they have no money?" Confidently, it answered, "This is not Atlanta's way."

The argument then turned to finances; a public hospital was the most economical way to care for people. Having a hospital would be "better for the city, better for the railroads and manufacturers who care for their employees, and better for people of every class who feel the burdens that common humanity imposes."[23] In response, a reader seconded the editorial's appeal to economic interests and urged businessmen to contribute to the hospital. Pointing out that capitalists needed workers, he wrote, "Without the laboring classes progress would be very tardy, and in order to make this useful class of our citizens feel that their presence is appreciated by the wealthier classes, their interests should not be neglected." He bluntly asked of the city's business community, "What has been done by the owners of the many factories, foundries, machine shops and other institutions of our city, employing the thousands of working men for whose benefit this great asylum of succor is so much needed, should injury overtake them while in the discharge of their daily labor?"[24]

The appeals were hardly fruitful. By late autumn of 1890, Hirsch and his committee had received a $30,000 promise from the city, $20,000 from the sale of the benevolent home, and about $16,000 in financial pledges from a total of about twenty citizens. Nevertheless, the building subcommittee decided to charge ahead and hold an elaborate ceremony to place the cornerstone for the main administration building on Tuesday, December 23, 1890, the first anniversary of Henry Grady's death.

The show was impressive. Members of the masonic orders from Atlanta and West End met at ten o'clock at the corner of Broad and Marietta Streets to prepare for the procession to the hospital site. As the time for the parade approached, hundreds of citizens assembled downtown. Those joining in the parade took their places along Marietta Street, filling first the block behind the starting line, along the broad avenue to where the bronze statue of Henry Grady would later stand, and then further west.

When the parade kicked off at 10:30 that morning, mounted police led marchers down Marietta Street, took a left on Edgewood Avenue, and proceeded for a half mile to Butler Street. Immediately behind the police was a locally organized Zouave Band, a quasi-paramilitary brass band wearing uniforms modeled on those of France's renowned Zouave d'Afrique—fighters who gained global fame during the Crimean War. (During the late nineteenth century, actors dressed in Zouave costume would travel as part of Buffalo Bill's Wild West Show.) The Atlanta Zouave wore colorful red and blue outfits, with baggy trousers, white leggings, a short jacket, and a tasseled fez. The exotic mock warriors festively cleared the way for members of the hospital's building subcommittee followed by the mayor, the city council, a contingent of reporters, the "Masonic Fraternities," and then other fraternal organizations followed by whoever else wanted to march in the parade. It is easy to imagine Henry Grady would have delighted in the day's spectacle.

Half an hour after the parade started, the official ceremonies began with a prayer by the Reverend John Heidt, followed by the laying of the cornerstone. John Davidson, Grand Master Mason from Augusta, performed the task. The faces of the cornerstone, donated by the American Marble Company, carried the following inscriptions:

Erected in Memory of
Henry Woodfin Grady
He Whose Heart was so Easily Touched
By Other's Woes Would ask no
Fitter Monument

And on the adjacent face:

Cornerstone Laid by
John S. Davidson
Grand Master of the Georgia F.A.M.
December 23rd A.D. 1890 AL5800

As was customary in the ritual laying of cornerstones, relics were placed in a metal box inserted in the stone. For the Grady hospital, the relics would include personal items from Henry Grady and totems from the city. Donated by his widow, a portion of the original manuscript of Grady's last prepared speech—the one he gave in Boston—was placed in the cornerstone. As if to further infuse the hospital with the spirit of its namesake, the cornerstone also held a photograph of Henry Grady and a copy of a book containing a selection of his speeches and letters.[25]

As Grady's friends celebrated laying the building's cornerstone—which contained his beliefs in its core—they reiterated his ideas. In flowery remarks, Mayor John Glenn paid tribute to his friend in terms that might have embarrassed Henry Grady. His main point, however, resonated with his audience: that Grady's ideals would be realized in the hospital's service to his city. Patrick Calhoun, a renowned railroad attorney in Atlanta who at the time was a partner in the firm of Calhoun, King & Spalding, gave the keynote address.[26] Noting Grady's popularity, Calhoun proclaimed, "never has a private citizen in this republic been so mourned."[27] He then invoked Grady's principles to explain why the hospital was a suitable memorial. Grady's widow, Julia, and his mother, Ann Eliza, who were among the relatives, friends, and dignitaries attending the ceremony, must have taken solace from the speeches.

With the cornerstone laid, fundraising and construction continued for the next seventeen months. The $68,000 that the committee had raised by the time the cornerstone was laid remained more than $30,000 short of the amount needed to realize the hospital's modest plans. Faced with a challenge to raise that much money, Joseph Hirsch attacked the problem with gusto. Again, however, there was little to show for his efforts. Although some large gifts came in, they couldn't offset the spending for construction.[28] Money started to run out. At the beginning of May the general contractor stopped working on the project. Not having been paid for the work done in April, Darling Brothers simply couldn't afford to continue the project until they received more money.

The complex was fairly far along. The two brick buildings for the white wards were almost completed and the wooden wards for black patients had been erected. The main administration building was about half-finished. The project had gone too far for the city to stop. Samuel Inman asserted, "not only every citizen, but the city government itself, is under a moral obligation to see that the enterprise is carried through."[29] Yet, Hirsch and his committee still needed to raise nearly $30,000.

Hirsch went back to work. He proposed that the city council appropriate another $10,000 and lend the committee $10,000 more. He would raise the rest of the money from private contributions. Hirsch hoped that this fusion of public and private money would allow the building to be completed inside of the year. Through the spring and summer of 1891, however, the going was slow.[30] The city council had no money to give. Soliciting private citizens, Hirsch managed to bring in substantial gifts from a few people. Joel Hurt, for example, made his first contribution to the hospital ($500) on May 24, 1891.

Up until mid-May, however, fewer than 80 people in the city had contributed to the cause since Grady's death. Efforts to canvas residents from all walks of life brought little reward. The greatest exception to this was the Atlanta firefighters. In late May more than sixty of them pledged to help, most contributing fifty cents or one dollar to the cause. Although Hirsch raised enough money so that exterior work could restart that summer, by September he remained shy of the fundraising goal. The construction delay due to lack of funds, and the difficulty in raising the money, bothered but did not deter him.

Hirsch used nearly every means imaginable to raise money for the hospital. Under his leadership the committee sponsored a fund-raising performance of Gilbert and Sullivan's opera "The Pirates of Penzance," organized other concerts, held raffles, and appealed to churches, club women, charitable organizations, labor unions, fraternal organizations, businesses, and individuals.[31] Hirsch ignored no one and

Fulton Bag and Cotton Mills

As part of his profitable business, Jacob Elsas offered his employees houses for rent in a small "mill village" that he built near his Fulton Bag and Cotton Mill factory. (Today, Atlanta's Cabbagetown community embraces much of the original mill-workers' community.) He originally hoped to rent the houses to his workers at a profit. Many of the workers, however, had their own ideas of the good life and chose to live elsewhere. Like textile mill owners across the South, Elsas welcomed volunteer do-gooders who wanted to practice social work among the mill hands. In general, the workers were impoverished and had little formal education. Most of them hailed from the countryside and many of them changed jobs and moved frequently. At first Elsas tried his own hand at improving the lives of workers with a company-run welfare program. The workers' desire for autonomy (plus their suspicion of his motives) made it hard for the company to successfully conduct social work among the employees. In 1902, however, Elsas turned the program of uplift and betterment over to others.

Six mission-minded women lived and worked in Wesley House, a settlement house Southern Methodists established in the mill village.[42] Through his firm, Elsas, who practiced Reformed Judaism, donated ten percent of the Wesley House's annual budget. (The settlement house's budget ran to nearly $6,000 in 1914.) The company also provided the settlement house with rent-free space in a failed 56-room hotel in the mill village.

Seeing social service as an inherent part of Christian spirituality—and intrinsic to the church's mission to build the kingdom of God—the Methodist women sought to improve the lives of workers and their families.[43] Eager to promote middle class views of domestic life, they offered women in the mill community lessons on cooking, sewing, housekeeping, and sanitation. In addition to providing day care (at 5 cents per child per day), tutoring, and recreation, Wesley House also operated a health clinic and small infirmary in the mill village. Staffed by nurses and volunteer doctors, the clinic at Wesley House saw approximately 150 patients per month in 1914. The clinic charged five cents for each visit, but did not turn away people who could not pay.

While the company had its reasons for wanting a clinic near the mill, at first glance it seems odd that Atlanta's Methodist women saw the need to offer medical care to people who lived only one mile east of Grady. It makes more sense once one takes into account the mill workers' six-day workweek (usually lasting ten hours each day). They must have been exhausted. Certainly the health clinic fit within the larger program of the settlement house movement.

Unfortunately for his paternalistic aspirations, Elsas' Fulton Bag and Cotton Mills in Atlanta became the site of one of the most infamous labor conflicts in the American South.[44] A lengthy strike started in May 1914 and continued through the following winter. Elsas' workers wanted higher wages. They also wanted to limit their workweek to 54 hours. In addition, the United Textile Workers, which led the strike, tried to end child labor in the mills. Workers at the Fulton Bag and Cotton Mills also tried to join the union.

The labor strike gained national attention when the U.S. Commission on Industrial Relations sent representatives to Atlanta to gather testimony from workers in March 1915. The employees reported working long hours in the dark and lint-filled mills six days per week. They also claimed that many of the workers were children, a violation of a recently enacted federal law. The head resident of Wesley House, Miss Emma Burton, testifying on behalf of the company, denied that the Fulton Mills purposely resorted to child labor. She claimed that parents "misrepresented" their children's ages in order for underage children to earn money in the mill. She indicated that she worked with the company to ferret out child labor. Although she described living conditions in the mill village as crowded, in general she gave favorable reports about the company's operations.[45] The strike ended as a failure in May 1915.

cajoled nearly everyone in his effort to gain contributions for the hospital. Through the dramatic stop and restart of construction Hirsch repeatedly pleaded the hospital's cause. He also contributed from his own pocket. Given the initial enthusiasm with which the civic leaders greeted the project, and the early success in raising money, it surprises that the effort stalled fairly quickly and that the fund-raising for the project became such a struggle for Joseph Hirsch and his committee.

Robert Lowry, who helped Hirsch raise money, pointed to one source of the difficulty: "this is peculiarly a public institution and [interested citizens] feel that the city should pay for it." The people who were used to giving money had already been tapped. Lowry argued against trying to raise more money by popular subscription, noting that the funds would come from "the very class of people who will never need the hospital." Those who would need the hospital, Lowry said, "have not contributed and will not contribute except by taxation."[32] In short, the people should be willing to be taxed for the institution if the burden was equally shared. Hirsch returned to the city council for more money in September.

James W. English, Sam Inman, Dr. Cooper, Dr. Calhoun, and Jacob Elsas joined Hirsch's appeal to the council for funds. Captain English noted that because the city held title to the property, the citizens' committee was blocked from borrowing against the value of the land. Dr. Cooper noted "people are dying in Atlanta almost every day on account of not having the proper medical attention at the proper time." The hospital was a vital need for the city's residents. While the city had no money to offer, it authorized the Grady hospital committee to borrow $20,000 with the understanding that the city would pay the interest and pay off the loan through an appropriation the next year.[33]

By the time the hospital was formally dedicated on May 25, 1892, Hirsch and his committee had raised $104,000; they claimed to be only $400 short of the amount needed to fully equip the new institution.

(Later complaints about a shortage of equipment at the time of opening—including essential tools for surgery—indicate that the committee did not publicize the true extent of the financial shortfall.) Some needs for equipping the institution were met by non-financial gifts that arrived at the last minute. The Church of the Redeemer, pastored by Dr. A. F. Sherrill, outfitted two of the hospital's private rooms shortly before the dedication, while a Mr. Theo Schumann donated three blankets.[34]

It seems likely that the last dollars easily could have been raised from within the ranks of Atlanta's prosperous business community. Even visiting locomotive engineers attending a convention in Atlanta donated $300 to the cause. To rely on business and labor alone for the last-minute financial gifts, however, would not have been the Atlanta way. As happened throughout the city's history, Atlanta's civic leaders pulled off a public way to at once raise money and attempt to increase public support for their effort. To bring in the last dollars the Grady Committee held a benefit baseball game at Atlanta's Brisbane Park—a fitting method given Henry Grady's presidency of professional baseball's Southern League.[35] With the money in hand, the hospital was almost ready to open. The day before it began accepting patients, Grady held an open house for the women of Atlanta. About 2,000 of them visited the new facility that day, many taking time to decorate the building with fresh flowers. With this final touch of color, the new Henry W. Grady Memorial Hospital was ready to meet many of Atlanta's health care needs.

While businessmen dominated the drive to create Atlanta's charity hospital as a memorial to Henry Grady, physicians would have to live with (and sometimes even live within) the new institution. Clearly having much at stake, local physicians joined in planning for the future hospital. Oddly, however, Atlanta's physicians did not hold their first formal meeting until only a few months before the building's scheduled dedication ceremony. Although they played a leading role in raising public awareness of the need for a charity hospital during the spring of 1888, physicians happily left much of the organizing work to others. Doctors, however, took charge of formalizing the hospital's internal procedures after the board of trustees named a medical board for Grady in March 1892. Composed of physicians from the community, this board would oversee the medical rules and practices at the hospital.[36]

Gathering for its first meeting on the evening of March 11, 1892, at Dr. Hunter Cooper's office, Grady's medical board unanimously elected Dr. Abner Calhoun as its president. The board selected their host for the evening, Dr. Cooper, as vice-president. A proven medical politician, four years earlier Dr. Cooper had chaired the organizing committee for a city hospital and in 1889 he had served as president of the Atlanta Society of Medicine. At the same meeting, Grady's medical board chose Dr. William S. Elkin as its secretary. Like the other physicians, Dr. Elkin practiced medicine in the center of the growing city. Well-established and thoroughly respected by his colleagues, Dr. Elkin had been president of the local medical society in 1884 just as Dr. Calhoun had been in 1880.[37]

Headed by some of Atlanta's most distinguished physicians, Grady's new medical board quickly created a subcommittee to investigate how other hospitals organized their medical staffs. The board would spell out regulations for Atlanta's new charity hospital only after finishing that survey—a kind of differential diagnosis for hospital rules. Drs. Cooper, William Armstrong, and W. Perrin Nicolson coordinated the study of other hospitals. (The latter two served as president of the local medical society in 1874 and 1890, respectively). They started their study at a time when physicians, trustees, and hospital administrators across the United States eagerly explored the best ways to organize a hospital. There was, however, no national consensus on hospital standards or procedures. Grady's medical board would have to create its own guidebook. Without the physicians' active involvement, Grady hospital would not have been prepared to start caring for Atlanta.

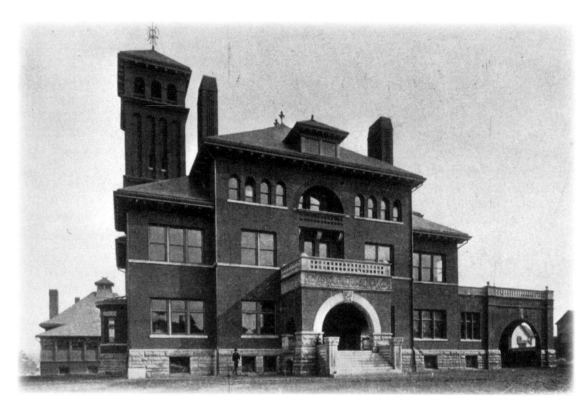

Grady Memorial Hospital (circa 1892)
The patient wards are located behind the main building; one can be seen on the left.

Building Patterns
1892–1917

Today marks a new era in the history of our city—an era of prosperity and growth that will far exceed the measure of our past achievements. Every city should take care of its sick and suffering. Atlanta is marching upward and onward, and is setting a pattern for the world to imitate.

—Mayor Hemphill, May 25, 1892

Grady Memorial Hospital opened its doors to patients on June 2, 1892, a week after the formal dedication, heartily supported by Atlanta's citizens and featuring the latest in hospital design. The hospital's layout was supposed to create a well-ordered, sanitary environment for the modern practice of medicine. The largest of its buildings, the main administration building, visually dominated the hospital grounds.[1]

The three-story red brick and stone building is 120 feet long. When it opened, two hallways intersected in the center of the building to divide the main floor. Along these corridors were a matron's room, a dining room for officials and convalescents, the director's consultation and reception rooms, a pharmacy, and an operating room. The surgical suite extended to the second floor where, from a circular observation area, as many as one hundred medical students could watch surgeons operating below them—for which the hospital charged students a small fee. (In 1904, the hospital added a new operating room attached to the original one on the building's northeast corner.) The second and third floors of Grady's main building provided beds for up to ten patients who paid the hospital's fees out of their own pocket. Six of these rooms for "private-pay" patients featured fireplaces that may have been added primarily as a decorative feature since the hospital's main building had a central heating system. The top floors of the administration building also contained quarters for resident physicians and for the hospital's nurses. In addition, the building originally featured a porte-cochere for ambulances.

Two small ward buildings, each measuring 32 by 42 feet, stood adjacent to the main building. Both contained a small kitchen and dining room, linen closets, laundry facilities, and attached bathrooms. The hospital dedicated one of the wards to treating special cases—usually people with a contagious disease. Grady also featured independent sick wards housed in long, rectangular buildings "made of brick or Indiana limestone except colored wards, which are in effect temporary buildings."[2] Each ward held twenty beds for patients, segregated by race and sex. Two of the three wood frame buildings on Grady's campus housed black patients; the other held offices and administrative departments. A small building erected near Pratt Street served as the hospital's morgue. Grady also had a short railway system, approximately one-eighth of a mile long. The hospital used this shortest of short lines to transport food from the hospital's central kitchen to buildings on the medical campus. Because the outbuildings were not connected to the central heating system, the little railroad also carried coal to the three frame structures.

City officials expected Grady to play an important role in healing the ill and injured, and they were optimistic about the hospital's ability to save lives. In its annual report at the end of 1892, six months after Grady's opening, the Relief Committee of the Atlanta City Council predicted "hundreds of lives will be saved each year [by Grady], for the fact, many wounds and diseases cannot be treated successfully unless we observe strict hygiene, cleanliness and proper nursing of the patient. It is impossible for hundreds of poor to afford this, [who] therefore die of septic wounds [when] their lives could have been saved in a properly kept hospital."[3] The elected public officials recognized the life-saving power of a clean, well-run hospital. They also understood that without such an institution, hundreds of the city's residents would die—essentially from neglect.

Grady Hospital's First Patient

Mr. Allen Kimball, a local railroad employee, was the first patient admitted to the new hospital. Entering Grady the day it opened, Kimball would stay with the hospital for the rest of his life. Following his successful treatment, Kimball, an African American, joined Grady's staff, working as an orderly and an ambulance driver until he died in 1931. Interestingly, Grady turned away the first person to seek treatment at the institution. It rejected him for two reasons: first, he was not a resident of Atlanta and, second, he was chronically ill. Originally, Grady rejected "incurables" as a matter of policy. The hospital's administration feared that treating such patients would cost so much money that the institution would go out of business.

Medical Schools and Grady Hospital

Located across the street from Grady, Atlanta Medical College provided medical staff for the new hospital. The oldest of the city's three medical schools, it competed aggressively with the others for students and faculty. This competition made ready access to hospitals crucially important for medical schools. While it mattered in attracting pupils, it was especially significant for teachers. Professors of Medicine needed to be able to treat what they referred to as "clinical material." The assumption was that having a large number of patients to choose from would help a medical school give pupils and teachers the best chance to learn, teach, conduct research, and improve the practice of medicine. Providing Grady with its medical staff was a feather in Atlanta Medical College's institutional cap, helping it attract students and retain faculty. Certainly, treating the city's poor at the charity hospital gave the medical school ample access to sick patients. The importance of having a steady supply of patients makes it understandable that other medical schools wanted their faculty appointed to Grady's medical staff.

The Georgia College of Eclectic Medicine and Surgery hoped to give its professors access to the patients at Grady. Chartered in Forsyth, Georgia, in 1839, the Georgia College of Eclectic Medicine and Surgery moved to Macon before reestablishing in Atlanta in 1883.[4] Having taught in the city for almost a decade, its faculty could reasonably expect permission to teach at Grady. After all, four years earlier Atlanta's physicians had agreed that the city's charity hospital would be open to all medical schools. Grady's administration, however, rejected Georgia Eclectic's request. They claimed that adding faculty and students from a second medical school would create discord. The hospital's board agreed, vaguely asserting that giving hospital privileges to faculty and students from another medical school ran counter to the hospital's best interests.[5] This ended the first of many "turf battles" that would reappear regularly in coming years.

In 1898, the two leading medical schools in Atlanta, Atlanta Medical College and Southern Medical College, joined forces to create The Atlanta College of Physicians and Surgeons (ACP&S).[6] The college named Dr. William Kendrick, a strong advocate of Grady's mission, as its dean, with Drs. Abner Calhoun, William Perrin Nicolson, and Floyd McRae among its faculty. Over the coming years each of these physicians would continue to give Grady strong support. Under their leadership, ACP&S immediately became the city's preeminent medical school. What that meant, however, would soon be open to debate. Embracing a new, more scientific and systematic approach to medicine shortly after the start of the twentieth century, interested people and well-endowed institutions in the United States started asking serious questions about medical practices and education. The Carnegie Foundation, funded by the famous

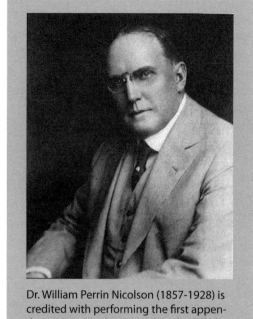

Dr. William Perrin Nicolson (1857-1928) is credited with performing the first appendectomy in Grady Hospital (in the fall of 1892). The operation may have been the first appendectomy done in Georgia.

steel magnate Andrew Carnegie, was among the most vigorous of these.

Late in the first decade of the twentieth century, the Carnegie Foundation commissioned Abraham Flexner to evaluate the quality of medical education in the United States and Canada.[7] Flexner did thorough research, visiting every medical school in each nation. (In one undoubtedly hectic month Flexner inspected thirty schools in a dozen cities). In January 1909, Flexner looked into Atlanta's three medical schools. They failed to impress him except in ways that were ugly. He succinctly summarized his findings about the College of Eclectic Medicine and Surgery, the suitor Grady rejected a decade earlier: "nothing more disgraceful calling itself a medical school can be found anywhere." Its laboratory, he reported, "occupies a building which, in respect to filthy conditions, has few equals, but no superiors, among medical schools."[8] Its clinical facilities were essentially non-existent. Harsh as they may seem, Flexner's descriptions of Atlanta's medical schools were more accurate than callous.

Flexner remarked on the nominal entrance requirements for applicants wishing to attend the new Atlanta School of Medicine (ASM), which organized only four years earlier. Like other Southern medical schools of its kind, it accepted students who had completed two years of high school. Even this minimal requirement, however, was easily waived for those with fewer years of formal education. A person who had only attended grammar school could be admitted to ASM if someone associated with a school, any school, testified to the applicant having "adequate scholastic attainments." This waiver turned out to be the rule rather than the exception. In the class that entered ASM in 1908, seventy-three percent came based on such an "equivalent."[9] Its laboratory equipment was "slight," although it had some good equipment, including an x-ray machine.

ASM also had two wards in the basement of the school, providing twenty beds. While those saw use, the school depended heavily on Grady for clinical teaching. Unfortunately, Grady was fairly ineffective for teaching ASM's students because the hospital was far enough away that the school's students did not "conscientiously attend."[10]

Abraham Flexner's kindest remarks about medical education in Atlanta were reserved for the Atlanta College of Physicians and Surgeons—even though it appeared to have more flaws than merits. Its nominal entrance requirements meant that it too enjoyed an inferior student body. Fortunately, it speedily sifted the wheat from the chaff. Seventy percent of the class of 99 pupils that entered in 1908 flunked out or dropped out within the first year. For Flexner this served as "statistical proof" that the students

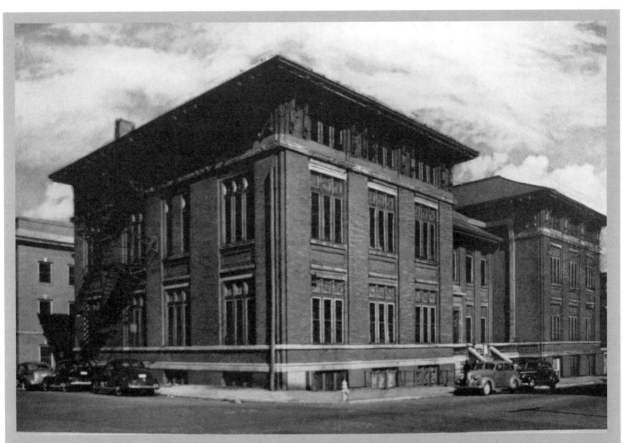

The original Atlanta Medical College, built in 1857, was torn down in 1906. Andrew Carnegie donated $40,000 for the construction of the new Atlanta College of Physicians and Surgeons building, and he spoke when its cornerstone was laid on April 7, 1906. This building became the Negro Division of Grady after World War I. The building was demolished in 1961.

who enrolled at ACP&S were remarkably ill prepared to study medicine.[11] Of course, the same data indicated that the faculty took their jobs seriously and did not generously hand out the "gentleman's C" in order to pass meager students.

Flexner did manage to compose a few other kind sentences about Atlanta College of Physicians and Surgeons. For example, he allowed that the school had good equipment, describing ACP&S as "perhaps the best equipped of all the schools of its grade…." He concluded, however, that with no full-time instructors in any of the laboratory sciences and an academically weak student body "the equipment cannot be used at its real value." He also praised ACP&S for its association with Grady Memorial Hospital. Yet, he thought the school made poor use of the hospital. ACP&S students did not take full advantage of access to Grady's clinical facilities in part because patients had to give their consent before students could receive "bedside instruction" in the wards. When they were granted permission, Flexner observed, "students are so unappreciative of their opportunities that attendance in the wards is very irregular."[12] While as many as six students could be accommodated at Grady's bedside clinics, on average only two students attended those sessions. Ever the pragmatic optimist, Flexner concluded that despite its dire condition, medical education in Atlanta could be saved. He prescribed consolidating the Atlanta School of Medicine and the Atlanta College of Physicians and Surgeons "to form the medical department of the University of Georgia."[13]

The Flexner Report about medical education in North America gained national attention soon after it rolled off the presses in 1910 and quickly earned substantial

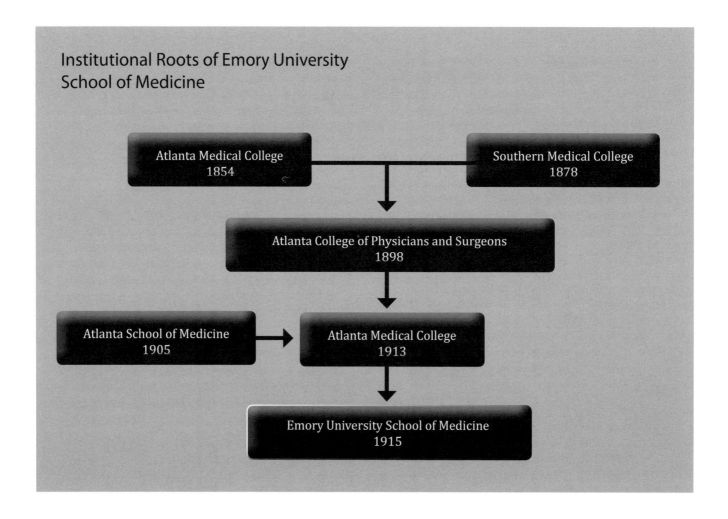

influence. Flexner's observations and recommendations affected the structure of American medical education for decades to come. One of the most widely reported reforms Flexner proposed involved closing some medical schools—mostly intellectually modest ones. Wide influence is attributed to the Flexner Report because as many as one-fifth of the 160 medical schools in North America closed or merged in its wake.

Three years after the Carnegie Foundation published Flexner's research, The Atlanta College of Physicians and Surgeons combined with the new Atlanta School of Medicine. The merged medical school took its name from the oldest of the predecessor schools—Atlanta Medical College. Like the Atlanta College of Physicians and Surgeons (and the original Atlanta Medical College), the new Atlanta Medical College (AMC) became intimately involved in the life and work of Grady. As part of its bid to win an "A" ranking from the American Medical Association (AMA), the new AMC needed to be connected with a hospital. With fourteen of its faculty already on Grady's medical staff, the school sought to control all of the clinical instruction in the hospital from each October through May. (The "control of clinical work" from June through September would belong to the seven members of the hospital's medical staff who were not on AMC's faculty.) Once again the Georgia College of Eclectic Medicine and Surgery asked for clinical privileges for its students, and this time it was approved.[14]

In his landmark report, Abraham Flexner urged medical schools to enhance their academic standing by affiliating with an established university. Unfortunately, Atlanta's medical schools had significant trouble heeding Flexner's suggestion because the city lacked a university. Some civic leaders, however, started planning one thanks to a dispute among Methodists in Nashville. Opened thirty-five years earlier by leaders in the Methodist Episcopal Church, South, Vanderbilt University was in the midst of a dramatic identity crisis when Flexner's report appeared. Vanderbilt, which had a medical school since it opened, wasn't concerned about ties between medical education and the university. It was fighting a religious war that had been declared several years earlier when, in 1905, Methodist bishops lost power in running the school. Nine years later a ruling by the Supreme Court of Tennessee would end hostilities at Vanderbilt. With the school once and for all separated from the denomination, the opening of a new Methodist school elsewhere in the South was assured.[15]

Anticipating such an outcome, one of the theologically archconservative bishops who served on Vanderbilt's board, Warren A. Candler, had started thinking about organizing a new Methodist university in Atlanta, where he served as bishop. His argument for choosing Atlanta may have received a boost among his confederates after Bishop Candler's brother, Asa Candler, the president and primary stockholder of the Coca-Cola Company, offered to donate one million dollars to the cause. In a hurry to fashion the university, the Candlers were able to move the main campus of an established Methodist college in Oxford, Georgia, to Coca-Cola's hometown. The old Emory College, on whose board Asa Candler sat, and where earlier Bishop Candler had been president, gave the new university instant roots in southern Methodism. It also provided an established academic institution for Atlanta's medical schools to court.

With the business-minded Bishop Candler serving as chancellor, Emory University showed ambition at the start. Like Vanderbilt, the new university wanted to have its own school of medicine. It worked out well, then, that in 1914—the year Tennessee's Supreme Court ruled on Vanderbilt's ties to Methodism—the Atlanta Medical College was scouting for an academic partner. The existing medical school and the nascent university soon entered into formal negotiations. Drs. William Elkin, Wilmer Moore, and Frederick Paxon spoke for Atlanta Medical College while Asa Candler, the Reverend Plato T. Durham (Dean of the Candler School of Theology), and William D.

Thomson (an attorney who would become Dean of the Emory University School of Law) represented Emory.

The talks between the medical school and the university led to Emory absorbing Atlanta Medical College and re-chartering it as the Emory University School of Medicine. With the deeding of its buildings to Emory on June 28, 1915, Atlanta Medical College effectively ceased to exist. The medical faculty and the university's leadership heartily endorsed having Dr. William S. Elkin continue to serve as Dean, which he would do for another decade. Thanks to the history of mergers among medical schools associated with Grady, absorbing Atlanta Medical College meant that Emory's medical school controlled the hiring for two-thirds of Grady's medical staff positions. (Physicians in private practice held the other posts.) Soon Emory's medical school would take sole control of Grady's black wards and oversee Grady's outpatient departments.

Superintendents of Grady Hospital

The Short, Unhappy Career of Dr. Albert Fensch

A German immigrant, Albert Fensch moved to the United States at an early age. Described as "a gentleman of cultured manners and a liberal education," he held diplomas from two medical schools and worked in several different branches of medicine.[16]

The Cotton States and International Exposition, Piedmont Park, 1895

Three years after the opening of Grady Hospital, President Grover Cleveland pressed an electric key in his library that inaugurated the exposition. Over 25,000 people were present at the opening on September 18, 1895. It closed December 31, 1895. The exposition cost three million dollars.

In probably the most formative experience in his career, Dr. Fensch practiced medicine at numerous army hospitals during fourteen years of military service. As an army physician, he served in the American west and was present at the capture of Geronimo. Among his accomplishments as an army doctor, he helped organize the hospital at Fort McPherson near Atlanta. Dr. Fensch left military service to become Grady Memorial Hospital's first chief executive, leading a staff of eighteen employees when it opened in 1892.

Under Dr. Fensch's guidance Grady ran smoothly—at least for the first three weeks. By the end of June, less than one month after the hospital admitted its first patient, the nursing staff threatened to go on strike. Dissatisfied with their salaries, the nurses wanted an immediate pay increase. The hospital's administrators averted a crisis by raising the nurses' salary to a minimum of $20 per month. Dr. Fensch had survived the first major crisis to confront Grady Memorial Hospital. The next one would erupt soon enough.

Within a few weeks of the nursing pay dispute an intense and disruptive conflict developed between Superintendent Fensch and Dr. H. L. Gill, the head House Physician. The hostility between the two men started after a patient complained to Dr. Gill about one of the nurses. Without first consulting Superintendent Fensch, Dr. Gill spoke with the nurse about the patient's complaint. Doing so put Dr. Gill in Superintendent Fensch's doghouse. Apparently, Dr. Fensch believed Dr. Gill should have sought the superintendent's approval before speaking to the nurse in question. The two men's intense verbal combat ended when the two physicians stopped speaking to each other—which they did in a matter of days. The clash ultimately led each to resign from the hospital's staff on the same day, October 31, 1892. Dr. C. J. George, a member of the house staff, would serve as acting superintendent for the next two months.

The Shorter, Even Less Happy Career of Dr. Thomas Kenan

Following a search that lasted several weeks, the board elected Dr. Thomas Kenan, a local physician, as superintendent of Grady hospital effective January 1, 1893. Dr. Kenan was born in Milledgeville, Georgia, the son of Augustus Holmes Kenan, an attorney and prominent politician who served in the Georgia legislature, signed the Confederate Constitution, and was a congressman in the Confederate States of America. Tall and thin, Dr. Kenan was a Confederate veteran who had practiced at the state's insane asylum in Milledgeville during the 1870s and 1880s. He had lived in Atlanta for four years when he was elected to head Grady hospital.

Looking for someone who could manage the hospital well, the board was more interested in finding a person with "good business tact" than in hiring a physician.[17] In Dr. Kenan they thought they had found a perfect combination. Given his experience as a surgeon "on board a man-o-war" and a reputation for being "a strict disciplinarian" the board expected there would be "no wrangling among those under him."[18] Within six weeks of his appointment, Dr. Kenan provided the board with a letter of resignation. The problem, from his perspective, was that he lacked authority to fire anyone or, for that matter, hire anyone. In short, the superintendent was powerless to effectively supervise the institution. As he told a reporter, "it is useless for a man to try to run a place of that kind unless he is given the power."[19] Apparently divided over whether to give more authority to the superintendent, the board waited until its regular meeting at the end of February before accepting Dr. Kenan's resignation.[20]

Dr. Tomlinson Fort Brewster

Dr. Tomlinson Fort Brewster, who became Grady's new superintendent on March 1, 1893, would guide the institution for the next fifteen years. Born and raised in Cherokee County, Georgia, Tomlinson Brewster earned his medical degree from Jefferson Medical College in Philadelphia. After completing his schooling, Dr. Brewster settled in Harris County, just north of Columbus, Georgia. The energetic Dr. Brewster was a leader in his rural community where, over the next thirty years, he did much more than practice medicine. Elected to the state legislature, Dr. Brewster became so fond of Atlanta (where the legislature convened) that he moved there in the late 1880s. In Atlanta Dr. Brewster sold life insurance in addition to practicing medicine. He also became actively involved in Central Presbyterian Church (located across from the State Capitol).

During Dr. Brewster's tenure, Grady followed through on the original plan to start small and expand slowly, adding a new department every few years in the first twenty years. In his decade and a half at the helm, Dr. Brewster oversaw the opening of a children's ward, the start of Grady's school of nursing (for whites only), and the creation of a maternity ward. Some of Grady's founders had pushed the hospital to include a maternity ward at the start, but the trustees rejected the idea. Perhaps simply getting the institution going generated enough complications to satisfy board members. Their languid approach to expansion also was tied to financial battles.

With barely enough cash on hand to build the hospital, Grady struggled to get adequate funding from the city for operating expenses. In his annual report to the city council, the President of the Board of Trustees of Grady Hospital reminded the city's elected officials that, "when the Grady Hospital was completed and turned over to the city, its appointments lacked completion in several details, because of the scarcity of funds."[21] Among these "appointments" were surgical instruments. While public hospitals in other cities provided this equipment, the devices used in the surgery department at Grady were the property of individual surgeons. Eventually surgeons like Dr. L. Sage Hardin donated their equipment to the institution.

Perhaps some city leaders were surprised at the cost of delivering medical care. By the hospital's fourth year in operation, discussions about city spending for the services at Grady intensified. That summer, the Board of Aldermen heard their colleague Joseph Hirsch threaten to shut down the hospital unless the city increased funding. Hirsch insisted that the $30,000 the city had spent to run Grady the prior year had been utterly inadequate. Without a larger budget, he said, the trustees would be forced to close the hospital. When the Board of Aldermen failed to reach a decision as their June session ended, Hirsch agreed to table the matter until the next budget meeting. When the finance committee met in October, Hirsch successfully argued for more money. Certainly it was not the last time that Grady would face financial catastrophe.

Another serious fiscal crisis took place several years later in Dr. Brewster's term as superintendent. In August and September 1903 the city council's finance committee notified the mayor that Grady was spending money too quickly. It warned that without a sharp cut in expenditures the hospital would run out of money before the year's end.

The meeting that Grady's board held to develop a response involved "a series of sensations." Dr. Thomas Longino, a physician, alderman, and ex officio Grady trustee, harshly criticized the hospital's medical board while other trustees attacked the hospital's management.[22] In addition, there were vague reports of "something said" about blacks being fed at city expense and nurses being paid too much. Unable to find a way to cut costs, the trustees invited suggestions from the city's finance committee and even recommended Alderman Inman become a Grady trustee. Shortly after the meeting, Dr. Longino publicly suggested Grady abolish its paying patient service.[23] If it enacted his idea, Grady would only serve charity cases. Since the pay-patients produced revenue that went straight to the city rather than into the hospital's coffers, their absence would not directly affect Grady's finances. It is unclear how abolishing the paying patient service would have reduced operating expenses if charity cases simply replaced the fee-paying patients. Judge George Hillyer, meanwhile, offered a plan of his own that he promised would cut costs at Grady.

Judge Hillyer commanded respect among the city's leaders. The son of a congressman, he captained a Georgia regiment in the Army of Northern Virginia and participated in the battles at Fredericksburg and Gettysburg. More significantly for the debate over Grady and city taxes, Hillyer carried authority because he had served as mayor of Atlanta from 1885 to 1887. In the context of a vigorous debate over city taxes in 1903, Judge Hillyer suggested the city privatize Grady—likely the first (but certainly not the last) time a politically prominent figure did so publicly.

Arguing that the city hospital was not a "natural monopoly" in the way of, for example, the water works, Hillyer urged the city to lease the hospital to a private group.[24] This, he suggested, would remedy relatively rapid growth in city spending for public relief—the amount had risen dramatically from about $6,000 when Hillyer was mayor to $45,000 in 1903. Thirty-three thousand of those dollars in the city's budget, however, went to Grady, an institution that did not exist during Hillyer's term in office.[25]

Even excluding expenditures for Grady, Atlanta's spending for relief had doubled in sixteen years, rising from six to twelve thousand dollars. Hillyer clearly was correct that when the money spent running Grady was included, the city's relief expenditure had greatly outpaced tax revenue. Yet, it is unclear how the city would have saved money through privatization except by drastically changing the character of the hospital or by returning to under-reimbursing hospitals for charity cases. (In 1900, Grady's average daily cost to the city was $1.13 per patient, fifty percent more than the 75 cents per day the city reimbursed St. Joseph's at the time Grady opened.)[26] It is likely that reimbursement from the city would have been a private group's primary source of operating income. Given Grady's central mission as a charity hospital, fees would generate little revenue. Thus, reducing salaries and some services together with cutting costs for food, linens, and laundry would have been likely routes

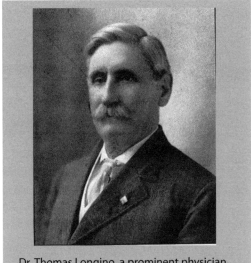

Dr. Thomas Longino, a prominent physician and politician, had been mayor of West End before becoming an alderman in Atlanta. He served as a surgeon in the Spanish-American War. He died in 1911.

to profitability. It is probable, however, that Judge Hillyer was less interested in how a private group would prosper than he was in keeping taxes low. Indeed, reducing taxes seemed to be Judge Hillyer's chief mission. Privatizing Grady, however, also meant a return to an older view of what city government was supposed to accomplish.

For most of the nineteenth century American city governments relied on small budgets and low taxes in order to accomplish relatively little. Their primary job was to construct public works rather than democratically distribute services. The main way they kept taxes low was by keeping as many services as they could out of general funding. Instead, they paid for public improvements through special assessments levied on property owners who would benefit from a specific improvement in infrastructure. Because of the charter reform of 1874, Atlanta would be pushed toward an assessment system when it tried to expand public services in the 1880s. The special assessment system would apply to paving streets and providing water service on the theory that a property owner with a brick street or with access to city water benefited directly from that improvement.

While public services in Atlanta remained unevenly distributed, adopting the special assessments system meant that residents who got city services began to pay a larger share of the costs than they had when improvements were paid for out of the general fund. This assessment system, however, could not work with poor relief or charity medical care since, by definition, the charity case could not pay for services received.

Charity medical care stood at odds with the direct pay-for-services approach to city financing. For one thing, the benefits of charity medical care were diffuse. While it helped the recipient directly, it also benefited the city as a whole. One aim of general hospitals like Grady was to cure the working poor and return them to economically productive labor.* Another aim was to prevent servants who were ill from infecting their employers. The benefits Grady offered for the common good led Atlanta to allocate funds for Grady from the city's general budget. In short, the mechanism for funding Grady was to assess everyone and allocate the revenue to charity. By definition this was a form of redistributing wealth—and it was a redeployment that served a clearly defined set of public purposes.

Judge Hillyer's hope to privatize Grady in order to reduce taxes was more in tune with an approach to city government that had been left behind a generation before. In his proposal, which did not go anywhere with the city council's special taxation committee, Hillyer seemed to admit the need for Grady; he did not, however, acknowledge that when he was mayor the city failed to adequately reimburse private hospitals for public charity cases. In making his privatization proposal in 1903, Hillyer seemed to have forgotten that the city's miserly payment to private hospitals prompted physicians and other civic leaders to fight for a city hospital in 1888. As a public hospital Grady would take care of the poor, a mission then seen as benefiting the entire community. Being a publicly owned hospital also meant Grady would be accountable to the citizens. Yet, as Hillyer's comments during the budget crisis of 1903 make clear, Grady's nature as a public institution could be a subject for debate whenever people fought over city finances.

A case concerning emergency care during Dr. Brewster's tenure illustrates another aspect of Grady's identity as a public hospital. It also exemplifies a debate at the time about who was responsible for payment to treat injuries caused by a corporation. As the fiscal crisis was hitting Grady and the city of Atlanta during the summer of 1903, James McWhirter, a well-known citizen who was in the marble and granite business, had the misfortune of having his arm broken in a trolley car accident. Having rushed off to Grady, accompanied by other "reputable citizens," McWhirter was forced to wait to see a physician—but not because Grady had more critically injured patients to deal with first.[27]

Although there were enough physicians available for McWhirter to be seen by a Grady doctor, someone at the hospital decided McWhirter ought to be seen by a physician who worked for the Georgia Railway and Electric Company. (The trolley line had contracts with private physicians to provide medical care for people injured in accidents involving its equipment.) The company's physician, Dr. John Hurt, did not show up after being called to Grady; after a considerable wait Mr. McWhirter visited his personal physician for treatment. Surely a sense of great urgency had led McWhirter to seek help at the hospital in the first place. Its refusal to care for him ran counter to Grady's reason for being. The central idea had been, as a newspaper editorial characterized it, that all who came to Grady immediately became "the ward of the city," regardless of their ability to pay.[28] Obviously McWhirter could have gone home

---

*Among Grady's 1,482 patients in 1900 whose occupations are known were 218 laborers, 108 cooks, 69 houseworkers, 64 laundresses, 34 farmers, 33 seamstresses, 30 factory hands, 18 dressmakers, 18 housekeepers, 16 carpenters, 13 tailors, 13 firemen, 11 bookkeepers, 9 machinists, 8 mechanics, 8 butchers, 7 cabinetmakers, 7 electricians, 6 stonecutters, 5 candy makers, 5 blacksmiths, 4 milliners, 3 printers, 3 masons, 2 boilermakers, 7 teachers, 5 clergymen, 24 prostitutes, a lawyer, an actor, a journalist, and a legislator.

and called for a company doctor to visit him there if that was what he wanted. According to the editorial writers, identifying the party causing the injury should not have been at issue. Instead, they argued, emergency patients should be attended to first; concerns about responsibility for payment could come later. In the context of the city's (and Grady's) fiscal crisis in 1903, it appears concern over money could have affected patient care.

Dr. Brewster faced one of his greatest administrative challenges in the spring of 1905 when the hospital's nurses revolted against their supervisor. The superintendent of nurses was a northerner, Miss Margaret A. McGroarty. She had been trained at Bellevue Hospital in New York where, according to Joseph Hirsch, she was educated "under the strictest discipline." Mr. Hirsch lauded Miss McGroarty's effort "to organize, systematize and gently but firmly discipline the nurses of Grady hospital."[29] The nurses in Atlanta, however, found her ways offensive, describing her as being "too harsh, domineering, and dictatorial." They were especially unhappy because, they claimed, she assigned nurses she disliked to the black wards for months at a time. Among Miss McGroarty's alleged outrages, she scolded a nurse "in the presence of negro patients" because the nurse had "rebuked a negro orderly who would not obey her instructions."[30] The nurses in training would not accept her upbraiding the white nursing students in front of their black patients. The superintendent saw their protest as insubordination, "difficulties that should not exist in a well-regulated hospital."[31]

On Saturday, March 4, more than one-third of Grady's thirty-three student nurses marched into Dr. Brewster's office, resignations in hand, threatening to quit unless Miss McGroarty was fired. When Dr. Brewster took no action, a dozen student nurses walked out. As it turned out, Miss McGroarty had tried to resign the day before, but board president Joseph Hirsch rejected her attempt. Finally, on the following Wednesday, March 8, the board accepted her resignation—which she made conditional upon the twelve nursing students who had walked off the job being fired, which they were. Two days later the dismissed students begged the hospital's medical board for reinstatement. In order to return they had to publicly confess that the medical board had been right to fire them and agree to have their "terms of service" extended by several months as a punishment. They would work as nursing students for six extra months in order to have the right to return to school. In other words, they accepted a half-year's labor as their fine.[32]

Some physicians initially resisted the reinstatement of the nurses. Dr. Floyd McRae and two other members of the medical board, Dr. James B. Baird and Dr. William S. Elkin, objected vigorously. Noting he had operated on several patients on the day of the walkout, Dr. McRae termed the student action "inhuman."[33] Agreeing with Dr. McRae, Dr. William P. Nicolson said, "this desertion of the patients was not only an act of insubordination, but it was an act of inhumanity as well."[34]

Dr. Nicolson, who chaired the committee on medical matters, explained that only after he heard all the facts did he come to believe the nurses should be allowed to return. He claimed that a member of the hospital's medical staff had advised the nurses that their strike would cause no ill effects to the patients. The Grady pharmacist, Dr. F. Lewis Eskridge, had sided with the nurses and signed a blistering public notice lambasting Mr. Hirsch and the hospital's medical board. The board fired Dr. Eskridge. It was later revealed that the house surgeon, Dr. Charles R. Andrews, had dictated the letter. When Dr. Andrews and another physician tried to resign, the hospital rejected their effort, deciding to fire them instead.[35]

As the proceedings wound down, Mayor Woodward added his two cents. He asked that in the future the hospital hire only southern women to be superintendent of nurses. The board of trustees and the medical board quickly affirmed the mayor's request.[36] This row was unusual, but it indicates the kind of political waters Superintendent Brewster navigated.

During his fifteen years at the helm Dr. Brewster fostered a positive working relationship between Atlanta Medical College's faculty and students and Grady's staff and other doctors. Dr. Brewster retired after developing Bright's disease (nephritis) in 1907. He died in 1910 and was buried in an unmarked grave in the Central Presbyterian Church section of Oakland Cemetery. In 2003 a marker was placed over his grave site.

Mr. James J. Meador

Following Dr. Brewster's departure, the hospital appointed Mr. James J. Meador superintendent. Mr. Meador, born in 1838 in La Fayette, Alabama, was one of eight children. He served in the Confederate Army through the Civil War and was wounded in the First Battle of Manassas. After the war's end Meador moved to Atlanta and entered the wholesale tobacco business. He was a founding member of the Board of Trade (1866) and the Atlanta Chamber of Commerce (1871). Mr. Meador also served as a city councilman from the second ward at the time Grady was being founded. In 1877, he opened a successful life insurance business, which he operated until being named Grady's new superintendent in 1907. Unfortunately, the highly respected businessman's tenure as Grady's chief lasted less than one year. He died at the hospital on October 11, 1908. Like his predecessor, he is buried at Oakland Cemetery. After Meador's death, Ms. Anna Y. Bridges, a nurse on the Grady staff since 1903, served as acting superintendent for several months.

Dr. William B. Summerall

Dr. William B. Summerall moved to Atlanta in 1903 in order to work for the city. For four years, from 1904 to 1908, he oversaw the city's contagious disease hospital, which primarily isolated smallpox patients from the rest of the city's residents.[37] He earned a well-deserved reputation for being a progressive and accomplished physician devoted to improving public health. Like other leading doctors of his day, Summerall strongly advocated inoculating infants against smallpox. It didn't surprise when Grady's board tried to lure Dr. Summerall to become the hospital's new chief. Dr. Summerall, however, rejected the board's initial attempts, apparently because the pay was too low. (They were six hundred dollars apart.) Determined to land Dr. Summerall, Grady's board found half of the additional money in its budget and asked the city for the other $300 in order to meet his salary demand. With the city's promise to provide the additional money, Dr. William B. Summerall became Grady's new superintendent at the start of April 1909.

Dr. Summerall promised to give the public the best possible service, treating rich and poor alike. Given few of the wealthy were likely to enter through the hospital's gates, his promise may have been a rhetorical flourish underscoring a strong commitment to giving the indigent first-rate care. In any case, to achieve his goals, he urged Grady's board of trustees to expand the hospital's capacity from 100 to 250 beds. In his view, the hospital barely had enough beds to treat all of its emergency patients. More beds would help Grady better serve Atlanta. In addition, Dr. Summerall pushed the board to create a separate ward for private-pay patients of the medical school faculty associated with Grady.

Hardly among Atlanta's poor, private-pay patients came to Grady only because their physician practiced there, a custom that Dr. Summerall encouraged. Creating a new ward specifically for them would allow Grady, in theory at least, to ease the ongoing transition of moving medical treatment for middle class patients from home to hospital. With a ward of their own, wealthier patients would be relieved of mingling with the poor in a public space. Putting private-pay patients on their own ward would continue segregating patients by class, just as in its original design the hospital segregated wealthier patients in private rooms. Grady's patients would not be divided by race alone.

Dr. Summerall wanted to attract more patients who could pay for their own treatment for one simple reason: to subsidize the cost of treating charity cases. He needed more money largely because Atlanta's city government continued to underfund Grady. There was never enough money to operate the hospital adequately. Grady consistently needed additional resources to improve facilities, add new medical equipment, and hire physician specialists. The inadequate backing haunted Grady during its first two decades. The city's small annual budget appropriation for Grady paralleled its meager reimbursement of Atlanta's private hospitals for indigent care before Grady opened.

Dr. Summerall's plan for getting around the city's miserly funding followed the precedent that The Johns Hopkins University Hospital established in Baltimore a generation before: have paying patients subsidize the cost of charity care offered at the hospital. Atlanta's government, however, rejected the scheme. Apparently city hall wanted every dollar it could get from Grady. So the hospital's revenues continued flowing into the city's general fund.

Despite the budgetary constraints, Dr. Summerall made enough progress in easing the hospital's financial woes to invest in new equipment. These purchases were needed if the hospital was going to stay abreast of innovations in medical science and technology. If it fell behind the times, patients would die for budgetary reasons, not because diagnostic equipment or treatment options were generally unavailable. Similarly, shortchanging the hospital on equipment would limit the training of medical students at Grady. The urgency of the matter, and the pressure of keeping up with recent medical and surgical advances, made finding more money an endless plague upon Dr. Summerall's office.

In 1910, Atlanta's voters approved a $100,000 bond issue to pay for the hospital's expansion and under Dr. Summerall's guidance Grady undertook its largest construction project since opening. After holding an architectural competition, the board selected Harry Leslie Walker's design for the new hospital. A native of Oak Park, Illinois, as a teenager Walker briefly worked for Frank Lloyd Wright. Following study at the Art

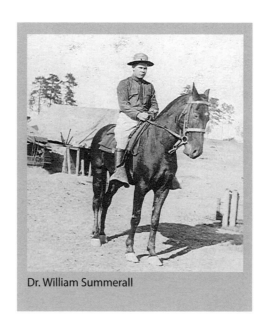

Dr. William Summerall

Institute of Chicago, Walker graduated with a B.S. from M.I.T. in 1900. He then moved to Atlanta to start his architectural practice. Working with Dr. Summerall and the building committee, Walker's firm (King and Walker) quickly fleshed out the plans for the new Grady facility. The bids from contractors were opened in November and hospital leaders laid the cornerstone weeks later, on December 29, 1910.

When the facility was completed less than two years later, the new building at 56 Butler Street had room for 110 white inpatients. Among its more notable features, the structure contained a large, open solarium on each floor so patients could enjoy the outdoors as much as possible. In an era before centralized air-conditioning systems were plausible for hospitals, the solarium offered an important means of ventilating the building. In this, as in other aspects, the new building reflected the most current thinking about hospital layout and design.

Dr. Summerall had thought deeply about how building design could enhance the hospital's function as a place of healing. In creating the new facility, designing for cleanliness was one of his top considerations. On the theory that germs hid from cleansers in cracks and crevices, the hospital's interior featured smooth surfaces throughout. The

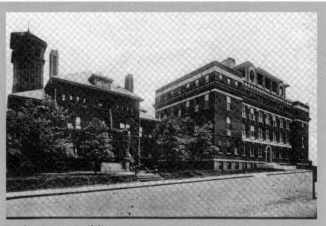

Butler Street Building, 1912
The Butler Street Building is shown on the right with the original Grady Hospital on the left. Construction began in 1910 after city voters overwhelmingly passed a $3 million bond issue (by 8,409 to 66). The bond issue designated $100,000 for the new 110-bed hospital.

floors were made of a type of marble thought not to crack. Where that material could not be used, the builders laid down "battleship linoleum," described as "smooth, noiseless, and germ proof."[38] The walls also were designed for easy cleaning. The electric lights were made of "porcelain-covered brass" and the windows featured "dust-proof grooves" to keep out dirt.[39] The two operating rooms had a ten-foot square skylight above a glass sheet that kept out dust. Specially designed electric lights placed between the glass and the skylight allowed for surgery to be performed at night. The operating rooms also had adjacent areas where surgeons changed their clothing and sterilized their hands.

The edifice had plenty of ventilation and light in part because there were no solid interior walls. Every room had windows and a transom above each door. While it may have brought in a good bit of dust on its own, the ventilation system fit in with the most recent technology. Two large fans on the roof brought fresh air to chutes running through the building. The air supply in each room, however, was independently controlled. In addition, patients could be taken in their beds to galleries on the southern end of the building for access to direct sunlight and fresh air. The hospital also featured the most modern plumbing, a newsworthy feature in a city full of privies. The faucets were run by knee-levers so that "when a surgeon or nurse sterilize their hands, infection is not gathered by touching the pipes again."[40] In keeping with the germ-free ideal, no pipes ran through the floor by the toilets. Suspending the plumbing overhead allowed workers to clean floors thoroughly.

While Dr. Summerall devoted much thought to building for cleanliness, he also considered design elements to help the building last. Thus, making the building fireproof was one of Dr. Summerall's central goals. While he did not fully succeed, some of the features Dr. Summerall insisted on helped reduce the threat of fire. These included minimizing the use of wood in the structure by adopting reinforced concrete for the building and using shale brick for the facing. Only the doors and window trim in the new structure were made of wood.

From top to bottom it was reportedly the most modern and complete hospital building in the South. A single elevator at the center of the building ran from the basement to the roof. Similarly, dumb-waiters ran from top to bottom, allowing for quicker delivery of food and supplies to every floor. A laundry chute ran to the basement, which held a sterilizer for mattresses and towels in addition to the laundry. Kitchens, baths, a drunk tank, the ward for prisoners, the hospital drug store, and a laboratory also occupied the basement level. The lab included an area for bacteriology and an x-ray room. Administrative offices, a library for physicians, a lecture hall, and a small ward occupied the first floor. The wards for men stood on the second floor, the wards for women on the third floor. The north end of the fourth floor held two operating rooms. The larger of them (20 feet by 20 feet) had seats allowing sixteen students to observe procedures. The rows, built one above the other, began six feet from the operating table. Much of the south end of the fourth floor was reserved for private rooms for patients paying for their own care. In all of this, the design was intended to make the hospital better for patients and physicians.

The new building certainly helped Grady keep in step with Jim Crow. Dedicating the new facility to treating white patients allowed Superintendent Summerall to transform the old "white ward" into space for treating the hospital's growing number of black patients. The new building became "White Grady." Gradually the old building changed into "Black Grady" (but not until November 1912 when two of the white wards in the old building were "ordered opened for the use of colored patients to accommodate the overflow [in the black wards] so as to relieve the congestion").[41] In southern terms, the building was up-to-date in every way. Unfortunately, the definition of a "modern hospital" has a way of changing rapidly. Within two years of the building's completion, reports about its use showed Dr. Summerall's medical theory about hospitals being slapped hard by financial reality.

Isma Dooly, who covered women's issues for the *Atlanta Constitution*, painted an ugly picture of the city hospital in a story published in April 1914. Ms. Dooly's report in the *Constitution* was part of a publicity campaign civic leaders organized to promote passage of a $750,000 bond issue designed to pay for more improvements at Grady. The proposed bond included $150,000 for a new facility for white patients who paid their own bills. The bond money also would upgrade Grady's other facilities, especially the black hospital. An active participant in the Grady Hospital Aid Association, Ms. Dooly had long helped Grady. Her personal views may have spurred what seems like hyperbole in the news story. For example, she wrote, "I have been in the squalid quarters of poor negroes, but I have never seen anything which more deeply wounded my sense of what is due humanity than what I saw in the Grady hospital the other day."[42] Yet, her expose was more than a simple pro-bond puff piece.

It eloquently demonstrated that Grady's physical condition and overcrowding were threatening Atlanta's public health.

Ms. Dooly could honestly report what Grady was lacking. Grady did not have an area for contagious diseases like whooping cough, the leading cause of death for children in Atlanta at that time. Indeed, Ms. Dooly reported that two-thirds of the deaths in Atlanta in 1912 and 1913 came from infectious and contagious diseases. Yet, Grady had "no facilities for the treatment of measles, meningitis and other infectious and contagious diseases."[43] Its only isolation ward was a small building that housed adults with sexually transmitted diseases. Grady not only lacked many facilities found in America's more progressive hospitals, its quarters proved incredibly overcrowded. Even the new White Grady building was filled beyond its intended capacity. Because the charity wards were full, many indigent patients were housed in the private-pay wards on the fourth floor. As a result, many private pay patients were shut out—a costly practice for the city.

In 1914, Grady still lacked adequate space to house its nursing staff. A small ward on the first floor of the new White Grady offered some space for nurses. Others were consigned to an old building off of the back of the hospital grounds, next to the morgue. Two of the nurses, Ms. Dooly reported, lived in a linen closet. The working conditions for other employees were beyond miserable. The hospital's original kitchen building was in disrepair, its walls falling down, the ceiling loose, and there were mud-puddles on the floor of the room where supposedly sanitary meals were prepared for four hundred people each day. The dining area for the hospital's eighty black employees consisted of an unventilated ten-foot by twelve-foot room immediately off of the kitchen grill area. These were the conditions in the new, modern, up-to-date White Grady; conditions were worse elsewhere at the Gradys.

Ms. Dooly painted a remarkably disturbing portrait of Black Grady. The facility was so congested that patients were placed in

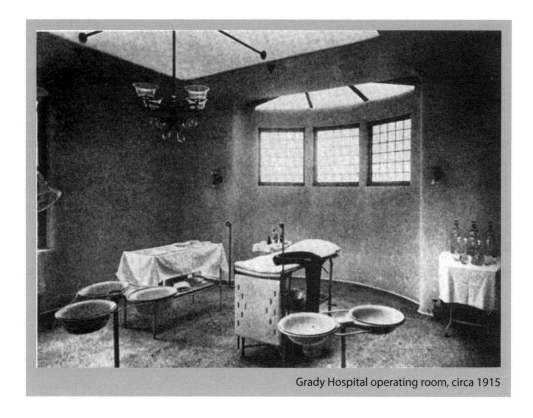
Grady Hospital operating room, circa 1915

hallways and on porches. Grady's black wards were overcrowded, lacked adequate light, and had splintered floors and falling ceilings. Black Grady was turning away as many as 20 people per day because there was no room. In fact, the hospital could care for only half of the eligible indigent population.

Every bed in the women's ward at Black Grady was occupied. Ms. Dooly reported, "there is no maternity ward for negro women, and negro children have been born on the doorsteps of vacant houses. Women bearing children have been picked up off the street and taken to strangers...."[44] Given that a red-light district ran behind the hospital, newspaper readers may have shuddered in proper Victorian horror at the thought of poor but respectable women bearing children in brothels. (A year later the "colored maternity ward" consisted of one bed in a small room.)[45]

As for the outpatient clinic, Ms. Dooly claimed she could not in good conscience fully report all that was wrong "in a paper supposed to go outside of the city and urge strangers to come in."[46] She did note, however, that the clinic building where patients were diagnosed was completely jam-packed. On the day she visited, the clinic building meant for fifteen to twenty patients held from fifty to sixty people—many of them with communicable diseases. She reported that in the first three months of 1914, two of the clinic's patients had been diagnosed with smallpox. The crowded waiting area was a place where diseases could be transmitted easily.

The one emergency operating room in the outpatient clinic was perhaps the only space in the hospital where Jim Crow barriers could not be firmly upheld. The emergency operating area was so crowded, Ms. Dooly reported, "it is not unusual for a white patient to be on one table, a colored patient on another."[47] Economic necessity had become the mother of de facto racial desegregation, likely a horrifying prospect to white newspaper readers in a state that enforced Jim Crow laws. The three-quarter-million-dollar bond issue would go a long way to helping Grady better fulfill its mission to care for Atlanta.

The campaign was heavily promoted across the city. Civic boosters argued that without an improved, modern, professional Grady, Atlanta would be hamstrung in competing for funding of medical research from northern philanthropic foundations. (An unnamed northern "welfare foundation" was said to be considering creating a one million dollar endowment for medical research work in a Southern city.) Without a Greater Grady containing "ample, modern and expansive laboratory, clinical and hospital facilities," Atlanta would lose out.[48] Advertisements supporting the bond issue were presented on screen at the movie houses, business leaders organized a get out the vote campaign, and the city's preachers gave support for the issue on the Sunday before the election. The *Constitution*, boosting the effort, gleefully claimed, "there is scarcely an organization of importance in the city which has not put its stamp of official approval upon the bond issue."[49]

The impressive efforts of Ms. Dooly and Atlanta's civic leaders fell short as the bond issue of 1914 failed to gain the votes of two-thirds of Atlanta's registered voters, the state requirement for passing a bond referendum. City residents who voted on May 5, 1914, supported the measure by nearly eight to one; yet, it was not enough. Despite winning a majority of the city's registered voters, the $750,000 bond issue failed.[50] Even with the loss, some observers interpreted the heavy vote in favor of the bond issue as a clear expression of the community's support for improving Grady. Others, however, including Robert L. Foreman, an insurance executive and the son-in-law of Evan P. Howell, thought the working class had opposed the bond issue. In Foreman's view, the working class was sick of being forced to bribe attending physicians 1% or more of the value of a burial insurance policy in order to get a death certificate (which insurance companies required before paying off on a policy).[51]

A year after the bond referendum, a committee of labor leaders inspected the hospital to assess whether their membership should support yet another proposed bond issue. The proceeds from the next bond referendum dedicated to Grady, $350,000, would pay for a new building for white patients, replace the wood-frame firetraps housing the black wards with a concrete building, establish a true "maternity ward for colored," create a dormitory for nurses, and build a new clinic. Led by Louie P. Marquardt, president of the Georgia State Federation of Labor, the union leaders were alarmed by what they saw during their visit on a Friday evening.*

In a report to the Atlanta Federation of Trades on August 11, 1915, the committee declared its visit "a revelation."[52] It found all of the wards incredibly overcrowded and noted both the black and white wards were "taxed beyond capacity." Committee members observed that the black wards were more jammed than the white ones because Grady had "less proportionate space allotted to the colored population." In Black Grady they found "cots placed in an endless row along the corridor."[53] Surprised to find sixty percent of Grady's patients were white, the labor leaders were horrified to find children with whooping cough and typhoid fever in rooms with adults. Charity cases occupied five of the twelve private rooms dedicated to White Grady's paying patients. Dr. Summerall had confided to the labor leaders that patients at the outpatient clinic "did not receive the care and attention they should" because of overcrowding, but the hospital was doing the best for them that it could under the circumstances.[54] The labor leaders also learned that the hospital's ambulance service made an average of nearly eighteen calls per day. Worried that someone else might need a hospital bed more than the patient who called for the ambulance, the driver and physician on call often refused to bring patients to Grady because of overcrowding. The driver and doctor on board were, in effect, rationing hospital care.

---

*Other members of the labor investigating committee included W. J. Wooding, William Robinson, George M. Bryant, Thomas Ball, and Clark Puckett.

Charles Summerall

Dr. William Summerall may have left Grady Memorial Hospital for military service thanks in part to the influence of his brother, Charles, who, in turn, owed the start of his own distinguished military career to his physician sibling. Two years older than Charles, Dr. Summerall persuaded his younger brother to study for the West Point entrance exam and then tutored him with success. Charles later would return to his alma mater as a teacher of artillery tactics. Before then, however, Charles served as aide de camp to Major General William M. Graham first at a military camp in Atlanta and then while General Graham commanded the Second Army Corps during the Spanish-American War. In the brief period of America's involvement in World War I, Charles Summerall went from being a major to major general. After commanding an artillery brigade at Cantigny, he became 1st Division commander during the fighting in the Argonne. Later in the conflict he was appointed commander of the V Corps. After the Great War ended, he commanded the 1st Division. From November 1926 to November 1930 he was Chief of Staff of the United States Army. General Summerall (he became a four-star general in 1929) was an important innovator of modern artillery technique, and his efforts laid the groundwork for the outstanding American field artillery used during World War II.[113]

In 1914 the clinic treated 28,000 patients, more than four times the number cared for only five years earlier. Hospital records confirmed continued overcrowding. On the day before the labor committee visited, July 29, 1915, there had been 309 in-patients—124 patients over capacity. In the new White Grady, a room on the first floor designed to be a sterilization chamber was being used instead to house two ambulance drivers. The small area (25 by 42 feet) on the first floor designed to be a patient ward was still being used as a nurse's dormitory. With twenty-two beds jammed into the space, the nursing students had no privacy; they also had no place for recreation.

Dr. Summerall's living arrangements were little better. The labor leaders reported, "the hospital chief, a white man, can only be accommodated in living quarters over the stable" which he occupied with his wife and child.[55] Under those conditions, Dr. Summerall continued working to improve the hospital in every possible way. The shortage of money continued to hamper his effort, especially when the $350,000 bond issue the local labor union leaders supported did not materialize.

An important part of Dr. Summerall's job was to provide the city of Atlanta with an annual report. The ones he wrote in the first years of his tenure were relatively straightforward; they, rarely veered from a matter-of-fact tone. The annual report he presented for 1916, however, is stunning. After eight years of fighting the city fathers, Grady's frustrated chief forcefully spelled out his diagnosis of the hospital's ailments: the operating budgets were insufficient and the voters did not provide bond funds for capital improvements. In a blistering attack, he blamed Atlanta's government and citizens for Grady's inadequate funding.[56]

Dr. Summerall's complaints about the city's meager financial support for the public hospital had plenty of merit. Having had four small fires since 1909, Grady's original building was a disaster waiting to happen. Summerall pointed out the obvious: A rapidly rising number of patients (in line with Atlanta's expanding population) overwhelmed Grady's worn-out facilities. There simply were not enough beds. At times during 1909, 1910, and 1911 the hospital placed tents on its lawn to provide shelter for the patient overflow. While the new building on Butler Street eased the space crunch, Grady's need to expand medical services continued. In 1913, a year after the Butler Street building opened, the hospital averaged 157 patients per day. Within three years the number surged to 273 per day—75 patients beyond capacity. Having literally run out of beds by the end of 1916, the hospital resorted to placing patients in chairs in the halls.

The staggering number of patients overwhelmed the hospital's physical and fiscal resources. Grady's kitchen, laundry, and operating room equipment were outdated. More than that, the high level of emergency calls stretched its ambulance service to the limit; the number of trips nearly doubled between 1910 and 1915. Outpatient clinic visits more than tripled between 1910 and 1916, rising from 11,421 patients to 35,472 in six years. Remarkably, the $1.72 daily cost to treat an inpatient at Grady held steady from 1910 to 1916 as Dr. Summerall worked feverishly to contain Grady's operating expenses. The fast-growing demand for services, however, pushed the hospital to increase capital investment in space and tools.

Six years after voters had passed the $100,000 bond that paid for Grady's Butler Street building, the hospital was desperate for money to make capital improvements. Fixing up its worn out areas, creating more space for treating patients, and buying a broad range of new equipment would all cost money that the city did not provide in its annual appropriation for Grady. The failure to pass the bond issue in 1914 and the futile attempt to develop financing in 1915—despite the important political support of Atlanta's labor unions—left Dr. Summerall more than frustrated. Thus, at the end of 1916 the nearly fed-up Dr. Summerall insisted Atlanta either raise taxes or issue bonds in order to remedy Grady's dire infrastructure problems.

Deeply frustrated with the city's paltry financial support, Dr. Summerall gave no quarter to the astute businessmen at the city's helm. Neither did he absolve ordinary citizens. He bluntly noted that Atlanta's lack of funding hindered Grady from fulfilling its mission. The public hospital depended financially on its owner, the city of Atlanta. In essence, if the city government refused to increase Grady's budget (or authorize voting on a bond issue), Grady would be incapable of treating all who sought its help. More than that, the city had been unable to pass a bond issue of adequate size to make capital improvements to Grady. In addition, citizens rejected raising the city's tax rate. (Dr. Summerall claimed Atlanta had the lowest tax rate in the country for cities of its size.) Ultimately, Dr. Summerall blamed the citizens of Atlanta. He wrote, "The answer is raise the tax rate or issue bonds. It does not rest with the mayor, or the general council, or the department boards to do either." At the end of his sixteen-page report he asked, "will the people do it?"[57] Frustrated as he was when he wrote the annual report for 1916, he hung on as Grady's superintendent for the next year and a half.

Dr. Summerall left Grady in August 1918 (although his departure officially would be in November) in order to join the Medical Corps of the Army. A veteran of the Spanish-American War, Dr. Summerall was commissioned as a captain and served as an administrative officer for a base hospital. Following the war he served with the Public Health Service until February 1922 when he took over as head of the Baptist hospital in Atlanta. He died September 5, 1939, at the age of 74.

During Dr. Summerall's tenure, Grady's board of trustees remained powerless to squeeze enough money out of the municipal government to turn Grady into the kind of hospital Dr. Summerall envisioned. Despite their frustration with the city, many of Grady's trustees took an active interest in the institution and supported the hospital with substantial financial gifts. While the city government acted stingily, from the outset Grady enjoyed the support of an energetic board of trustees.

An Active Board of Trustees*

James Warren English

James Warren English, a prominent Atlanta businessman, served on the original board of trustees of The Henry W. Grady

---

*The members of Grady's original board of trustees were Joseph Hirsch, John T. Glenn, Robert D. Spalding, Thomas B. Neal, Jacob Elsas, William L. Moore, Robert J. Lowry, Captain James English, and Samuel M. Inman.

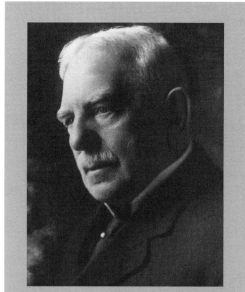

James English (1837-1925) was an important supporter of Grady hospital and friend of Henry Grady.

Memorial Hospital. Born in Orleans Parish, Louisiana, in 1837, English was orphaned when he was fourteen years old. After apprenticing himself for five years to learn the trade, English established a carriage-making business in Griffin, Georgia, in 1856. He joined the Confederate Army just a week after the Civil War started. Deployed to Virginia, English participated in many of the great battles fought by General Robert E. Lee's Army of Northern Virginia and eventually he served as a member of General Lee's staff. At war's end, English moved to Atlanta and married Emily Alexander.

English enjoyed an outstanding career in business and local politics. Among his many accomplishments, English built 500 miles of railroad line connecting Atlanta to the coalfields of Alabama and beyond. He also founded the Atlanta Terminal Company, builders of the Atlanta Terminal Station (1905) in the city's downtown. English served as a director of the Central Georgia Company and of the Atlanta West Point Railway Company. An important New South financier, English was active in local banking. He helped organize the American Trust and Banking Company in 1890, created the Fourth National Bank, and served as vice-president of the Atlanta Savings Bank. Elected to Atlanta's city council in 1877, English chaired its Finance Committee and led a committee representing the city's interests in discussions to transfer Georgia's state capital from Milledgeville to Atlanta. Elected Mayor of Atlanta in 1881, English implemented an electric fire alarm system, a modern police signal system, and a paid fire department for the city. English also owned and operated the Chattahoochee Brick Company, which he started while a member of Atlanta's city council (three years before becoming mayor). His business methods there have invited the greatest criticism of his career.

Leasing the right to the labor of convicts from the state of Georgia, the local counties, and the city of Atlanta gave English the nearly-free labor that allowed his brick factory to be profitable. The vast majority of leased convicts in the South at the end of the nineteenth century were young black men convicted of ambiguous crimes like vagrancy or minor offenses like hitching a ride on a freight train. Paying the state of Georgia a small sum entitled Captain English to benefit from a convict's labor for one year. (County and city convicts usually worked for shorter terms, depending on the amount of their fine or the length of the sentence.) In return, English's companies were supposed to provide the convicts with adequate food, clothing, and shelter.

The Chattahoochee Brick Company failed miserably in all three areas. The food was rancid, the clothing minimal, and the shelter crowded and dirty. The evidence remains in the testimony former convicts and employees presented to an investigative commission the Georgia legislature organized in the summer of 1908. The commission found that the convicts leased to English (reportedly he controlled 40% of the convict laborers in Georgia) worked in brutal and miserable conditions. Subject to regular beatings of twenty lashes or more from a leather whip while stretched out over a barrel, convict laborers could be bought and sold, traded from one business to another with impunity. Convict labor in the South then amounted to, as Douglas A. Blackmon persuasively argues, *Slavery By Another Name*.[58]

These convict-laborers were the men upon whom at least one physician from Grady would conduct medical experiments at the turn of the century. It is highly unlikely that anyone sought permission from the men being experimented upon.* In any case, James English, who saw the slavocracy end at Appomattox, lawfully used convict labor as a ticket to joining the plutocracy. Yet, Captain English also used his substantial power to give the hospital crucial support from the start.

In a city without big-league reformers — Atlanta did not have a Jane Addams like Chicago or a Frank Parsons like Boston—charity asked few questions.

The local intellectuals who offered remedies for the evils of the day would come out of Black Atlanta. Those with great minds like the intellectual W. E. B. DuBois and John Hope, the president of Morehouse College, thought carefully about how to improve society. Black Atlanta also had active philanthropic women whose Neighborhood Union brought uplift, education, and health care to poor black neighborhoods. Eager to achieve democracy, their effort to remake the city would be limited by their skin color.

White Atlanta had a rising business class that was eager to make money but generally recoiled at the prospect of remaking society. Within it, of course, were a few philanthropists who held to a nineteenth century equation of charity with social betterment. Like so many of Grady's early trustees, Captain English believed in self-help for the poor. He also understood the significance of the charity hospital for his city and was willing to help make certain that no person who had the potential to be economically productive

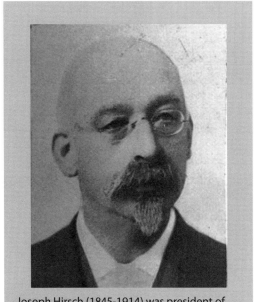
Joseph Hirsch (1845-1914) was president of Grady hospital's board for 20 years. He was a remarkable businessman and philanthropist.

should die of neglect. His strong support was crucially important to Grady's birth and early survival.

Captain English died at age 88 on February 15, 1925, and rests in Oakland Cemetery.

Joseph Hirsch

Joseph Hirsch, another early supporter of the hospital, served as the president of Grady's board practically from the start. Born in Germany in 1845, Hirsch came to the United States when he was fifteen years old. Initially arriving in New York City in 1860, the young man soon moved to Marietta, Georgia, and then to the nearby town of Acworth. During the Civil War the teenage Hirsch served in the Confederate Army's 11th Georgia Infantry. Two years after the war ended, Hirsch and his brother, Morris, established the M & J Hirsch Company in Atlanta.

---

* Horrifying as this sounds today—and as it was at the time—it is important to place it in historical context. The standards of medical ethics were far different at the start of the twentieth century than they are at the start of the twenty-first century. In 1901, when Grady's Dr. Claude Smith conducted medical experiments on a convict-laborer at Captain English's Chattahoochee Brick Company, the idea of patient consent was still new. It had been established only a few years earlier by the famed Dr. Walter Reed.

That firm became the starting point for Joseph Hirsch's outstanding career as a businessman and philanthropist. The brothers' venture grew rapidly, soon becoming one of the leading wholesale and retail clothing establishments in Atlanta. In addition, Joseph Hirsch also served as president of a paint company and as director of a bank. His civic and philanthropic work included service as a member of the Atlanta Board of Education, affiliation with B'nai B'rith, and helping found the Hebrew Orphans Home. A member of the Odd Fellows, Hirsch also was a close friend of Henry W. Grady.

His relationship with Grady may have led Hirsch to spearhead the drive to build Atlanta's new charity hospital, but his own ethos propelled him to spend two decades as the president of Grady Memorial Hospital's board of trustees. Friends and other contemporaries affectionately called him "the Father of Grady Hospital." No one among the wealthy did more to relieve the physical suffering of the city's underprivileged. Few native-born Southerners had such a finely honed sense of responsibility for giving the masses a chance to pursue in full health the promise of American life as did the Jewish immigrant from Germany. After his death in 1915, the *Constitution* reported, "His magnificent contribution to the Grady hospital and his unremitting efforts on behalf of that institution have made it a lasting monument to his memory and his services will be gratefully remembered as long as the Grady hospital continues to perform its mission of charity."[59] With Hirsch's death Grady lost one of its earliest and most ardent supporters. Through his selfless commitment to Grady, he helped ensure the establishment and continuing existence of the hospital.

The medical board of Grady Memorial Hospital passed the following resolution upon the death of Joseph Hirsch: "It is but justice to the memory of Mr. Hirsch to say, that he was the chief and moving spirit, in the inauguration of Grady Hospital; being untiring in this philanthropic effort, and contributing most liberally of his time, and money, in its establishment."[60]

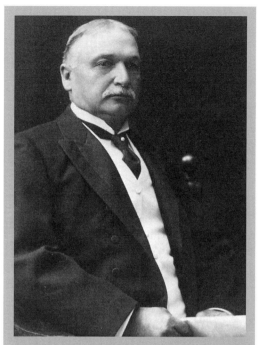

Samuel Inman (1843-1915) never held an elected political office in Atlanta but was considered "Atlanta's First Citizen." His career included banking, cotton, railroads, and serving on the boards of numerous civic organizations including Grady Memorial Hospital.

The Board of Trustees passed a separate resolution to memorialize Mr. Hirsch: "For a quarter of a century he has been the untiring friend and supporter of the Grady Hospital. By this means he has done his great work in relieving the sick and destitute of our city and has helped to bring health and strength to the helpless and suffering and poor. When Atlanta had no hospital, he started the movement to establish one – a place where the sick people and those who were injured and unable to help themselves could find relief from their suffering and be healed in their sickness. He was the prime mover in founding this City Hospital and joined by others of our prominent, benevolent citizens, the movement he gave life, inspiration and beginning to, culminated in the Grady Hospital. … He was a friend of the sick, the suffering, the poor and the orphan. His good works do follow after him and his deeds of benevolence and charity stand forth now as his monuments."⁶¹

Within six months of Hirsch's death, Samuel Inman, another longtime friend of Henry W. Grady and supporter of Grady hospital, also died.

Samuel Inman

Samuel Inman was born on February 19, 1843, in Dandridge, Tennessee. In 1859, having graduated from Maryville College, Inman traveled north to enter Princeton University. He withdrew from that institution two years later to join the Confederate Army. (He served in the First Tennessee Cavalry for four years.) Despite his not having completed the university's academic program, Princeton awarded Inman a diploma after the war. He was one of four members of the class of 1863 upon whom the university's trustees conferred degrees despite the war ending their academic progress.

Two years after the war, Inman relocated to Atlanta from Augusta, Georgia. Together with his father he established a firm specializing in the buying, selling, and exporting of cotton. S. W. Inman and Son eventually became one of the largest and most widely respected enterprises of its kind in the world. Its fantastic success also helped make Inman one of Atlanta's wealthiest residents. His philanthropy rather than commercial prosperity inspired Henry Grady to call Inman "Atlanta's First Citizen."

Samuel Inman's many civic achievements included helping to start the Georgia School of Technology, where he served on the board of trustees for many years. He was also a principal figure in creating the Confederate Soldiers Home, raising $35,000 to enlarge Agnes Scott College, and funding the reopening of Oglethorpe University. Inman also was the principal donor for a new seminary for the Methodist Episcopal Church. (It was predecessor to Emory University's Candler School of Theology.) In addition to being a member of the original committee created to establish Grady Hospital, Samuel Inman chaired a subcommittee that secured money

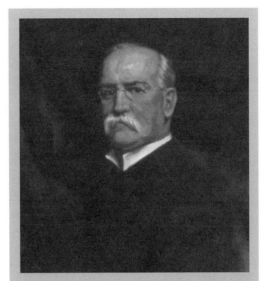

Dr. Abner Calhoun (1845-1910) was one of the most important physicians on the Grady Hospital volunteer staff and one of the greatest physicians in Atlanta's history.

from the sale of the old benevolent home to help pay for Grady's construction. Samuel Inman was a member of Grady's board for several years. He died on January 12, 1915. Businesses were closed, Georgia Tech suspended classes, and flags throughout the city were flown at half-mast during his funeral service.⁶²

The Medical Staff

Dr. Abner W. Calhoun

Dr. Abner W. Calhoun, who played a crucial role in establishing Grady, was born about thirty miles southwest of Atlanta in Newnan, Georgia, in 1845 to Dr. Andrew and Susan Calhoun. Abner Calhoun left home when he was sixteen years old in order to join the Confederate Army. Serving with fellow soldiers from Georgia in the Army of Northern Virginia, he suffered severe wounds at least once. After recovering from his injuries he remained on active duty until he witnessed General Lee surrender to General Ulysses Grant at the Appomattox Court House on April 9, 1865. After the war he attended Jefferson Medical College in

Philadelphia, graduating in 1869 at the top of his class. Dr. Calhoun returned to Atlanta following special training in diseases of the eye, ear, nose, and throat at hospitals in Vienna and Berlin. The first Eye, Ears, Nose, and Throat (EENT) specialist in Georgia, Dr. Calhoun enjoyed a thriving private medical practice. He also served as professor of Eye and Ear Surgery in Atlanta Medical College. Dr. Calhoun later became President of the Atlanta College of Physicians and Surgeons. An active scholar, Dr. Calhoun made many important contributions to the field of ophthalmology. In 1890, Dr. Calhoun reported successful cataract surgery on 135 patients. Two years later he reported 904 cataract surgeries on patients ranging in age from three months to 94 years old.[63]

Throughout his professional life Dr. Calhoun devoted much time and many financial resources to giving free medical treatment to Atlanta's poor. Upon bestowing an honorary L.L.D. degree on him in June 1890, officials at the University of Georgia introduced him as the doctor who probably provided more free care than any other physician in the South. At his own expense he created a clinic for indigent patients in the basement of the Atlanta College of Physicians and Surgeons. Active in many of the city's civic organizations, Dr. Calhoun also served on the city's board of health and the Atlanta Board of Education. Among his many accomplishments in public health, Dr. Calhoun successfully argued that all school students in Atlanta be required to have smallpox vaccinations. Although he lacked the political ambition to follow the advice of friends and run for mayor, Dr. Calhoun had enough acumen and interest in business to serve as a director for both the Third National Bank and the Georgia Railway and Electric Company.[64]

After a two-year illness, Dr. Calhoun died on August 21, 1910. He is buried in the Calhoun family mausoleum at Oakland Cemetery. In 1923, the Calhoun family gave a $10,000 gift to the Emory University School of Medicine to establish the Abner Calhoun, M.D., Medical Library. A gift of $32,000 followed in 1926.[65] On April 4, 1946, 101 years

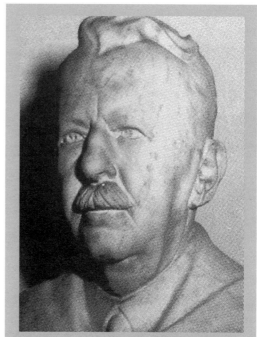

The marble bust of Dr. George Noble (1860-1932) is located at the Academy of Medicine in Atlanta

after his birth, the Academy of Medicine, located on West Peachtree Street in Atlanta, dedicated its auditorium to his memory. (At the occasion, his grandson, Dr. Abner Calhoun Withorn, unveiled a portrait of Dr. Calhoun.)

Dr. George Noble

Dr. Noble was born in Atlanta on February 25, 1860. After graduating from Atlanta Medical College in 1881 he continued his studies at Bellevue Hospital and at Woman's Hospital in New York City. A specialist in women's diseases, he may have been the first surgeon in Georgia to intentionally and successfully remove the cancerous uterus of a pregnant patient. He was a member of Grady's original visiting staff and practiced at the hospital for 26 years. In 1905, he helped organize the Atlanta School of Medicine, serving as Dean and Professor of Abdominal Surgery. When the Emory University School of Medicine formed, it named Dr. Noble Emeritus Professor of Clinical Gynecology.

During his life, Dr. Noble received numerous honors, including an honorary degree from the University of the South. He was a leader in many professional societies and served as president of both the Medical Association of Georgia (1896) and the Atlanta Society of Medicine (1897). He died on October 29, 1932.[66]

To Become the Model of a Modern Hospital

In its first decades, the leading physicians, trustees, administrators, and supporters of Grady hospital actively pushed to make the institution one of the best charity hospitals in the nation. (Their choice fit in with Atlanta's drive to establish itself as the leading city of the New South.) As interpreted by its proponents, Grady's quest for excellence meant adopting the most recent approaches to disease and diagnosis. In order to achieve excellence, Grady needed to adopt the best new practices and technologies—a constantly moving target. Dramatic gains in scientific understanding and medical knowledge led to rapid innovation in medical equipment and procedures, complicated the organization of knowledge, and made the practice of medicine more intricate.

Medical understanding of the role proper hygiene played in controlling the spread of contagious diseases was still in its infancy at the end of the nineteenth century. The work of Louis Pasteur seemed still to be more widely admired than understood. Indeed, for much of the latter nineteenth century the germ theory of disease had a hard time winning acceptance in American medicine. Similarly, it took American physicians a generation to accept Joseph Lister's innovations in antiseptic surgery. First published in the 1860s, Lister's research into the role of disinfectants in preventing infection during surgery evolved over the next several years.

At the time Grady opened, American physicians only recently had begun appreciating the benefits of aseptic surgery. With the introduction of sterilized dressings and rubber gloves in the 1890s, surgery became increasingly sanitary, at least when performed in the hospital. Better understanding of germs and bacteriology, together with the new sanitary practices and products, helped make the hospital a safer setting for practicing medicine. The hospital was becoming something other than a warehouse for the ill or a supply source of patients upon which to conduct medical research or use as "material" for teaching. The scientific (followed by medical and then public) acceptance of the germ theory of disease, and the medical community's fresh understanding of the necessity for aseptic surgery helped transform the character of American hospitals. So did the adoption of new technologies.

Grady bought its first x-ray equipment in 1909 when the diagnostic tool was relatively new. Wilhelm Roentgen had discovered the x-ray in 1895 in Germany. A decade later it was becoming part of the panoply of equipment transforming American hospitals. Adding the radiology machine to Grady' existing arsenal—including its important pathology laboratory—enhanced Grady's capacity to use the most modern medical techniques. Ironically, the machinery's novelty may have prompted anxiety among patients; some worried that hospital employees, especially interns, were using the new machines without knowing exactly what they were doing. Their concern may have been heightened as Grady adopted rapid improvements in x-ray medical technology. Grady replaced its first x-ray machine within three years at a cost of $1,500. In addition to getting a new machine in 1912, Grady hired Dr. John Derr as a full-time radiologist. Having a specialist at hand may have helped assure patients that the hospital would properly supervise interns using the equipment. Grady's hiring of a radiologist also is indicative of American medicine's increasing specialization at the start of the twentieth century.

New technologies and practices like radiology helped alter the role of the hospital in American medical care. By the early twentieth century the best diagnostic equipment could be found only in hospitals.

The physicians in private practice could not afford to duplicate the hospital's services. Because of its role as the home for medical tests and procedures, x-ray machines, and other new tools, the hospital's importance for medical diagnosis and treatment only increased. Pathologists in hospital laboratories examined blood under a microscope and used tests to confirm the presence of bacteria in a patient. In addition, hospital laboratories gained importance as centers for scientific discovery. The ability to understand and use scientific innovations may have helped improve public health as much as it raised the social status of physicians. A convalescent care center for the poor only a few decades earlier, American hospitals started becoming diagnostic centers for everyone during the first decades of the twentieth century. That helps explain why hospitals began to attract a new class of inpatients.

By the turn of the century, more middle-class Americans were starting to find hospitals socially acceptable. This was because the hospital's identity as an institution was being transformed thanks to improved sanitary conditions and new technologies, especially diagnostic equipment. By the start of World War I the hospital was broadly accepted as a place for surgery and emergency care. Not until the 1920s, however, would middle class Americans begin to accept the hospital as a proper place to bear children or be treated for serious illness. For example, it was only at the end of the 1920s that Wesley Memorial Hospital at Emory University reported having as many inpatients for medical treatment as it did for surgery. "The significance of this," wrote the hospital's director, "is that it indicates the increasing tendency to hospitalize patients to purely medical care, a situation which was not true a relatively few years ago."[67]

The hospital's adoption of the fruits of modern science was not inevitable. Dr. Summerall, for example, made a conscious choice for Grady to have the newest and most effective medical technologies for the benefit of its patients, physicians, professors, and medical students. His decision was driven by medical considerations rather than simply by the logic of the market. The vast majority of patients were charity cases with highly restricted options for where to be treated. While having the best equipment might attract more paying patients, the revenue they generated—which went directly into the city treasury instead of Grady's budget—would not justify adopting new technologies based on finances or

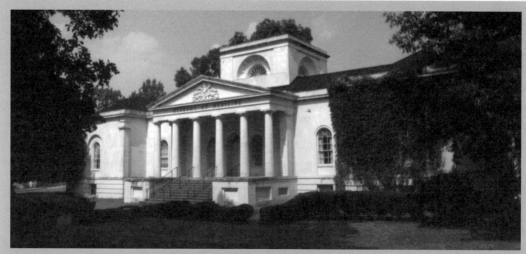

Academy of Medicine is located in midtown Atlanta. It was designed by Philip Shutze and R. Kennon Perry and was dedicated in December 1941.

capturing market share. American hospitals were not paying homage to the dictate of markets. Similarly, Grady did not embrace new technologies solely to benefit medical school programs of research and teaching.

While the adoption of the latest scientific equipment and practices was primarily for the patients' benefit, adopting fresh innovations helped Grady achieve the aim of its supporters and trustees—for Atlanta to have one of the leading public hospitals in the nation. It also fit the ethos of the medical profession—to heal the sick in the best way possible. At the same time, new diagnostic tools like the x-ray, improved treatments for cancer, and surgical innovations were professionally exciting. In these new tools and procedures the quest for scientific innovation and novelty met the hope for effective treatment. Together they generated a genuine sense of possibility among physicians that the art of healing could be made both more effective and more broadly accessible. That makes it easy to see why physicians had so much at stake in Grady's decision to adopt the latest equipment and procedures.

Founding The Grady School of Nursing

On March 24, 1898, the State of Georgia granted a charter for the Grady Hospital Training School for Nurses. The school named Miss Adah Patterson, a graduate of Johns Hopkins, as its first director. In that role she guided development of the school's two-year diploma program. Within a year of her arrival, the school accepted 19 women as students (out of 130 applicants). Once enrolled, the women in the nursing school lived in a dormitory on the hospital's second floor.

On May 16, 1900, the Grady Hospital Training School for Nurses graduated its first class of six students. Three of the young women, the Misses Parker, Tibbs, and Tygart were from Atlanta. Miss Finley was from Fairmont, Mississippi, Miss Worley from Lynchburg, Virginia, and Miss Daughtry was from Norfolk.

Nursing students gained new educational opportunities in obstetrics with the opening of Grady's first maternity ward in 1904. Its arrival also led the school to add a third year of study to its curriculum. At the same time, Grady's nursing school adopted more rigorous admission standards. Applicants were compelled to provide a letter from a clergyman testifying to her being of "good moral character." This was not as vague as it might seem at first glance. Hospital administrators generally defined moral character in terms of sexual activity. An applicant also needed to provide a letter from her physician attesting to good health. At the time nursing schools wanted to be certain that students did not carry either syphilis or tuberculosis. The school also set age limits for its students, supposedly not considering anyone younger than 21 or over 35 years old. There were no educational requirements, but at the end of the second month of school the students were tested on their ability to read, write, add and subtract, understand fractions and percentages, and take notes in class.[68] Limited resources, especially the severe shortage of student housing, probably did more than tighter standards to keep the school's enrollment small. In 1904 the school accepted fifteen women (out of 156 applicants), four fewer than in its first year.[69]

Grady's Ambulance Service

In 1899, when the ambulance service made nearly 2,000 calls (including 270 for accidents), Grady owned three horses and one ambulance. More significantly, it answered calls in an area covering 26 square miles.[70] Ten years later, in 1909, the number of calls to the ambulance service had risen by twenty-five percent. With such a heavy demand for ambulance services over such a broad territory it is little wonder that the hospital's superintendent wanted to add two lighter, more modern vehicles to the ambulance department.

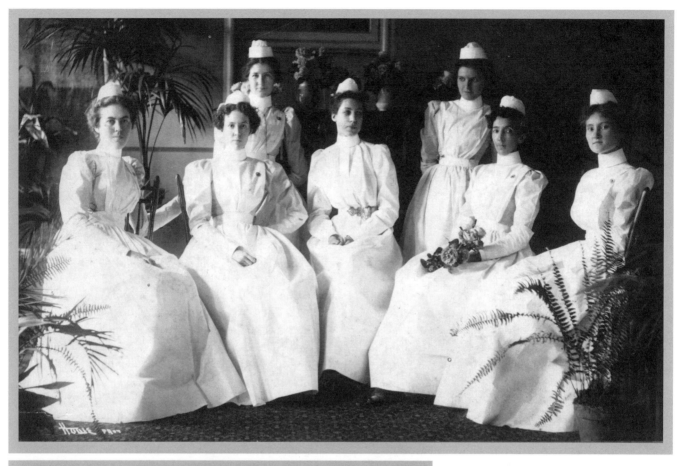

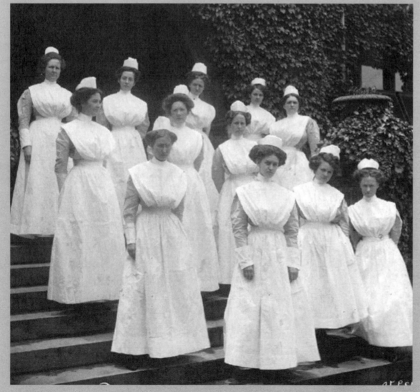

Grady School of Nursing

Above: Class of 1900

Miss Ada Finley, Miss Fannie Tibbs, Miss Algie Tygart, Miss Gwendolyn Worley, Miss Estelle Daughtry, Miss Lella Parker, Miss Rogers (superintendent of the school)

Left: Class of 1911

At a hospital board meeting in October 1909, Charles Northen, a board member and nephew of a former governor of Georgia, suggested that the hospital purchase its first motorized ambulance.[71] He believed that the hospital's horse-drawn ambulances would be unable to handle an anticipated increase in emergency calls (keeping pace with population growth and the arrival of motor vehicles). Since some private motor ambulances had begun serving Atlanta, at least intermittently, and were used in other cities, Mr. Northen's proposal was hardly radical. The board of trustees appointed a committee to look into the matter, naming Mr. Northen as its chairman. By February 1910 the hospital's medical board had endorsed Grady's purchase of an "automobile ambulance."

Several months later, in April 1910, Dr. Summerall reported that the hospital's four horses had reached their limit. It was time to either acquire a motorized ambulance or more horses before the heat of summer arrived.[72] Northen's ambulance committee won more time to study the matter, exhaustively researching ambulance manufacturers. When the trustees met on January 31, 1911, more than a year after Northen raised the subject of buying a motor ambulance, Dr. Summerall blasted the board for not having acted. Putting his demand for the vehicle in defensive terms, Summerall suggested critics would assail the city's hospital—and thus its trustees—for not having modern equipment.[73]

The hospital finally ordered a thirty horsepower ambulance from The White Company in April 1911, at a cost of $2,800.[74] Its arrival that summer prompted the building of a garage—at a cost of $283.50—and shopping for insurance coverage.[75] On October 11, 1911, shortly after the vehicle arrived but before insurance was purchased, the ambulance stalled on the railroad tracks at a crossing in Kirkwood on Atlanta's east side. The occupants were a patient going home following a surgical procedure, a physician, and the ambulance's driver, Allen Kimball (the first patient admitted to Grady Memorial Hospital). As it stood stalled on the tracks, the ambulance was hit by a train, which threw the ambulance body fifty feet from the chassis. The train then pushed the chassis another 100 feet down the track before coming to a stop. Remarkably, the patient and the two other accident victims all survived. With the new machine a wreck, Mr. Fred Patterson, director of H. M. Patterson Funeral Home, one of the leading white-owned funeral homes in the city, offered Grady free use of his motor ambulance until the hospital could repair its vehicle.[76]

Medical Innovation at Grady Hospital

Following through on an idea credited to Mrs. Clark Howell, in July 1894 a group of women organized the Grady Hospital Aid Association to formalize the auxiliary and the charitable work that women had been performing at the hospital.* Holding their first meeting at a bastion of the civic elite, the Capital City Club, the women wasted no time. Even before their first formal meeting they convinced Jack Slaton, an attorney and future state representative and governor, to secure a charter for incorporating the group. The spirited social lioness Mrs. Nellie Peters Black, who only a few years earlier played a crucial role in creating King's Daughters Hospital, chaired its executive committee—which was a who's who of Atlanta's white women. The committee chairs included Mrs. W. A. Hemphill, wife of the former mayor, Mrs. Morris Rich, whose husband ran the city's great department store (she headed the committee on clothing), Mrs. Henry W. Grady, and Mrs. Robert J. Lowry, wife of the banker and civic leader. These women were aware of the class implications of their formally assisting the charity hospital, an alertness shown in public pronouncements that the aid association would be made up "of no special class, but embraces all classes."[77]

---

*The founders of the ladies auxiliary included Mrs. Henry W. Grady, Mrs. Robert Lowry, Mrs. Nellie Peters Black, Mrs. Samuel Inman, and Mrs. Morris Rich.

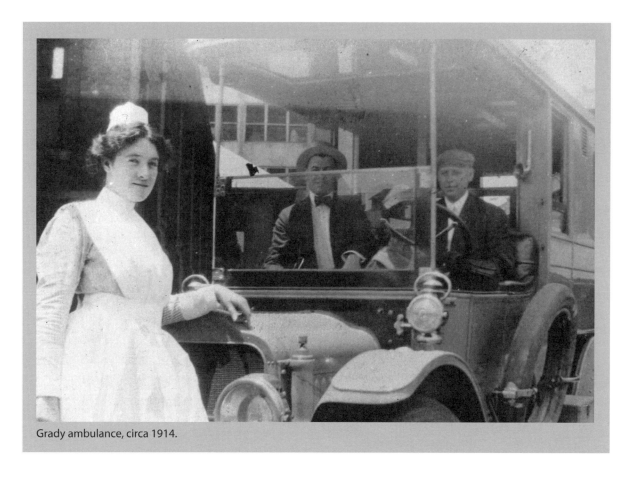
Grady ambulance, circa 1914.

Three hundred-fifty women joined within the first three weeks, leaving little doubt that the effort attracted broad support. With Mrs. Samuel Inman as its first president, the new organization sought to "extend the workings of the Grady hospital until it takes its place among the leading institutions of its kind in the country."[78] The scale of their ambition for the city and its institutions paralleled that of the city's male civic leadership. The women's group, however, had their own set of interests. In practical terms, they organized themselves in order to establish a children's ward and a maternity ward at Grady.

For nearly all of the nineteenth century American physicians had treated children at home rather than in hospitals. In the century's last decade, however, an increasing number of physicians had come to support establishing children's wards. Giving children their own space in the hospital isolated them from older patients. It also suggests that an important new approach to American medical practice was gaining ground: giving different groups of people specialized care. The hospital claimed Grady's was the first children's hospital ward in Georgia and perhaps the entire South. (The children's ward movement was new enough that one Atlanta newspaper earnestly but mistakenly reported the planned ward was intended to house orphans.)

Among other accomplishments, the women's aid association funded, built, and equipped a ward for white children on the Grady campus. Raising over $5,000 from friends, churches, local school children (who contributed nearly $1,500), and public sales and festivals, the women were able to fully fund the building and all of its furnishings. The woman's auxiliary purchased land adjacent to the Grady campus for the children's ward. They also ran the building committee, overseeing the building's design and construction. Chaired by Mrs. Robert J. Lowry, the children's ward building committee included several other socially prominent women along with four male physicians, Drs. Elkin, Cooper, Hardin, and R. D. Spaulding.[79] They created a building with separate wards for boys and girls along with four private rooms. In May 1897, less than three years after organizing, the aid association presented the city with the new ward. Their success helped "extend the workings" of the hospital along the most modern lines of the modern hospital movement.[80]

Yet, only a few months after the children's ward opened, the "Woman and Society" page of the *Constitution* bemoaned the city's indifference toward Grady. A few women were interested, but, the writer observed, "the lack of universal interest in the hospital, both on the part of those whose duty it is to be interested, as well as the citizens of Atlanta at large, is one incredible, and one which does not speak well for that spirit of loyalty and charity that should belong to the city in regard to its charitable institutions."[81] The scolding of the city continued as the columnist claimed that "as a rule, one of the prides of every large city is its hospital, and yet with the exception of a very few people, there is not that interest manifested in the Grady hospital that there should be."[82] Although a fairly large number of women belonged to the ladies auxiliary, only a few visited the hospital or volunteered there. The article about the citizenry's involvement with Grady clearly was meant to inspire greater volunteerism. Independent of the newspaper's urging, a separate group of women organized themselves not only to assist Grady but, more broadly, to help the less fortunate.

Calling themselves the "Order of Old-Fashioned Women,"* eight of Atlanta's "young matrons" took it upon themselves to organize for charitable purposes and at the same time proclaim their objection to the modern club woman. Unlike the reform-minded women associated with the Grady Hospital Aid Association, the "old-fashioned women" had little use for the lectures and presentations common to women's clubs. Designed as a social club, the Order of Old-Fashioned Women lacked standing officers or formal structure. Their gatherings reportedly were modeled after the sewing circles of their grandmothers' generation when, as one journalist noted, "to 'speak out in meeting' was deemed a sin."[83] The old-fashioned women got together to play rather than learn about or discuss social problems or reforms. The little group's ironic protest against modern womanhood soon took hold beyond Atlanta, spawning subsidiary organizations in Nashville and Augusta.[84]

The playful approach of the Order of Old-Fashioned Women could not, however, obscure the fact that it was a society with a serious purpose—helping others. It was led by some of the most prominent women in the city, including Mrs. Wilmer Moore, Mrs. Robert Maddox, Mrs. Morris Brandon, Mrs. Preston Arkwright, and Mrs. Henry Inman. To raise money for their good works they relied on fund-raising events typical for their time, including various sales and small entertainments like cakewalks. One of their most lucrative ventures was a comical dancing carnival held at the Atlanta Opera House. Having gathered several thousand dollars through these ventures, the women with the light-hearted approach dedicated themselves to supplying Grady with a maternity ward.[85]

At the time, most upper class women wouldn't think of bearing their children in the hospital. Aware that the poor lacked the privacy and comforts at home that wealthy women enjoyed, the old-fashioned women sought to create a space where poor white women could give birth. The old-fashioned women were, in fact, on the cutting edge. First invited to cooperate in creating a maternity ward with the clubwomen of Grady's ladies' auxiliary, the old-fashioned women soon took the lead.[86] The aid association bought land adjacent to the existing Grady complex for the maternity ward. (When they sought to tender it to the city, a dispute briefly arose about the best use of the site

---

*The founders of the Order of Old-Fashioned Women included Mrs. William Moore, Mrs. William Ellis, Mrs. Julian Field, Mrs. Morris Brandon, Mrs. Robert Maddox, Jr., Mrs. Thomas R. R. Cobb, Mrs. Robert Foreman, and Mrs. Henry Inman.

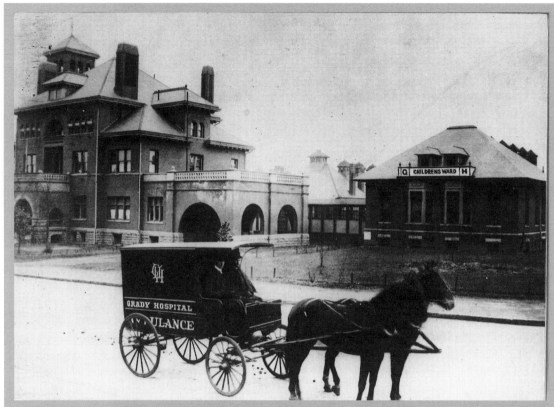

Children's Ward, 1896
Children primarily received care in their homes, usually from a family member. The opening of the ward was a remarkable step forward. The driver of the ambulance is Allen Kimball. Kimball was the first patient admitted to Grady Hospital when it opened in June 1892.

with hospital officials argued that housing for nurses was a more urgent priority.) The Order of Old-Fashioned Women's maternity ward opened in 1904 on the site donated by the Grady Hospital Aid Association.

Just as caring for a child in a special ward was becoming an important medical practice in the 1890s, establishing isolation wards also represented the best in medical science. Funding from a public source rather than the charity of women allowed Grady to build an isolation ward. There the hospital's physicians cared for patients with highly communicable diseases like smallpox, scarlet fever, measles, and tuberculosis. While it did not fund the new ward in full, Atlanta's city council appropriated $5,000 to help pay for the unit. Perhaps council members did not fully appreciate the importance of isolating patients carrying highly contagious, airborne diseases. These, of course, were just the kinds of diseases that might easily run rampant in a crowded city. Other debilitating diseases, just as prevalent in the city as in the countryside, required different remedies.

Hookworm

The work of Dr. Claude Smith, a pathologist at Grady and demonstrator of pathology and bacteriology at Southern Dental College, offers a notable example of how physicians used hospital laboratories to investigate causes of infectious diseases. In 1901, Dr. Smith was among the small number of American scientists investigating the role of parasites in human illness. He suspected that a parasite afflicted people in the South. In an effort to prove his theory, Dr. Smith examined stools from twenty convict-laborers working in clay pits at Captain James English's Chattahoochee Brick Company. In looking at the samples at Grady's lab, he discovered that two convicts suffered from hookworm, a blood-sucking parasite. In the next phase of his investigation, Dr. Smith performed a simple experiment. He applied soil containing hookworm larva to the wrist of a prisoner free of the disease. After one hour he removed the soil from the man's wrist. Dr. Smith saw that the skin had become red and swollen; he also observed that the patient had intense itching at the site. Close examination later revealed that the man had eggs from the parasite on his wrist.[87] Significantly, the number of hookworm eggs in the patient increased over the next few days.[88]

Dr. Smith demonstrated through his experiments that hookworm spread through contact with the soil and deduced that hookworm was endemic in Georgia. Indeed, it seemed to be a southern illness.[89] Considering the results of his research, Dr. Smith concluded physicians and others urgently needed to diagnose, treat, and cure people suffering from the debilitating illness. Dr. Smith made his findings public in an address to the 53rd annual meeting of the American Medical Association held at Saratoga Springs, New York, in June 1902.[90]

If they had paid it any attention, hookworm would have been exactly the sort of disease to worry civic and business leaders in the New South. It brought its victims more than itching skin; it resulted in anemia, chronic fatigue, and sometimes death. Perpetually tired workers did not suit the image of the region that New South promoters wished to present. They wanted Yankees to see the South as salubrious, an area with healthy workers waiting for northern capitalists to invest in railroads, mines, factories, and commerce. Unfortunately, the northern press consistently described southerners as lazy. Dr. Smith's research could have helped New South boosters deflect that criticism. Instead of being lazy, the stereotypical poor, gaunt Southern "cracker" suffered from a treatable illness. For Dr. Smith to have helped change northern minds, however, his work needed a broader audience than it received.

Only a month before Dr. Smith presented his findings, another scientist had reported the results of his own research to a meeting of the American Gastroenterologic Association. Trained in zoology in Germany, Charles Wardell Stiles had investigated parasites in livestock for a decade but only recently started looking at hookworms in humans. At the meeting of gastroenterologists Stiles announced his discovery that the hookworm present in North America was a distinct specie, different from the one identified in Europe sixty years earlier. (Other researchers learned later that the hookworm he identified—Uncinaria americana, also known as Necator americanus—had migrated to North America from Africa during the time of the slave trade.)

Even before starting that work, Stiles had preached that hookworm infected southerners. He was not alone. A number of researchers found hookworm in Florida, South Carolina, Georgia, Alabama, and Louisiana as much as twenty years earlier. The observations of these physicians remained tucked away in medical journals, finding little publicity and generating no sense of urgency. While European doctors knew about those discoveries, most physicians in the United States remained oblivious to hookworm's presence in the South.

Charles Wardell Stiles had gone on a research tour across the South looking for evidence of hookworm. According to the historian John Ettling, "[w]ith the haste of a man certain he has come across something genuinely important, Stiles organized his findings and put them into print."[91] Stiles' conclusions greeted a highly disinterested public when they were released on October 24, 1902. It seemed likely that his research results, at best, would become little more than a professional secret. Six weeks after publication, however, on December 5, 1902, the New York *Sun* reported that Charles Wardell Stiles had discovered the "germ of laziness." It took a journalist, Irving C. Norwood, to transform Stiles' discovery of a species of hookworm into the finding of a germ. Norwood's flair for a phrase catapulted

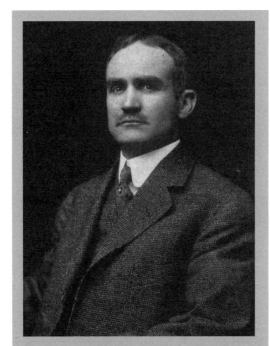

Dr. Claude Smith (1873-1951), a pathologist at Grady Hospital, came to the conclusion in 1901 that the parasite hookworm was endemic in Georgia. His efforts and those of others played a significant role in the eradication of the problem in the lives of thousands of citizens.

news about hookworm onto the front page of newspapers across North America and Europe. Initially the public greeted the reports of Stiles' research with skepticism and derision. Despite the early reception, Norwood's creative description of Stiles' discovery eventually became an invaluable contribution to publicizing the disease's existence.[92]

Although not accorded the publicity, credit, or funding for further research that Stiles won, Dr. Smith's research contributed to human understanding of a widespread and devastating disease—one with important social and economic ramifications. Among his significant accomplishments was showing that southerners became infected through ground itch, debunking the dominant theory that the practice of eating dirt caused hookworm.[93]

In 1909, a small but very well-funded group started a major war against the parasite and its impact on southerners.

The newly formed Rockefeller Sanitary Commission for the Eradication of Hookworm Disease made controlling hookworm in eleven Southern states its primary goal. The Rockefeller Commission was modeled on the Puerto Rico Anemia Commission, co-founded in 1904 by Drs. Bailey Ashford, Walter King, and Pedro Gutierrez Igaravidez. Five years earlier, in 1899, Dr. Ashford, a military physician, had discovered that the blood-sucking intestinal parasite hookworm caused the anemia that was ravaging Puerto Rico. He reported that hookworm lived in contaminated soil and that the disease is both preventable and curable. The Puerto Rico Anemia Commission implemented treatments and preventive techniques that would reduce the mortality from hookworm in Puerto Rico by 90% in the following years. It was a notable example for the Rockefeller Commission to follow.

Funded with one million dollars, the Rockefeller Sanitary Commission was one of the many philanthropic endeavors to which John D. Rockefeller devoted his time after retiring from the company he started, Standard Oil. The sanitary commission's ambitious goal was to take its crusade against hookworm around the globe. To publicize the public health hazard hookworm posed, the sanitary commission spurred massive educational programs in the South. Teaching people about hookworm was only a first step. Testing for hookworm disease, and treating it, soon followed. By the time the Rockefeller Sanitary Commission closed shop in 1915, health professionals had treated tens of thousands of Georgians for the parasite. Although its incidence diminished, hookworm remained a problem in Georgia. In 1922 it was reported that 15% of the juniors at Emory's medical school had hookworm.[94]

Two drugs proved effective in treating the illness. First, Chenopodium (*Chenopodium ambrosioides*) oil obtained from the American wormseed paralyzed the intestinal parasite. This allowed patients to excrete the organism easily after a dose of castor oil or magnesium sulfate. Second, a medication called Thymol, an antiseptic extracted from the oil of thyme, also proved effective. Using this medicine to treat a patient cost about fifty cents at the time Dr. Smith engaged in his research.

Dr. Smith's persistent investigational work, together with the wide-scale public health education efforts resulting from the research he, Charles Wardell Stiles, and many others conducted since the 1880s count as significant achievements in American medical history.

Accusations of Mismanagement at Grady

Holding Grady Accountable for Refusing Patients

Thanks to its status as a public hospital, Grady was subject to a level of scrutiny that private hospitals (both for profit and non-profit) avoided. City ownership also made the charity hospital accountable in ways that private hospitals were not. Because it was answerable to Atlanta's citizens, Grady seemed unable to have solely internal problems. What happened there was public business and the city's residents took advantage of their right to share in the hospital's public life. When they noticed, the city's newspapers eagerly reported the conflicts associated with Grady. The hospital also was subject to political interference.

In 1897, Milton Camp, a member of Atlanta's city council, charged the hospital with mismanaging the care of its patients. He reported finding an ill man in the lock-up at the police station who had been taken off of the streets, apparently suffering from an overdose of opium and morphine. Thanks to councilman Camp, the man came under the care of one of the city's ward physicians, Dr. Charles D. Hurt, a surgeon and Professor of Materia Medica and Therapeutics at the Atlanta Medical College. Dr. Hurt called for an ambulance to take the man to Grady. Arriving with the ambulance, Dr. Strickland, the hospital's house doctor, refused to accept the patient. According to Camp, the doctor declared the overdose victim an unsuitable case for the hospital. In his view, Grady rejected the "unworthy poor."

For generations middle class Americans had distinguished between the "worthy poor" and "unworthy poor." Drug addicts were counted among the unworthy. Impoverished people who suffered injury or illness but led "morally upright" lives usually won the status of "worthy poor." This moralist distinction rather than medical necessity sometimes became a basis for determining whether to treat an ailing person.[95] At Grady, however, a person's moral rectitude wasn't supposed to matter. The hospital of last resort in Atlanta was supposed to be fully inclusive; anyone could come to Grady. Being a public hospital, Grady could not actively neglect or turn away anyone. Thus, the councilman's complaint against Dr. Strickland seems justified. Angry at the way the "morphine eater" was treated, Camp wanted an investigation, perhaps to confirm his own views about Grady's failing. The problem, he claimed, was "in sending out with the ambulance these young and inexperienced physicians."[96]

In another case, Dr. James Gaston, a local physician, reported on a Grady physician's refusal to admit an elderly black man suffering from gangrene. The doctor at Grady rejected the patient out of concern that the wound's infection was contagious. Because at that moment no isolation rooms were available, the doctor turned the man away. Doctor Gaston responded by renting a room for the man in a house on Edgewood Street where he amputated the man's gangrenous leg, thereby saving the patient's life. After this incident, both Dr. Gaston and Mr. Camp spoke out against the hospital. Dr. Gaston's complaint involved more than the hospital's refusal to treat the sick. He also objected to the hospital excluding physicians who were not associated with the Atlanta Medical College. Gaston charged Grady's administration with discriminating against homeopathic and eclectic physicians. These doctors, Gaston claimed, were "practically debarred" by Grady's management.[97]

As a result of these events, the city started investigating Grady in August 1897. Publicly welcoming the inquiry, hospital officials defended Grady's policy to reject "incurables." Their argument rested on seemingly practical economics; the sheer number of such patients could easily overwhelm the institution's meager financial resources. Although councilman Camp considered dropping the investigation, Joseph Hirsch, the chairman of Grady's board, together with Dr. Brewster, the hospital's superintendent, asked the city council to appoint a special committee to conduct an investigation.

At the city council's public hearings about Grady, several local physicians charged the hospital and its staff with incompetence and neglect of duty. Denying the accusations, the hospital claimed the physicians testifying against the institution were retaliating against Grady for denying them privileges to practice there. Other witnesses accused Grady of poor bookkeeping and of overpaying for supplies. After the hearings and more investigation, the city council cleared Grady. The council, however, concluded that the city needed to have a stronger voice in hospital management. As a step in that direction, it requested that the hospital send monthly reports to the council.

Did Grady Properly Supervise Medical Education?

In 1907, Dr. Thomas Longino, a city councilman and former mayor of West End, charged Grady with grossly neglecting patients. Dr. Longino claimed that the attending staff failed to supervise interns properly, especially during surgery.[98] Attributing the problems to inadequate oversight, Dr. Longino insisted that the city appoint a new board of trustees. It is unclear that the businessmen on Grady's board of trustees could have identified improper supervision of interns during surgery. They would have to rely on physicians following rules set by the hospital's medical board. In defending the hospital, Dr. John Earnest noted that the same regulations in force at most hospitals in the United States governed Grady's interns.

The Grady administration rejected Dr. Longino's criticism as unjust. In their defense, hospital officials noted that only medical school graduates who passed a rigorous exam became interns at Grady. In addition, the hospital emphasized that an experienced physician supervised each intern. Using these arguments, Grady quieted the controversy. With councilman Longino's effort to have the city appoint a new board of trustees for Grady thwarted, the matter seemed resolved. It would not be long, however, before Atlanta's medical schools turned Grady into a professional battleground again. Changes in medical education in Atlanta set the stage for another set of accusations against Grady.

Friction among the faculty of the Atlanta College of Physicians and Surgeons (ACP&S) had prompted several of the school's best teachers to resign in 1905 and open a new medical school, the Atlanta School of Medicine (ASM). Within two years, charges and counter-charges between the two medical schools concerning access to, and care for, patients at Grady became a public issue.

In December 1907, several members of the Grady medical staff with ties to the new ASM proposed banning all medical students from visiting patients at Grady.[99] If successful, the gambit would do more than end fifteen years of practice at Grady; it would also throw a wrench into the competing teaching program of ACP&S. With their own students blocked from being trained at Grady, the ASM's faculty had launched a fairly bold offensive against the older medical school. Not surprisingly, staff physicians affiliated with the ACP&S—including Drs. Calhoun and Nicolson—fought back. They argued students should continue being involved in caring for patients. Faculty from both medical schools knew that students could learn much from watching an experienced physician in practice. Indeed, by that time staff physicians taught medical students at hospitals in every major city in the United States. As happened often, the public became involved in the hospital's affairs.

People outside the medical field tended to make one of two arguments against student ward rounds. First, medical students might make patients feel uncomfortable. Second, they might spread diseases among the inpatients. Mrs. Nellie Peters Black, who remained an active supporter of Grady and its mission, argued on both grounds against medical students seeing patients. Invoking the golden rule ("do unto others as you would have them do to you"), she asked, who would want strangers to observe a doctor's examination of them? She worried that the presence of students could upset the patients. She also was anxious that students would unknowingly infect patients with fresh germs.

Judge E. C. Kantz shared Mrs. Black's opposition to student ward rounds. He believed students might embarrass the hospital's patients. (Judge Kantz also believed medical schools should operate their own hospitals.) While these two respected Atlanta residents entered the fray in support of the upstart medical school, other leading citizens defended the hospital's practice of student ward rounds.

Dr. William Goldsmith, a prominent Atlanta physician who had been president of the Atlanta Society of Medicine in 1899, observed that no patient had ever registered

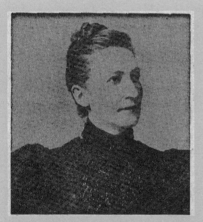

Mary Ellen (Nellie) Peters Black

Born in Atlanta, Nellie Peters was the daughter of Mary Jane and Richard Peters, a prosperous couple who rose to civic leadership after the Civil War. (Mr. Peters donated the original four acres of land for the Georgia Institute of Technology.) Nellie Peters received her education at Brooke Hall in Media, Pennsylvania. Upon graduation her parents offered her a choice of gifts to celebrate the occasion; she could have either a diamond or a horse. She chose the horse and named it Diamond. Living in Atlanta, she was frequently seen riding Diamond in the poorer sections of the city, lending a helping hand to the impoverished.

In 1877, Miss Peters married George Black, a lawyer, farmer, and member of the United States Congress. He was also a widower with seven children; the marriage to Miss Peters produced three more children. In 1882, George Black suffered a severe stroke; he died four years later.

In 1888, Mrs. Black returned to Atlanta and quickly re-entered civic life. She was an organizer of civic institutions and a joiner of clubs. While she belonged to the trendy social clubs founded in her time—the Daughters of the American Revolution, the United Daughters of the Confederacy, and the Colonial Dames—her heart was with the groups dedicated to social reform and improvement. A leading light in the city, she was as close as Atlanta came to having its own Jane Addams.* She stood for service to the poor, improving children's health and education, the admission of women into the University of Georgia, and a host of other causes. She helped organize the first mission to the poor in Atlanta, the Holy Innocents Mission on Tenth Street, helped start the Visiting Nurses Association in Atlanta, and was a founder and President of the Georgia Federation of Women's Clubs. A strong advocate for children, she was elected President of the Free Kindergarten Association in 1894, a post she held for twenty years. Her decades of work paid off in 1919 when the public schools in Atlanta finally adopted the kindergarten. Although she lived in Atlanta, her family maintained a farm in Gordon County. She took over the farm's management in 1897 and quickly became an outspoken advocate for agricultural improvement and rural reform. She was the Progressive's progressive, an organizer of people into clubs that advocated for and provided social betterment.[114]

Her impact on Atlanta, and Georgia, is still being felt thanks to her remarkably thoughtful contributions to the public good.

*Jane Addams (1860-1935) was an American social worker and humanitarian. After visiting Europe in 1882 and 1888, she returned to Chicago and established a neighborhood center among immigrants. Day nurseries and even college courses were offered. She was associated with the first eight-hour workday for women, child labor laws, juvenile courts, and housing reform. In 1931 she shared the Nobel Peace Prize with Nicholas Murray Butler, the President of Columbia University.

a complaint about medical students at Grady. He suggested disgruntled physicians whose students could not make patient visits had fabricated the "crisis." Dr. Goldsmith pointed out that the hospital's original design included a surgical amphitheater that allowed medical students to watch and learn from doctors performing operations. Adding a third leg to his argument in favor of keeping medical student ward rounds, Dr. Goldsmith appealed, in essence, to Atlanta's civic pride. He reeled off a list of hospitals in other New South cities—including Nashville, New Orleans, and Charleston—that allowed students to make ward rounds. The implication was clear: banning students from making ward rounds at Grady would consign Atlanta to the status of second-rate city.

Ultimately Atlanta's Board of Alderman voted to allow medical students to continue making rounds at the hospital. (The motion carried by a vote of 6 to 5.)[100] Following the aldermen's lead, the city council also approved continuing student rounds at Grady. (The council passed the measure by a vote of 18 to 5.) The city's permission for students to keep making medical rounds resulted in part from negotiation. In order to prevail, hospital administrators gave some ground to the complaining faculty from the Atlanta School of Medicine. Their most important concession gave faculty from both medical schools parity within the hospital's walls.

The Atlanta Race Riot of 1906

Extreme racial violence broke out in Atlanta during the first days of autumn in 1906.[101] The seeds for what became a murderous rampage by whites were sown earlier that summer during a heated primary campaign for governor. Both of the leading candidates promoted white supremacist views. Of the two, Hoke Smith, a lawyer and former columnist (and part-owner) of the *Atlanta Journal*, was the more outspoken. Smith's leading opponent was Clark Howell, the son of Captain Evan P. Howell, the man who had hired Henry Grady to work for the

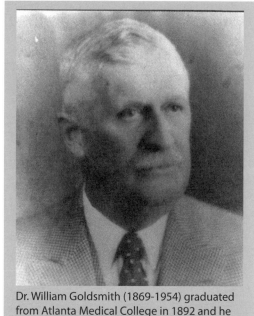

Dr. William Goldsmith (1869-1954) graduated from Atlanta Medical College in 1892 and he became an outstanding general surgeon.

Constitution. Following Grady's death the younger Howell became managing editor of the newspaper, a position that helped him as he pursued an active political career. First elected to Georgia's House of Representatives in 1886, at the age of twenty-three, he became Speaker of the House in 1890 and Georgia's Democratic National Committeeman in 1896. Clark Howell was president of Georgia's state senate when he decided to run for governor in 1906.

At that point, sixteen years after Henry Grady's death, the New South looked very familiar to those acquainted with the Old South. Romanticized notions of the Lost Cause came from the lips of New South orators and were carved into stone on courthouse squares across the region. Those statues of Confederate soldiers, gun at the ready, seemed to protect the revival of a form of Southern liberty thought to have died at Appomattox. Having become codified in law in the last decade of the nineteenth century, the race-based rule of Jim Crow had hardened in Georgia since Grady died. During that decade and a half, politicians like the agrarian firebrand Tom Watson found that highlighting racial divisions produced more votes.[102]

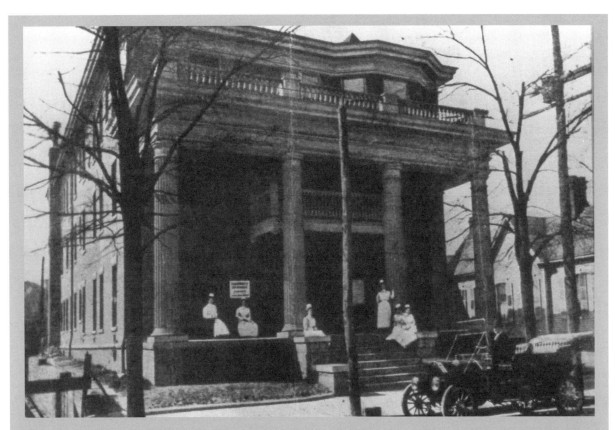

Georgia Baptist Hospital started in a small rented house on Courtland Street but moved to 69 Luckie Street (above) because of the need to expand. In 1913 the Georgia Baptist Convention purchased the Tabernacle Infirmary for $85,000. It continued to operate on the Luckie Street site for several years before moving to a larger facility.

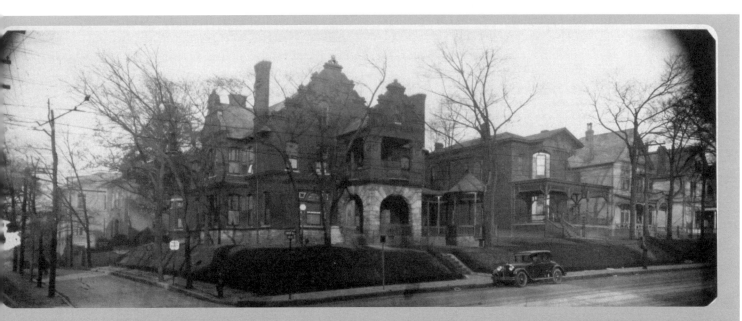

Amster's Sanatorium was founded in 1904. It was a 16-bed facility primarily for patients of Dr. Floyd McRae. It originally was the home of business executive Charles Swift and his wife, Lena, who built the house on Capitol Avenue in 1875. After their deaths it served as a rental property until Dr. and Mrs. Ludwig Amster purchased the fifteen-room mansion for their sanatorium. The property would later become part of the site for Atlanta-Fulton County Stadium.

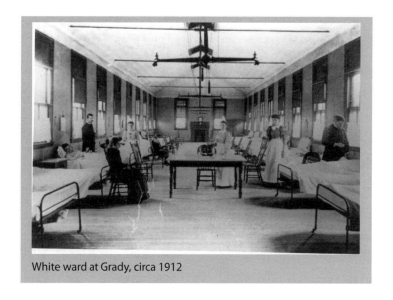
White ward at Grady, circa 1912

In the gubernatorial campaign of 1906, the two leading candidates each tried to capitalize on white fears about blacks. Hoke Smith, who had been Secretary of the Interior under President Cleveland, actively favored passage of an amendment to the state constitution that would more effectively disfranchise black citizens than they already were through the poll tax and whites-only primary. (A state report claimed that more blacks than whites paid poll taxes in thirty-three of Georgia's counties.)[103] His desire to extend white racial domination seemed to know few boundaries. In an especially direct statement Mr. Smith declared, "we will control the Negro peacefully if we can, but with guns if we must."[104] Clark Howell's greater moderation in tone reflected only a more modest approach to keeping black citizens from voting. He objected to the proposed amendment because it might rob poor whites from voting while handing the ballot to educated African Americans. Howell warned that if passed, the measure Hoke Smith supported would only cause blacks in Georgia to become better educated. There were other crucial issues in the campaign, especially regulation of railroads, agrarian reform, and Smith's crusade against the Democratic political machine that Howell represented. Nevertheless, the newspapers associated with the two men, like Atlanta's other newspapers, highlighted racial concerns.

Where many crusading northern newspapers engaged in muckraking, some of Atlanta's dailies specialized in race baiting. In the midst of the heated campaign, the city's newspapers insisted white residents exert greater control over black citizens. Two newspapers, the financially ailing *Atlanta Evening News* and the *Atlanta Georgian*, gave especially lurid and detailed allegations of black men assaulting white women. With reports of sexual assaults and the heated race-based political campaign capturing headlines, racial tension in the city rose. On July 30, newspapers accused a black man of raping a white fourteen-year-old girl. That evening a posse of white vigilantes hunted down the man on the south side of the city and shot him to death. In August, the virulently racist Smith won a solid victory in the Democratic Party primary.

The racial tension continued to develop for several weeks after the election. The week of September 17th saw an escalation of newspaper-driven hysteria, as "scattered and largely inconsequential incidents between Negro men and white women were transformed by the press and public discussion into 'an intolerable epidemic of rape.'"[105] On September 22, local newspapers reported several assaults by black men on white women. Publishing extra editions that afternoon, the newspapers raised questions about the virtue of the white "men of

Fulton." Would they stand by idly or would they defend white women against what the papers characterized as predators?

It was a Saturday. People had gotten their pay and some had gone in search of liquor. Primarily led by young white working class men—joined by plenty of middle class and wealthier men—mobs of whites attacked blacks throughout downtown. They pulled people off streetcars and beat them to death. A black man in a barbershop was shot to death at point blank range. Another was stoned and then tossed to his death from a bridge. Mobs paraded black bodies through the city's streets, even dumping three fresh corpses at the feet of Henry Grady's statue on Marietta Street. Then a mob of several thousand whites attacked several hundred black men who, trusting they could find safety in numbers, had gathered on Decatur Street near downtown. Their hopes dashed, the black men fled after a brief attempt to defend themselves. So many injured people were carted off to Grady that the hospital could not hold any more victims. Its 110 beds were full, its hallways crowded. With Grady overflowing, wagons took the newest victims to the police station until it also overflowed.[106]

Mayor Woodward, Police Commissioner James W. English, and other city officials could not effectively control their city. Even directing fire hoses at the roving mobs of white men did not dampen the racial hostility. In black neighborhoods, people sat on their porches with guns in their hand ready to defend themselves. Hundreds of blacks fled the city. Others that night were, for their own safety, locked-in at the places where they worked. Not until close to 3 a.m., when the militia and a rainstorm each arrived, did the night's violence cease. In the cool light of Sunday morning shocked citizens gathered in churches to pray, even though none of the city's leading ministers would address the crisis in their sermons that day. That night racial violence broke out again, as it would the next night. The racial discord that began on Saturday evening would not be brought under control until Tuesday.

The final number of casualties is unknown since family and friends carried many of the victims away. At least thirty-two blacks and three whites were killed and at least seventy people were wounded (sixty black and ten white). Hundreds of black citizens, perhaps as many as three thousand, fled the city during and after the riot. Over 500 men arrested for rioting were forced to pave streets in Atlanta for several weeks; most were released from jail by that November.

Alex Walker, a black citizen, was sentenced to life imprisonment for the shooting death of police officer James Heard, the son of Judge Heard. No white received such a sentence for the killing of a black citizen. Twenty whites were indicted for rioting, but the charges were reduced to a misdemeanor. George Blackstock, a white man, was sentenced on October 21 for assault and battery on an African American, the most severe charge brought against any white citizen. The Atlanta race riot won coverage in newspapers around the world and damaged the city's reputation and threatened to severely disrupt business.

A "Committee of 1,000" formed immediately after the riot. Meeting at 4 p.m. on that Tuesday, it took on reconstructing the damaged city. A subcommittee led by Captain James English, called the Committee of Ten, was designated as the final authority over

Great Atlanta Fire

On May 21, 1917, a fire developed in a small warehouse Grady used as storage depot. Located just north of Decatur Street between Fort and Hilliard Streets, the storage unit contained hospital supplies. Starting between some mattresses, the fire spread rapidly across three hundred acres just northeast of downtown, destroying 1,938 homes and rendering 10,000 people homeless before firefighters finally brought the flames under control. Known as the "Great Atlanta Fire," it resulted in property losses of $5,500,000 but, amazingly, only a single fatality.[115]

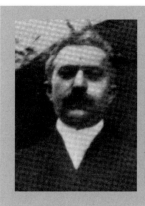
Dr. Ludwig Amster (1864-1936) was born in Vienna, Austria and immigrated to the United States. He graduated from the City of New York Medical Department in 1888. He and his wife, Flora, moved to Atlanta in 1894. He decided to specialize in gastrointestinal disease and established his sanatorium for this specialty. After retirement he returned to New York. He died in Rockaway, New York, in 1936.

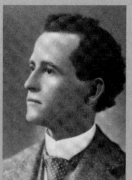
Dr. Floyd McRae, Sr. (1861-1921) graduated from the Atlanta Medical College in 1885. His reputation for care of abdominal wounds was nationally recognized by the time President William McKinley was shot in 1901. Dr. McRae was called for a consultation but the President died before the trip could be made. He was also an active member of the Grady Hospital volunteer staff.

the reconstruction effort. Forced into a corner by circumstances, white civic leaders began seeking dialogue with black leaders like the Reverend Henry Hugh Proctor, pastor of First Congregational Church. The desire to provide racial peace, if not reconciliation, helped push Atlanta's white and black civic leaders together. In the wake of the riot they forged a working relationship that would govern race relations in Atlanta for the next two generations. That coalition, dominated by whites, would have an impact on Grady's development over the coming decades, especially when white civic leaders sought black support for initiatives designed to help the hospital.

A City of New Hospitals

Several hospitals opened in Atlanta during the first decade of the twentieth century. The Baptist Tabernacle Church (Third Baptist Church) opened an infirmary on Courtland Street in 1901. The small facility would grow into Georgia Baptist Hospital, which eventually turned into one of the largest hospitals in the state. The next year, Presbyterian Hospital opened at Central Place. Three major medical institutions were founded in Atlanta in 1904. Seventh Day Adventists opened a hospital on South Boulevard. Local Methodists chartered Wesley Memorial Hospital in the same year and began accepting patients in a renovated building near Grady at the corner of Courtland Street and Auburn Avenue the next year. Also in 1904, Dr. Ludwig Amster opened a private sanatorium at the corner of Capitol Avenue and Crumley Street.

Dr. Floyd McRae, Sr., soon joined Dr. Amster as a partner in the venture. The two physicians would later rename their institution the "Piedmont Sanatorium."

The new hospitals helped relieve some of the overwhelming congestion at Grady. In 1905, all of Atlanta's new hospitals accepted charity patients whose cost of hospitalization was partially subsidized by the city. (Physicians offered medical treatment gratis.) Yet, the city's continuing growth also meant that even with five new hospitals, Grady would stay very busy.

Two Influential Women

Annie Bess Feebeck

Annie Bess Feebeck, a former schoolteacher from Millersburg, Kentucky, entered the Grady nurses' training program in 1906. She had earned a Bachelor of Arts degree from Thornwell College in Clinton, South Carolina, and taught grammar school in South Carolina and Kentucky before coming to Grady. After she graduated from its nursing school in 1909, Grady hospital appointed Ms. Feebeck as its night supervisor. The next spring it promoted her to superintendent of nurses.

Her authoritative rule and fiery personality led to frequent conflicts with other staff members. In March 1913, two head nurses threatened to quit because of Ms. Feebeck's tendency to publicly rebuke the staff. A month later, she publicly censured student nurses for what she saw as inappropriate behavior. The following December two interns and several nurses

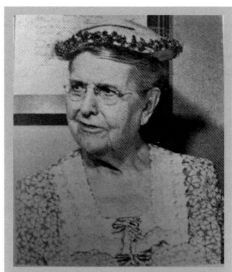

Annie Bess Feebeck (1881-1964) supervised Grady's nurses for many years. Feebeck Hall, a nurses' dormitory built during World War II at the corner of Armstrong Street and Pratt Street, was named in her honor.

accused her of harsh and abusive behavior. After inquiring into that episode, the hospital's administration censured Ms. Feebeck and forced her to make a public apology.[107]

Fourteen years later, in 1927, Miss Feebeck was on the hot seat once again. Nineteen nurses in White Grady gave a letter to Dr. Newdigate Owensby complaining about the way Miss Feebeck treated them. They also brought a petition to change the rigid rules under which they worked. The central issues centered on nurses dating interns and the kinds of punishment Miss Feebeck meted out to nurses. Following an investigation, White Grady's medical board recommended that "there be no social intercourse permitted between nurses and interns on duty, or while in hospital, on hospital grounds and in the vicinity of hospital or while either are in uniform."[108] The board explicitly declared, however, this did not mean a nurse could not date an intern if she so desired. Of course, it was well understood that the nurse would be fired if she married anyone. As for the punishments, the board indirectly suggested Miss Feebeck ease up a little. It also recommended the nurses have more privileges, including the right of student nurses to exercise outdoors between 7 and 8 o'clock in the evening.[109] These incidents suggest Miss Feebeck's strict rule over nurses was tempered by mercy from above. Miss Feebeck had the demeanor of a staff sergeant, a trait that may have been more useful for military service.

After the United States entered World War I, Miss Feebeck left Grady in order to join the Army Nurse Corps. She served as chief nurse at General Hospital Number 6, located at Fort McPherson near Atlanta. A few years after the war's end she returned to her post at Grady, serving as the director of nursing and nursing education until her retirement on July 1, 1944. During her career she served as the president of the Georgia State Nurses Association and of the Georgia Hospital Association.

Mrs. Ludie Andrews

Mrs. Ludie Andrews also played a remarkable role at Grady and in the history of nursing. She was born in 1875 in Milledgeville, Georgia, where she attended the segregated school in her community through the sixth grade. In 1901, at the age of 26, Mrs. Andrews applied for a scholarship to Spelman Seminary in Atlanta, one of the few institutions in the South offering higher education to black women. Mrs. Andrews graduated from that school's nurses training program in 1906. That same year she was appointed Superintendent of the Lula Grove Hospital and Training School for Colored Nurses operated by faculty from the new Atlanta School of Medicine. She served there until 1913 when the black nursing school shut down as the Atlanta School of Medicine prepared to merge into Atlanta Medical College. Several months later, in March 1914, after caring for two white patients with typhoid fever, Mrs. Andrews accepted an appointment from Grady to become its first Superintendent of the Nurses Colored Division. Three years later she formally organized Grady's nursing school for black women, the Municipal Training School for Colored Nurses, which was chartered on October 27, 1917.

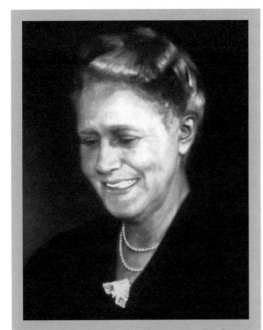

Ludie Andrews (1875-1969) became the first African American registered nurse in Georgia following a ten-year struggle with Georgia's courts, legislature, and the Georgia State Nurses Association.

When the State of Georgia first offered her accreditation as a registered nurse, she refused to accept because the state would not certify other qualified black nurses. Paying $200 in attorney's fees out of her own pocket, Mrs. Andrews continued her legal battle until she finally triumphed.[110] Thanks to her tenacity and courage, in 1919 the State of Georgia agreed to certify qualified nurses without regard to race. The following May, however, Ludie Andrews reported to the Grady hospital medical board that, "the state's nurses examining board refused to examine colored nurses from Grady Hospital."[111] The hospital's medical board referred the case to the chair of the hospital's committee on medical matters, who remedied the problem. In 1920, the school graduated six women—the first blacks in Georgia to become registered nurses.* These graduates were able to take the state examination for becoming registered nurses only because Ludie Andrews, for a decade starting in 1909, had fought for the right of black nurses to receive state certification as registered nurses.

Mrs. Andrews left Grady following conflicts with Superintendent Johnston; she became Superintendent of the Morehouse College Infirmary in 1920.[112] Eight years later the MacVicar Infirmary at Spelman College named her as its superintendent, a post she held until her retirement twenty years later. In 1943, she received the Mary Mahoney Medal for distinguished service to the nursing profession. At her retirement five years later, Morehouse and Spelman Colleges awarded her a Certificate of Merit for long and faithful service. Tragically, Ms. Andrews died in a fire at her home on January 6, 1969.

The Great War

The Great War among nations in Europe started in the same year that Atlanta's $750,000 bond issue failed. As the months passed, the United States' entry into the war seemed increasingly likely. In 1915, a German submarine torpedoed and sank the passenger ship S. S. Lusitania. Among the 1,100 dead were 128 Americans. On February 1, 1917, Germany began unrestricted submarine warfare against Atlantic shipping, including American vessels. Two months later the United States declared war against Germany.

To meet the medical needs of the rapidly expanding United States military, the American Red Cross urged medical schools to organize medical units for service overseas. Forty-seven members of the Emory faculty who worked at Grady went to war, most serving with the Emory Unit (Base Hospital 43).[113] Thirty-one of Grady's nurses also enlisted, nine of them joining the Emory Unit organized by Dr. Edward C. Davis. Born in Albany, Georgia, in 1867, Dr. Davis was a highly respected physician, member of the Emory medical faculty, and co-founder of the Davis-Fisher Sanatorium (later Emory

---

* The third graduating class of the Municipal Training School for Colored Nurses was the first to graduate since Georgia had begun to allow African Americans to become registered nurses. The members of the first class of Registered Nurses were Virginia Arnold, Fletcher Maye Calloway, Claire Harris, Lillie Mae Fambro, Lillian Thomas, and "Doch" Johnson.

Crawford Long Hospital) who had served as a physician in the Spanish-American War. After months of training, the Emory Unit left for Europe from New York on June 14, 1918. Within two weeks it was running a large hospital near Blois, France. There were 2,237 patients in the hospital on November 10, 1918, the day before the armistice ending the war was signed. Two members of the Emory Unit, Private Howard Candler Curtis and Camille Louise O'Brien, a nurse, lost their lives in the service. The unit served with distinction, treating 9,034 patients in its six and a half months of service at Blois. The unit deactivated shortly after returning to Atlanta in March 1919.[114]

Patterns

A set of patterns developed during Grady's first quarter-century. The quest of trustees, administrators, physicians, and staff to provide state-of-the-art hospital care to the city's residents was persistently frustrated by financial constraints. The regular failure of public bond issues to gain enough votes prevented the hospital's facilities from keeping pace with the city's growing population. As a result, outpatients faced delays in getting treatment and inpatients faced overcrowded wards. Consistently underfunded operating budgets impeded Grady's ability to stay abreast of new techniques and technologies that its patients and status as a teaching hospital required. Along with the advent of new systems for diagnosing and treating illness, Atlanta's growing population also drove Grady's need for more money. Because the income Grady earned went to the city's general fund, Grady could not increase revenue by bringing in more paying patients.

Grady's funding depended on politicians. One political reality was that for Grady to get more money, the city would have to increase taxes. The other political reality was that Atlanta's citizens and politicians, despite showing overwhelming support for bond issues, resisted increasing taxes for Grady's operating budget. Without more money from the city, Grady could only turn to private benefactors.

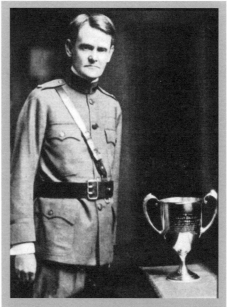

Dr. Edward C. Davis (1867-1931) served as a physician in the Spanish-American War and World War I.

Grady's status as a public hospital meant that almost anything that happened at Grady ended up in the public eye. Internal battles involving nurses, physicians, and administrators, questions about hospital administration, standards for admission and care, and nearly everything else came into public view. Under the right circumstances, what happened at Grady would become fodder for political debate.

Despite significant challenges—including internal conflicts and serious budget shortfalls—Grady did thrive during its first quarter-century. The municipal hospital successfully treated thousands of patients, chartered two nursing schools, trained hundreds of students from local medical schools, saw the Emory University School of Medicine form as successor institution to the schools that had long relied on Grady as their teaching hospital, initiated significant medical research, and made important contributions to public health in Atlanta and throughout Georgia. These too were notable patterns for Grady. By the time the Great War ended in 1918, Grady had laid a solid foundation on which it would continue to build in an increasingly urban and industrial New South.

Building Dreams
1918-1941

"We regret to say that politics in the medical fraternity and politics in general, have played a large part in the management of the complex system that now composes this great hospital."

– General Presentment, Grand Jury for Fulton County, October 1930.

Since the 1880s, Atlanta's medical community had hoped to make its city a regional center for medical care and research. Just as civic leaders boosted the chances of Atlanta becoming the dominant commercial city of the New South, its leading physicians looked for a way to make Atlanta the South's unmatched center for the business of medicine. Even Dr. Thomas S. Powell, one of the few physicians who had opposed establishing a public hospital in the city, supported turning Atlanta into the great medical center of the South. Among southern cities, Atlanta was well positioned to host a major regional medical center. Its nearest competitors were Johns Hopkins, 577 miles to the northeast in Baltimore, and Tulane University Medical Center, 425 miles to the southwest in New Orleans. With plenty of space to grow, boosters and impartial observers agreed Atlanta could become a major regional medical center.

In the early twentieth century, concerned physicians, civic boosters, and others looked for a workable way to turn the idea into reality. Some seemed to think the city's medical schools could give canopy for nursing the city's medical industry. Others thought that the city's hospitals offered a more logical starting point. A few years after becoming superintendent of Grady hospital, Dr. Summerall proposed "Greater Grady." Enlarging and enhancing the hospital, he argued, would transform Atlanta into a regionally dominant medical center. With the city's medical schools thoroughly discredited by the Flexner Report, it made sense for Grady to be the heartbeat of medicine in the city and region. There was no question that Grady was Atlanta's flagship hospital.

The campaign for the city's bond issue to improve Grady in 1914 had centered on creating Greater Grady. The failure to get enough voters to turn out for the $750,000 referendum for Greater Grady sent Dr. Summerall and civic boosters back to the proverbial drawing board. Each time they picked up the chalk, Grady's superintendents and civic leaders wound up with a similar picture. They continued to envision a Greater Grady where physicians and other medical researchers would treat patients, study diseases, teach medical students, and make pioneering breakthroughs in health care. With an improved Grady in place, they reasoned, northern philanthropic foundations would provide enough financial support for Grady to become a medical magnet. With their help, Grady would attract the funding and people needed to turn Atlanta into a leading center for medical care and research in the New South.

The dream of making Atlanta a great medical center was still far from becoming a reality as World War I ended, largely because of Grady's poor condition. Alfred Newell, an insurance executive and one of the hospital's trustees, noted the institution's disheartening state. "When the trustees, the medical board, the doctors, and the officers," he said, "are all united in a protest against the deplorable conditions [of Grady], they must be pretty bad."[1] Other trustees like Charles T. Nunnally, a powerful figure among the city's industrial and financial leadership, joined in Newell's lament. They could agree that the main reason for Grady's woeful condition was a shortage of money. Despite solid efforts, the city had not managed to pass a bond issue to fund the type of facilities Greater Grady needed.

An antiquated state law required two-thirds of registered voters to vote in favor of a bond referendum in order for it to pass (rather than a simply majority of those who voted). While the law hindered efforts to fund capital improvements through public bond issues, other constraints hindered local philanthropists. Just as the need for the city to create a city-owned general hospital was justified in 1888 because the task was more than a few wealthy individuals could accomplish, creating Greater Grady was too big for one or two local philanthropists to finance in 1919. The city council, with too few dollars for the rapidly growing city, appeared to be in no position to fill the void. In short, the dream of making Atlanta a great medical center continually clashed with financial limitations.

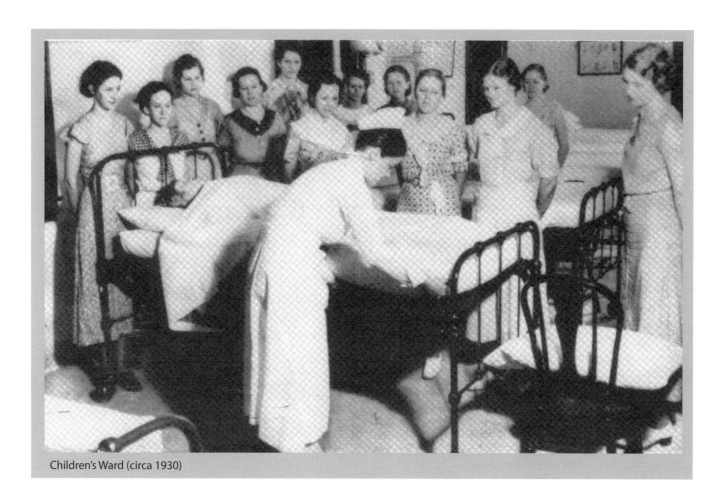

Children's Ward (circa 1930)

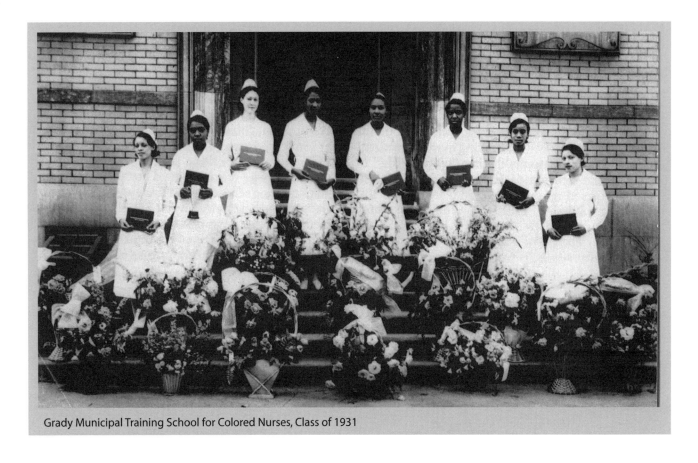
Grady Municipal Training School for Colored Nurses, Class of 1931

The ongoing conflict between hope and money would shape much of Grady's development for a generation after World War I. While promoters of Greater Grady hoped to expand the institution into a regional medical center, in the aftermath of the war the hospital was simply trying to meet the demands of the growing city.[2]

A New Black Grady

By 1910 the original "temporary" wards of Black Grady had fallen into utter disrepair. Dr. Summerall reported, "foundation timbers are decayed, floors are sagging and almost worn through in places, and the plaster on the walls is crumbling and falling off."[3] Within two years the two wards were no longer being used—in part because of their disrepair and in part because a shortage of students in Grady's nursing school prevented the hospital from accepting more inpatients.

In 1913, the new Atlanta Medical College (AMC) asked to use one of the old black wards for its paying African American patients. Located across the street from Grady, AMC frequently called on the hospital's physicians for help with emergency cases. Because Grady's facilities for treating blacks were so limited compared to the need, it seemed unlikely that surgical patients from the medical school could be admitted to Grady. That is why members of Grady's medical staff who were affiliated with AMC suggested that the school be allowed to rent one of the "abandoned colored wards" for its patients. Grady's board agreed to the proposal, but with the stipulation that all members of the medical staff—including those not affiliated with AMC—would have the right to place paying African American patients in the ward. The agreement also held that the city would pay nothing toward the cost of repairing and equipping the ward or for its nurses, maids, and orderlies. The city would only pay for the ward's heat, water, light, and laundry.[4] Although somewhat restored, the old Black

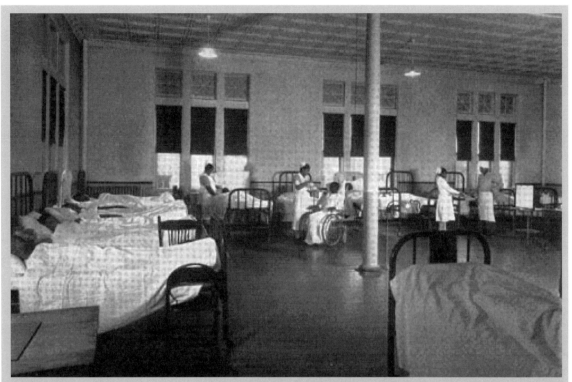
Black Grady ward, 1934

Grady wards remained woefully inadequate—as did the "new" Black Grady in the space White Grady left when its new facility opened in 1912.

In 1920, Emory University offered to make a substantial donation of property to Grady Memorial Hospital. Dr. William S. Elkin facilitated Emory's offer to give to Grady all of the buildings and grounds that the medical school owned directly across the street from the hospital.

The gift from the private school to the public institution came with three small but very important strings attached. First, while Emory provided the buildings, Grady would need to pay the costs incurred in turning them into suitable hospital space. Second, Grady was required to use the buildings for treating black patients. This would meet an important need since the hospital's black patients continued to overflow their dismal segregated space. The most important condition the university attached to its gift sparked little immediate controversy. Grady quickly accepted the demand that the Emory University School of Medicine fully oversee all patient care in the black wards. (Prior to 1920, medical staff unaffiliated with the medical school cared for black patients from June through September.)[5] Under these conditions, the hospital accepted the university's gift.

With the deal done, Emory turned over to Grady the old Atlanta College of Physicians and Surgeons building (c. 1906), located at the corner of Butler and Armstrong Streets. Grady finished converting the old medical school into a hospital in 1921, at a cost of $125,000, and then moved its black patients to their new quarters. Occupying three floors of the facility, the hospital's black patients enjoyed larger and more comfortable space than they had before. At the same time, Emory's medical faculty supervised their care, a fact that would annoy some people in White Atlanta during the next decade.

Emory's gift laid the foundation for a relationship that would shape Grady for generations, and, indirectly at least, set the stage for crucial changes to the area's health care environment.

The Municipal Training School for Colored Nurses

Grady's new hospital for black patients opened only one year after Grady's Municipal Training School for Colored Nurses graduated its first class eligible to be certified by the state of Georgia as registered nurses. A continuing shortage of white nurses had been a main reason for organizing the school. At the time Grady averaged 190 patients per day, but had only 36 white nurses. Because of the shortage, the hospital had removed white nursing students from the black wards early in 1914, replacing them with African American nurses supervised by African American head nurses.[6] Interestingly, the medical board proposed that the head of black nurses be relieved of any responsibility for the black wards; instead, black nurses would answer to the hospital's superintendent and the medical board. By the end of 1914 the board was pursuing a charter for a "Training School for colored nurses."[7]

Students at the school for black nurses reportedly followed the same curriculum as the students did at Grady's white nursing school. Hospital officials bragged that the only differences in the student's education involved uniforms, school pin, and graduation ceremonies. Whether or not the training of Grady's black and white nursing students could have been equal, it certainly remained separate. Many graduates from Grady's Municipal Training School for Colored Nurses found jobs at the Grady hospital dedicated to black patients. At the time, Black Grady and the Metropolitan Insurance Company were the only local businesses offering positions to black nurses. (Although Black Grady hired African American nurses, neither it nor Emory appointed physicians of color.)

Perhaps the most noticeable thing about Grady's nursing school for black women is that no member of its first graduating class had attended a public high school in Atlanta. Doing so would have been impossible for any of them. It would be four years after Grady's black nursing school graduated its first class that the city's segregated school system finally opened a high school for black students, Booker T. Washington High School. Thus it hardly surprises that students at the Municipal Training School for Colored Nurses generally had little formal education. Neither should it surprise that students at Grady's black nursing school faced intense racial discrimination.

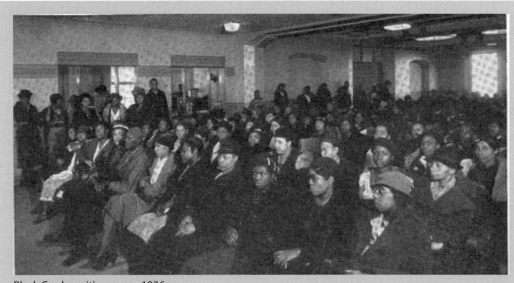
Black Grady waiting room, 1936

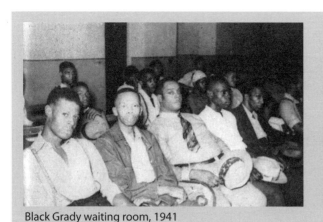
Black Grady waiting room, 1941

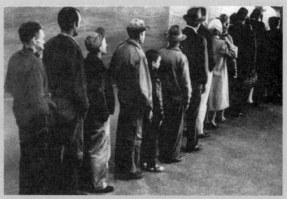
White Grady pharmacy, 1941

A report that The Rockefeller Foundation funded, and kept to itself for generations, provides compelling eyewitness testimony about the living and working conditions of students in America's black hospitals and nursing schools, including Grady's Municipal Training School for Colored Nurses.[8] As part of her research, the report's author, Ms. Ethel Johns, visited twenty-three black hospitals and nursing schools in the United States. A distinguished observer, the English-born Johns wrote frankly about the education, practical training, and lives of students she observed. In short, the education was minimal, the practical training was poor, and the lives of students included long hours, dismal housing, and a nearly penurious existence.

Ethel Johns considered the conditions for black student nurses at Grady among the worst in the nation—an extremely strong condemnation. Describing the living quarters for black nurses at Grady in bleak terms, Ms. Johns reported, "In two rooms in the basement I saw sixteen nurses trying to sleep. The beds were about two feet apart. There was no other furniture in the rooms. The atmosphere was fetid. The toilet facilities were inadequate."[9] With sixty students in 1925, Grady hosted one of the largest training schools for black nurses in the nation. Thanks to the hospital's superior equipment, Grady offered its nursing students a comparative educational advantage. If they knew about that, it might have offered little comfort to the school's students. They worked long hours, endured terrible housing conditions, and put up with harangues from the school's racist superintendent (Miss Feebeck).[10]

While its student housing was miserable, Grady's Municipal Training School for Colored Nurses was far from having the worst conditions in the nation. Nursing schools in the United States (for both whites and blacks) regularly exploited their students. Some schools, however, proved more awful than others. Ethel Johns lashed out most harshly at privately owned and managed nursing schools. In her view, black-owned for-profit schools tended to be the most ruthless in taking advantage of black nursing students, exploiting them to a greater degree than public institutions like Grady.[11]

While black nurses and nursing students faced harsh racial discrimination, other factors also help account for the way hospitals and schools treated them. At the time, nursing had little prestige among either black or white women. The distinguished historian Darlene Clark Hine observes that "pervasive stereotypes depicting nursing as a low status occupation affected career preferences of many black and white women."[12] During the 1920s most socially ambitious women preferred to enter teaching or social work. This was true for black women in particular. Ethel Johns reported, "in the South especially [nursing] is classed with personal service, a morass from which the negro woman … is trying to extricate herself."[13] At the same time, teachers faced with academically meager students were likely to steer them toward nursing as an occupation.

White Nursing at Grady Memorial Hospital

At the start of 1919, adequate housing for the white nurses at Grady was turning rapidly from an ongoing need into a crisis. A newspaper exposé by Eleanor Boykin reported that some of Grady's white nurses lived in "a stuffy little house" next to the hospital morgue. One of the rooms was six feet by twelve feet, "smaller by half," Ms. Boykin noted, "and much more dreary than the cells into which the inmates of the federal prison are put when kept in solitary confinement."[14]

During twenty years as chairman of the hospital's board of trustees, Joseph Hirsch frequently appealed to the city to build a new dormitory for nurses. Without better housing, the hospital would continue to have a shortage of nursing students.[15] Finally in the summer of 1912 the city council authorized $3,000 toward a design competition for a five-story home for nurses.[16] With the winning design by Blair Kern & Adams accepted, contractors had until March 1913 to submit their bids. Unfortunately, all five bids were almost triple the amount of money available from the city, $25,000.[17] By the time Hirsch died the next year, the dormitory project was stalled and the housing shortage for nurses was acute. Hirsch's heirs offered to contribute $10,000 for a dormitory if the city would allocate another $15,000.[18] Almost two years later, in January 1916, the city council appropriated $15,000. While architectural plans were drawn and the contract for construction let, work stopped when the city didn't turn over its money. In essence, the city continued to reject the gift even though it lost roughly $15,000 in revenue annually by housing some nurses in rooms designated for paying patients.

As World War I ended, the partially built dormitory project remained stalled. Doing personally what the city government refused, Mayor Asa Candler, whose sizeable fortune came from his substantial involvement with the Coca-Cola Company, donated $2,500 from his city salary toward the new home for Grady's white nurses. This was a significant step in meeting the pressing need, but it was still not enough to complete the project. A bequest of $30,000 from Charles E. Currier, president of Atlantic Steel Company, helped restart the project, but still more money was needed.

At the start of 1919, with nearly $50,000 spent on a project estimated to cost $180,000, it looked like there would be only enough money to keep construction going into the spring. Hospital supporters, however, might have become optimistic on New Year's Day when the city comptroller declared that

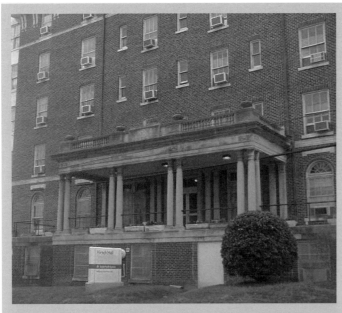

Hirsch Hall is named in memory of Joseph Hirsch, a friend of Henry Grady, and chairman of the Board of Trustees of the hospital for twenty years. Opened in 1922, the building served as a residence for nurses. It was demolished in 2011.

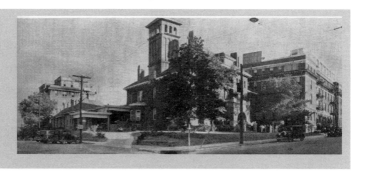

In this photo from 1935, White Grady is on the right and the original hospital is on the near left. The white hospital opened in 1912. Hirsch Hall is on the left in the background.

the city's finances were in excellent condition. With that good news, and a contribution of $25,000 from Fulton County that spring, Grady's trustees might have expected that the dormitory soon would be completed. Unfortunately, at the end of April the city council was forced to slash its budget for the year by $350,000 after yet another bond referendum failed to win support from two-thirds of *registered* voters. The budget cuts included $18,000 from Grady, of which $5,000 had been earmarked for the dormitory.[19] Construction stopped once more when the money that had been appropriated ran out in the middle of July.[20] An appeal to the city council for $50,000 was rebuffed, as was a desperate request to Fulton County for any contribution "from $5,000 to $75,000."[21]

The failure to finish the dormitory intensified Grady's severe nursing shortage. The crowded and dingy housing for white nurses, utterly lacking in privacy, was no more appealing than the adjacent neighborhood, the "Darktown" red-light district.[22] By the summer of 1919, Grady's white nursing school was down to thirty-six students, about half of what the hospital needed. There were no applicants, and few were expected. The hospital's terrible student housing made it difficult to attract students.

Asking the police board to "clean up" the area, the Reverend John Wyley Ham, pastor of the Baptist Tabernacle, claimed the neighborhood next to the dormitory prevented "girls of refinement" from applying to Grady's white nursing school.[23] Superintendent Johnston echoed the Reverend Ham, telling the police board that the surrounding neighborhood forced the nursing students "to live in a Hades on earth."[24] Although the police board agreed to instruct the Chief of Police, James Beavers, to "clean up" the neighborhood, it was unclear that the over-extended department—which had also been hit by budget cuts earlier in the year—would be able to devote much attention to the problem. Fortunately for the nurses, other advocates for Grady were looking past the neighbors.[25]

The nurses' housing crisis attracted attention from the City Federation of Women's Organizations. Chaired by Mrs. A. P. Coles, the federation of women's groups began to actively support the Ladies Aid Society of Grady Hospital. While the new group paid homage to Mrs. Lowry, who still headed the group that had been instrumental in building the hospital's maternity and children's wards, it would work directly with the superintendent of nurses, Miss Martha Giltner. A native Midwesterner, she had only recently become Grady's superintendent of nursing.[26] The fact that she was the fourth person to serve as chief of nursing in ten months suggests she had taken a challenging position.

On her fifth day at Grady, Miss Giltner sent a gracious letter to Superintendent Johnston explaining what was the matter with nursing at Grady. She informed him that the too few nurses serving at the hospital were terribly overworked. Worse, they didn't have a decent place to go to at the end of a long shift. The nurses' "un-hygienic, unhomelike, unheard of quarters, where such a thing as having privacy is unknown" was a hardship for the nurses. In addition, four Head

Nurses who "resigned to take much needed rests" would not be returning to Grady because they felt underpaid.[27] Nurses in private practice in Atlanta were earning about $30 per week; Grady offered a head nurse $75 per month.[28]

Miss Giltner had a radical suggestion for solving Grady's problem; she proposed it shutter some of the wards.[29] Given that Atlanta's population had grown to 200,000 residents and Grady had about 200 beds, eliminating 50 to 75 beds in the coming winter would be a radical step. Many nurses and physicians knew the need for hospital beds would grow as the seasons changed. In the prior winter the demand for beds at Grady outstripped supply as Atlanta, like the rest of the world, suffered through the Spanish Flu Pandemic of 1918—a wave of illness in which an estimated 3% of the world's population died.

The urgency of the upcoming flu season began shaping public response to Grady's nursing shortage and its root cause—poor housing for nurses. At the end of August, shortly after the City Federation of Women's Organizations became involved at the behest of nursing superintendent Giltner, a group of trustees and physicians made a public appeal for donations. Prompted by Grady's medical board, which originated the idea, the board of trustees formed a $150,000 fund-raising campaign for the hospital.[30] The money would let Grady complete the dormitory for white nurses and make other improvements.

The fund-raising movement was as effectively organized as any Liberty Bond drive and it generated a publicity machine that would have made George Creel, the head of United States propaganda during World War I, beam with pride.[31] Following Creel's lead, Grady's drive included the showing of short films at theaters and four-minute speeches given by volunteers. Led by J. R. Smith, a local businessman, the campaign appealed to the citizens' senses of pride and shame even more than to their fear of influenza. Putting the campaign in the context of the two million dollars needed to create Greater Grady, Dr. Garnett Quillian, the head of Grady's medical board, suggested that asking for $150,000 to meet Grady's immediate needs was hardly too much.

> An excerpt from the Grady Memorial Hospital Board of Trustee minutes of the meeting held June on 1, 1920:
>
> "Motion was adopted requesting Chairman of Committee on Hospital & Charities to introduce resolution at next meeting of [City] Council, permitting Superintendent of Grady Hospital to sell the two horses and the horse ambulance, not at the hospital, as they are useless."[187]

The drive organized committees of women and businessmen to canvass the city. Mrs. Ben Elsas led the women's committee, which included Mrs. Lowry as honorary chairman and prominent women like Mrs. Arnold Broyles, Mrs. Louis Regenstein, and Mrs. Samuel Candler Dobbs. A committee of civic leaders formed to inspect Grady and identify its needs included former mayor Asa Candler and well-known businessmen like Ivan E. Allen, Walter Rich, and W. W. Orr together with Rabbi David Marx. The group also sought and won endorsements from prominent organizations like the Fulton County Medical Society and the Atlanta Chamber of Commerce. As the campaign took shape, clergy supported the drive from the pulpit. Even the Atlanta City Council offered its support.[32]

Before the actual canvassing could begin, however, Mayor Key called a special session of the city council to consider "an emergency tax" of one-eighth of one percent. That would be enough to provide Grady with $150,000 and to raise an additional $70,000 needed to solve a financial crisis facing the city's public schools. After a bitter argument, the city council put off its vote for a week. In response, organizers of Grady's fund-raising drive called off the proposed campaign. By leaving "the responsibility of meeting the emergency of the city's hospital upon the city council," the campaign directors were adding pressure on the council to adopt the tax increase.

There appeared to be broad public support for the emergency tax. Clergy like the Reverend Ham and a variety of organizations, including the Atlanta Retail Merchants Association, the Presidents Club (consisting of the presidents of businesses and civic groups), and the Rotary Club, publicly supported the tax increase. When the city council met on October 6, it passed the measure by a vote of 21 to 8. Thanking the women of the city for their enthusiastic help and the Boy Scouts for their involvement, the campaign committee declared victory.[33] With the support of the taxpayers, the dormitory for white nurses would be completed. Ultimately the six-story, brick and concrete structure would cost more than $200,000. While much of the money was donated by the heirs of Joseph Hirsch, the majority of funds came from the emergency tax.

The new dormitory, named in Hirsch's honor, alleviated the housing shortage for white nurses. The need had been so great that student nurses started moving into the dormitory while it was under construction, as much as a year and a half before it formally opened in 1922. Located at 55 Coca-Cola Place, the new facility offered housing to ninety-six young women. There were sixteen private rooms and 40 double occupancy rooms. The building also contained several parlors, recreation rooms, a large auditorium, and a dining room. The space was so large it accommodated some of Grady's other pressing needs for space, including educational offices, classrooms, a library, and science laboratories. At the start of the twenty-first century, the building housed several of Grady's community outreach programs. (It was demolished in 2011.)

Labor Troubles

Labor unrest surfaced at Grady during the summer of 1919. On Monday, July 14, all but a handful of black employees at Grady refused to return to work unless the superintendent raised their wages to fifteen dollars per week.[34] The job walkout—the workers were not organized into a formal labor union—seemed likely to end quickly after the superintendent told the employees he would do what he could to increase their

Where Did We Put Those Towels?

On Thursday, April 14, 1921, a mysterious package was found in the garage of Mrs. Robert Lowry, a socially prominent woman who had long headed the Ladies' Auxiliary of Grady Hospital. The bundle in her garage contained an intriguing collection of "exquisite linen towels" embroidered by famous women from around the United States. Just what was a towel embroidered by Julia Ward Howe, containing the first line of her Yankee ode, *The Battle Hymn of the Republic*, doing in the garage of a Daughter of the Confederacy? The fault, perhaps, lay with Nellie Peters Black. In the early 1890s, Mrs. Black asked prominent women across the United States to donate personalized, embroidered linen towels to Atlanta's new charity hospital. Many women in addition to Julia Ward Howe responded, including Ms. Belva Lockwood, the first woman licensed to argue before the U.S. Supreme Court, Frances Willard, the famed social reformer, and Mary Day Lanier, the widow and editor of Georgia's favorite poet. After the towels arrived, however, the women on the committee deemed the linens "too valuable to be used" thanks to "their fine texture and valuable autographs." It probably never crossed the minds of Atlanta's striving women that such puffery would have outraged the democratic sensibilities of Julia Ward Howe. Mrs. Howe, who hoped to be remembered for her work on behalf of women's rights and prison reform, would never know that her efforts at embroidery were soon forgotten. The legatees to the feudal south had gathered the towels into a bundle, and it had lain in Mrs. Lowry's garage for many years. Following their discovery, the towels were to be sold at an auction benefiting Grady Memorial Hospital. Oddly, another stash of autographed linen towels from the early 1890s would be found at Grady in the early 1960s.[189]

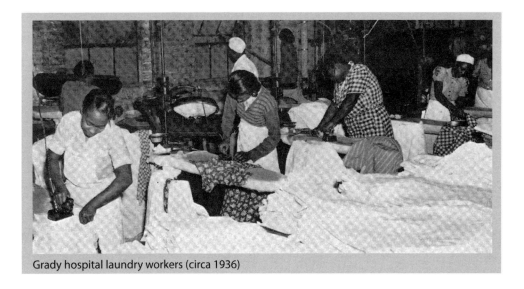
Grady hospital laundry workers (circa 1936)

wages. He warned them, however, he would do nothing until they returned to work. Getting permission from the chairman of the city council's Finance Committee, Superintendent Steve Johnston quickly devised a pay scale for workers. The hospital's chief offered to put the wages of the cooks, janitors, orderlies, and other jobs generally held by black men on a fixed scale, with pay raises given as their years of working at the hospital increased. He would pay them a minimum wage of ten dollars per week; the pay rose to $11 per week after three months on the job. Pay would increase again after an employee completed a half-year of service. Women would also get pay raises, although they would be paid far less. The women working at the mangle in the laundry room saw their weekly pay rise from $5 to $6 while ironers saw their wage increase from five to seven dollars. Maids were paid from five to seven dollars per week depending on their tenure at the hospital.[35] Superintendent Johnston's offer, however, fell short of the workers' demands (he proposed $12 while they insisted on $15), but he dug in his heels and refused to keep negotiating.

For help in dealing with the strike Johnston turned to Tom Landford, superintendent of the city stockade. As Johnston reported to the hospital's board, Landford provided "valuable assistance," helping to "quelch" the strike "by furnishing me prisoners both white and black in the laundry for several days."[36] To add insult to the workers who had walked off the job, Johnston raised the wages of three "of the old faithful negroes who stood by [him] and positively refused to strike" to $15 per week.[37]

The lessons for other black workers were clear. While in 1919 the law forbade leasing prisoners to a private corporation, nothing prevented prisoners from replacing municipal workers. Low-skill work at Grady was not safe from the threat of prison labor. The other lesson, equally clear, was that loyalty to the hospital's superintendent paid better than solidarity with fellow workers. Given that there were many labor strikes across the nation that summer, the work stoppage at Grady may seem unexceptional. Given the extremely limited power and position of black workers in Atlanta, however, and Grady's status as essentially the only hospital in the city to take a black patient, the strike stands out. It was far from the last labor walkout at Grady. For example, in the late spring of 1925, the hospital's orderlies went on strike. Their demands also would go unmet.[38]

The Great Baby Mix-Up Panic

In the spring of 1919, Grady became the setting for, and seemingly the culprit behind, a headline-grabbing panic that demonstrates the consequences of Grady's organizational failures and its severe shortage of nurses. A mother who had delivered an infant at Grady some months earlier insisted the child she came home with from the hospital belonged to someone else. Reports of her concern set off a chain reaction of anxiety among new mothers in the city. It might not have done so if it had been an isolated case. As it gained publicity, however, more mothers came forward to suggest that they too suspected something had gone wrong in Grady's maternity ward. The "baby mix-up" rapidly became the biggest topic of conversation across the city.

At about ten o'clock in the morning on May 22, 1919, Mrs. John Garner delivered a baby into the world. Later that night, Mrs. David Pittman also delivered a daughter. Trouble started brewing around 2 o'clock on the following morning. At that early hour Mrs. Garner asked to have her baby brought to her. Unfortunately, no nurses were immediately available to do as she wished. In the absence of a nurse, Mrs. Garner asked a maid named Lillie to bring her newborn. (At the time, Grady placed several infants side-by-side on a rolling table that was pushed through the ward to bring infants to their mothers.) Later that morning Mrs. Garner observed that the baby she had been given did not have an identifying nametag sewn on her sleeve at the wrist. She would later claim that even if it had been there, the tag would have been irrelevant because, she charged, the maid who gave her the baby from the cart could neither read nor write. Shortly before being discharged from the hospital, Mrs. Garner officially complained that the maid had switched her baby with Mrs. Pittman's newborn.[39] After looking into the events, Superintendent Johnston cleared the maid and proclaimed the babies were with their natural mothers.

Even after taking Mary Elizabeth home, Mrs. Garner continued believing the babies were switched. She became more unsettled as the months wore on. Finally she decided not only that the superintendent was mistaken, but that she needed to do something about the situation. To her it was clear that the girl she had come home with was not her true daughter. Reportedly, Mrs. Garner declared, "It's a poor mother that doesn't know her own child."[40] Viewing the matter from a different perspective, Mrs. Pittman quite agreed. Certainly the babies looked different from each other. Mary Elizabeth had blue eyes and red hair while Louise had brown eyes and black hair. Mrs. Garner claimed that the baby she came home with, the red-haired Mary, looked nothing like her other children, all of whom had brown eyes and dark hair.

In January 1920, eight months after the babies were born, Mrs. Garner hired an attorney and filed papers in court in effort to prove that Louise rather than Mary was her true baby. Tragically, Mary Elizabeth Garner died from pneumonia shortly after the case was filed.[41] At about the same time, Louise fell into a grate and suffered severe burns to her face. In the tragedy's aftermath, the Garners let the case lapse. In July, however, shortly after the Pittmans had another baby, the Garners went back to court. Judge George Bell was called upon to play Solomon.[42] After holding a hearing and examining evidence, including the testimony of the hospital maid, Judge Bell ruled that the case should go to trial to determine Louise's biological parents. Judge Bell was highly critical of Grady's system for tracking newborns.[43] Ultimately the courts decided that the Pittman family would keep Louise Madeleine until "she reaches an age to make a voluntary choice of her own deciding."[44] Sixteen years later, after visiting the Garner family in Macon, she decided to leave the Pittman's and live with the Garners, altering her name to Mary Louise Pittman Garner.[45]

New Governance

In the spring of 1921 the Atlanta city council began to consolidate its power. It started ridding city government and its agencies of all supervision by independent boards of citizens. The only exceptions were in cases where, like the public schools, the city charter mandated a citizens board of supervisors. As a result of the city council's action, its Committee on Hospitals and Charities assumed the function of Grady's board of trustees on May 1, 1921.

Nursing Troubles

July 1921 proved to be a tumultuous month at Grady. It was then that the hospital's medical board asked Miss Lillian Nelson, who had become superintendent of nurses a year earlier, to resign from the institution—which she did. A history of animosity between her and Superintendent Johnston led some people to suggest that he was behind the medical board's request. The superintendent, however, denied the allegation. For its part, the medical board cited Miss Nelson's lack of managerial experience as the main reason behind the move. They expected she would be unable to successfully handle an upcoming administrative restructuring in which one superintendent would lead both schools of nursing. Nurses and interns rapidly came to Miss Nelson's defense and threatened to walk out if the medical board forced her to resign. Consideration of the welfare of the patients (and the hospital) prevailed and the threatened walkout never took place.

On July 20 the city council's Committee on Hospitals and Charities accepted Miss Nelson's resignation.[46] Miss Annie Feebeck, the chief of nursing who resigned from Grady to join the military medical service during World War I, was named as her successor.

Although Superintendent Johnston denied that conflicts between him and Miss Nelson led to her being pushed out, the ill will between him and the nursing staff was evident. The hostility blew into the open when Miss M. A. Chesire, who had been a graduate nurse, charged Johnston with neglecting patients, nurses, and interns. She also claimed he had thrown lavish parties in his hospital "suite," tolerated the hospital's stewards insulting of nurses, and that he administered the hospital in a careless manner. She also complained that the hospital's food was terrible and frequently inadequate. Miss Chesire charged that the meals provided for nurses often consisted solely of boiled potatoes. Johnston strongly denied most of the allegations. He did admit, however, to having hosted dinner for the medical board when it held formal meetings at the hospital. He had also provided dinner when city council members and finance committee members met at the hospital. In his view, serving a steak and salad did not yet constitute a misdemeanor. In addition, Superintendent Johnston noted that Miss Chesire had been dismissed from the hospital for insubordination.[47]

Superintendent Johnston blamed local newspapers for inflaming the controversy. He identified a reporter from the *Atlanta Journal* and another from the *Atlanta Georgian* as being responsible for sensationalizing events at Grady. Johnston believed police beat reporters had been trolling the hospital's wards in search of tales to tell. With, in his view, at least two culprits identified, Johnston ordered reporters banned from Grady's wards.[48] Whatever the uproar in the local newspapers, no charges were filed against Superintendent Johnston.

Contagious Disease Hospital

Grady opened a new contagious disease hospital (on the corner of Coca Cola Place and Pratt Street) in 1922. For more than a decade Grady had treated people with various types of communicable diseases in the hospital's isolation ward. The new space allowed Grady to truly separate people with contagious illnesses from the public and other patients. Grady also devoted some areas in the new building to seemingly unrelated purposes. It is notable that the building's first floor held an infantile paralysis ward. Other areas in the building housed the city's health department. This seemingly tangential connection soon became more direct. Grady's contagious disease hospital expanded its responsibilities when the Atlanta Health Department began using it to detain patients with sexually transmitted diseases.

During the early 1920s, approximately 25 to 30 percent of Grady's patients suffered from syphilis, gonorrhea, or other venereal diseases.[49] At the time, patients with syphilis were treated with either a weekly intravenous injection of neoarsphenamine or an intramuscular injection of bismuth nitrate. Gonorrhea was treated with silver nitrate and later a colloidal silver preparation called Protargol. The contagious disease hospital often held people for two or three months of treatment. Despite the health department's efforts, sexually transmitted diseases continued to ravage the city. In 1936, 6% of pregnant white females and 23% of pregnant black females treated at Grady suffered from syphilis. (At a time of rampant hysteria in Atlanta about blacks infecting whites with syphilis, a New Deal program to test for syphilis was available to blacks but not to whites.)[50] By the early 1940s, the syphilis rates for patients at Grady were at 28% for black women, 24% for black men, 10% for white men, and 7% for white women.[51] The rest of Georgia had similar rates of syphilis infection.

The Steiner Clinic

Thanks to a generous bequest of $500,000 from Albert D. Steiner, a leading businessman in the city who died in 1919, Grady initiated a third major addition to its campus in 1922, the same year it opened Hirsch Hall and the Contagious Disease Hospital. In response to an overture from the executors of Steiner's will, Grady's board assigned members Charles T. Nunnally and Thomas C. Erwin to "confer with the Executors of the Steiner will and acquaint them with the needs of the Grady Hospital."[52]

Steiner had directed that the charitable fund endowed in his will should be used to "relieve the sufferings of the poor."[53] The best way to accomplish that, however, was left to the will's executors. Indeed, they were given broad leeway over how to use the "rest, residue and remainder" of his estate—the basis of the Steiner fund—to help the poor. After nearly three years of negotiations with Grady's board, Mr. John A. Hynds, an attorney representing the Albert Steiner Charitable Fund, proposed to the hospital's executive

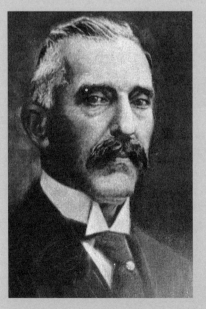

Albert Steiner

Albert Steiner was born in Austria in 1846. He immigrated to the United States the year after the Civil War ended and settled in tiny Dadeville, Alabama. Twenty years later he moved to Atlanta, where he became a successful businessman. Steiner had his hand in a variety of enterprises, including real estate, brewing (he was president of Atlanta Brewing and Ice Company), and banking (he was a director of the Fourth National Bank of Atlanta). A major leader in the city's religious, civic, and philanthropic life, Steiner was elected president of the Atlanta Hebrew Benevolent Congregation (later known as The Temple).

During his life he contributed generously to causes that helped the poor and the infirm, including a donation of $25,000 to the Scottish Rite Hospital for Crippled Children. In his will he would leave another $100,000 to that institution. While he provided significant gifts to family and friends, the bulk of Albert Steiner's estate went to the newly created Albert Steiner Charitable Fund. With $638,000 at their disposal, the fund's directors were charged with continuing Albert Steiner's remarkable contributions to the adopted city he loved.

Remarking on Steiner's will, the *Constitution* observed, "It is a notable tribute to a man's memory to have it said of him that he made the largest contribution ever left by a citizen of the state to the relief of suffering humanity.... No man ever left a more worthy will."[190]

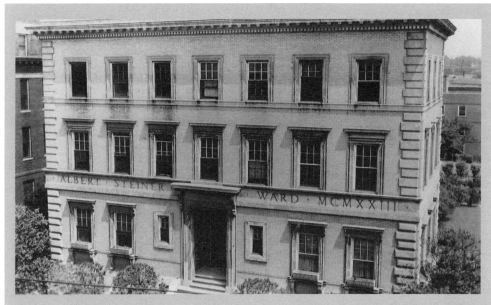
Steiner Clinic opened in 1923 and by 1930 had become the largest cancer hospital in the world.

committee that a ward for cancer patients, along with a general clinic, be built with money from the Steiner estate.

As it happened, both Mr. Steiner and his wife died from cancer. Perhaps that is why the executors of the fund, Joseph H. Hirsch, Henry Wellhouse, and Frank Liebman, sought to use the money to create a center devoted to research and treatment of cancer (and "allied diseases"). In addition, there was no specialty cancer clinic in Georgia at the time. Indeed, there were relatively few in the entire United States.

The first American hospital devoted to cancer patients had been founded in 1884, the same year it was revealed that Ulysses S. Grant had developed throat cancer. A little more than a decade later, Dr. Roswell Park established in Buffalo, New York, the first American facility for cancer research. Under the direction of Dr. James Ewing, in 1912 General Memorial Hospital for Cancer (formerly New York Cancer Hospital) developed the first hospital department in the United States devoted to treating cancer with radiation. The American Society for the Control of Cancer (which became the American Cancer Society) was formed in New York in 1913, only a few years after the founding of the American Association for Cancer Research (1907). With the help of these institutions, especially General Memorial Hospital and the American Society for the Control of Cancer, the executors of Steiner's estate developed sophisticated plans for Atlanta's first cancer hospital.[54] Thus, Mr. Hynds and the executors of the estate were asking Grady to implement a state-of-the-art program without peer in Georgia.

After the Grady committee accepted the offer, the Albert Steiner Charitable Fund and the city of Atlanta worked out a contract whereby the Steiner fund would pay to build and equip a hospital for cancer research and treatment. For its part, the city promised to administer and operate the institution in good faith. The Steiner fund's trustees only retained control over the right to hire and fire the house physicians who worked at the cancer hospital full-time. Steiner Clinic's visiting staff was made up of leading specialists in the city and its associate staff consisted of younger physicians; members of each took time away from their private practice to volunteer at the clinic. The contract between the city and the Steiner fund mandated that the cancer clinic make treatment of charity cases its first priority. Private-pay patients could be treated at the Steiner Clinic, but only as long as care of the city's poor took precedence. The money the city collected from private-pay patients at Steiner, according to the contract, was to be used to maintain facilities for the poor.

Soon after Grady's executive committee accepted the gift, the hospital's great supporter Jacob Elsas offered to give $50,000 to the hospital, of which $21,000 was to buy land for the new cancer clinic. He contributed the other $29,000 for Grady to enlarge its existing outpatient clinic, which was then named in his honor.[55] Jacob Elsas' gift allowed the Steiner Clinic to be devoted exclusively to caring for cancer patients.

The firm of Hentz, Reid and Adler designed the Steiner Clinic building. The firm's principal designer, the noted architect J. Neel Reid, had studied at the school of architecture at Columbia University and made the sojourn to Ecole des Beaux-Arts in Paris that was then customary for ambitious young American architects. Specializing in classical and Renaissance Revival designs, the firm created many notable houses for wealthy Atlantans along with a few commercial buildings. Located at 62 Butler Street, adjacent to other Grady property, the Steiner Clinic building was designed as a four-story (three fully above ground) reinforced structure with brick veneer. It contained 30 beds for patients when it opened in September 1924. The Steiner Clinic added 70 beds within a decade, making it the largest cancer hospital in the world at the time.

At its opening the Steiner Clinic had $70,000 worth of radium,* the second largest supply of any hospital in the world.[56] Radium's cost of $125,000 per gram made it virtually unaffordable for a physician in private practice. With 50 grams, the United States had the world's largest supply of radium; Marie Currie's Radium Institute had only 1 gram. By the start of the 1930s the price of radium had fallen to $70,000 per gram; it began dropping more rapidly several years later.

From the outset, the Steiner Clinic attracted individuals willing to pay for treatment. Although the clinic mostly served charity patients, it rapidly drew a large number of paying patients from Atlanta, and soon from throughout Georgia and the Southeast. Over time, however, it became so crowded that it would only accept patients who lived in Atlanta or Fulton County.

The Doctors' War

After Emory University's medical school began to coordinate patient care at Black Grady in 1921, physicians who controlled the care for patients at White Grady organized the Atlanta Graduate School of Physicians and Surgeons (AGS). Seeking arrangements with White Grady similar to those the Emory University School of Medicine had at Black Grady, the AGS, led by Drs. Frank Eskridge, Garnett Quillian, T. C. Davison, and Henry R. Donaldson, intended to use Grady's white unit for teaching post-graduate medical students.[57] Grady's overseers quickly gave the new school permission to use space in White Grady for teaching and to nominate members of their faculty for staff privileges at the hospital.[58] When the Elsas Clinic for white outpatients opened in April 1924, AGS essentially claimed the space for its own.[59]

In the spring of 1925, interns and staff at Grady began bickering over duties and pay. The interns and staff were concerned about how the leaders of AGS managed White Grady. They also worried that the four physicians who ran AGS had the authority to make staff changes in Grady's white unit without needing consent from the hospital's executive committee or the city council's Hospital and Charities Committee. The discord became so intense that the hospital's administration asked all of Grady's medical interns to resign by the start of October. Apparently AGS knew which staff members

---

*Marie Currie, a French physicist, discovered radium in 1898 in pitchblende – a radium and uranium-bearing mineral. There is about one gram of radium in seven tons of pitchblende.

it wanted to be rid of since it planned to reinstate half of the sixteen "resigned" interns. More than simply returning the favor, the disaffected interns sought to boot the AGS from White Grady. They were hardly alone. Fifty-nine members of the hospital staff signed a petition to support separating White Grady from the AGS.[60]

By the end of February 1926, physicians opposed to Drs. Eskridge, Quillian, Davison, and Donaldson had organized an effort to curtail the AGS physicians' power. The ensuing conflict between the two factions of physicians escalated to such intensity that local residents referred to the dispute as "the Doctors' War." Opponents of the status quo presented a proposal to the hospital to return control over staff changes to the hospital's executive committee. In another attempt to undermine the AGS's authority, the loyal opposition tried, for the first time, to give voting privileges at staff meetings to associate staff physicians. They also attempted to restrict the AGS's authority over the white wards by limiting candidates for a department's chief of staff to physicians who had served on Grady's staff for at least five years. In addition, they hoped to limit a department head's term to one year. In their defense of the way things were, supporters of AGS claimed the proposed changes would lead inexperienced physicians to control Grady. They also cautioned that, if adopted, the new rules would inflict enough harm on the hospital for the American College of Surgeons (predecessor to the Joint Commission on Accreditation of Healthcare Organizations) to remove Grady's "A" standing.[61]

Nearly two years of posturing finally ended when the parties to "the Doctors' War" reached a compromise in 1927. They agreed to allow associate staff to vote on all issues. They also decided that a chief of department would be retired after ten years of service. The compromise granted full use of the hospital, including the right to hold clinics at Grady, to former department chiefs. The city council's Hospital and Charities Committee would appoint the medical staff executive committee. Even with the two factions agreeing to the compromise, some physicians at Grady remained dissatisfied and attempted to reverse the new rules. The compromise that ended the Doctors' War held after a final skirmish at the end of April 1927.[62] It is hard to gauge the impact that the battle for control of medical care in White Grady had on white inpatients. It certainly distracted doctors and other staff who served Grady. The fight over internal controls probably affected the reputations of some physicians at Grady more than it did the health of the hospital's white patients. Even with the Doctors' War finished, however, battling over Grady continued.*

"A Disgrace to Any Civilized Community"

Grady's inadequate facilities angered the physicians who worked there. They could not hide their disgust during the annual dinner of the hospital staffs held in the fall of 1928. Dr. R. H. "Rube" Fike, head of the Steiner Clinic, declared, "when I say Grady is a disgrace to any civilized community I mean that its lack of proper facilities for treatment of the sick of Atlanta make it so."[63] Dr. James Paullin marveled at Grady's success under the circumstances and imagined what would be possible with up-to-date facilities. Noting that the city's physicians donated $1.5 million worth of free labor at Grady each year, Dr. Paullin pleaded that they have "proper facilities" in which to work.[64]

Dr. T. C. Davison explained why Grady's buildings and equipment were utterly inadequate. Reiterating what physicians had been saying for several years, Dr. Davison noted White Grady had not expanded since it opened; yet the demand for its services

---

* In 1927, before the final battle of the Doctors' War, the physicians at White Grady launched a new venture under the leadership of the AGS—a professional medical journal, *Archives of Grady Municipal Hospital, White Unit*. Apparently they ended the effort after publishing only one issue.

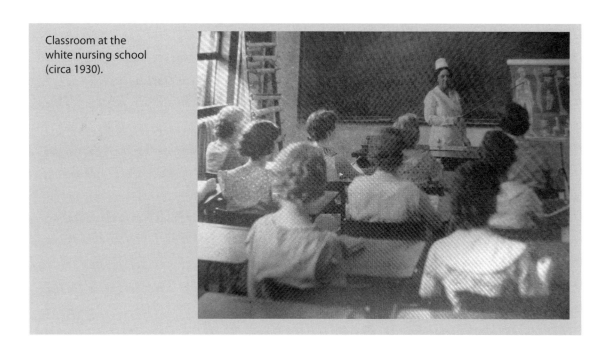

Classroom at the white nursing school (circa 1930).

had escalated dramatically because the city's population had doubled.⁶⁵ Some physicians believed that a new bond issue would give the city the financing needed for upgrading and expanding the hospital's equipment and facilities.

Joining their plea for a bond referendum in 1929, Dr. Davison claimed White Grady was "so congested that proper segregation is impossible."⁶⁶ He meant medical rather than racial separation. Patients with chronic illnesses and highly contagious diseases could not be separated out from others. There was inadequate space to isolate patients who developed meningitis or measles in the regular wards. "Tubercular patients, with other disease," he said, "are necessarily treated in the same wards with other patients." Endangering the lives of other patients was simply unfair.⁶⁷

Similarly, all types of surgical cases were mixed together in a general ward. Ideally, patients with different types of surgery would be placed in separate wards. The pediatric ward also lacked medical segregation. When measles, scarlet fever, or chicken pox broke out in the ward, the whole pediatric unit had to be quarantined and no new patients could be accepted until the illness ran its course. The contagious disease building had one floor dedicated to scarlet fever and the other dedicated to diphtheria. There was no place to isolate patients with other communicable diseases. As for Black Grady, Dr. Davison noted the black wards, which had moved from the old wooden buildings to their new quarters in 1921, were also severely overcrowded.

While many physicians looked to new financing and construction to ease the hospital's woes, others sought a broader solution. In 1928, Dr. Russell H. Oppenheimer, the Dean of Emory's medical school, had suggested a simple solution to the hospital's numerous problems: remove politics from the hospital by abolishing the city council's Hospitals and Charities Committee's oversight of Grady and returning its governance to an independent board of trustees.⁶⁸ Civic-minded citizens, he thought, would be less prone to interfering in the hospital's internal decisions. Doing so, he claimed, also would give the institution the more stable governance that he thought it needed. As it was, each year a new group of people was appointed to the council committee governing Grady. With some stability of membership, the board might prove more predictable in its leadership.

The Lesser Great Grady Fire

On June 20, 1930, two x-ray film cans exploded in Black Grady.[69] Fortunately, the hospital avoided a major catastrophe. While the fire was contained in one room, gas fumes and smoke filled the unit. Although the gas generated by burning x-ray film was similar to the phosgene gas used in World War I, no patients suffered ill effects. Several firemen, Grady staff, and newspaper photographers, however, did experience smoke inhalation. James Jones, a hospital orderly, heroically saved 20 patients. R. H. Cleveland, who did not work at Grady, carried another 15 patients out through windows. Officials estimated the damage amounted to $20,000. Rats chewing through the insulation around electric wiring caused the fire.[70] (A similar fire in May 1929 inside a hospital in Cleveland, Ohio, led to the deaths of 125 patients and staff.)

Two days after Grady's near tragedy, 59 staff physicians signed a petition to Mayor I. N. Ragsdale and the City Council requesting $125,000 to turn Black Grady into a more modern, fireproof hospital.[71] Joining in the chorus for reform, Superintendent Johnston spoke out again about the urgent need for the city to erect a better and larger structure for Grady. While that seemed unlikely to happen any time soon, Emory physicians at Black Grady and many other citizens pressed for improvements to the facility.

Control of Medical Care for Black and White

Shortly after the fire in Black Grady, Alderman G. Everett Millican, chairman of the Hospital and Charities Committee, recommended that Emory University operate White Grady in the same manner it ran Black Grady. Millican was not the first to offer the proposal. Three years earlier, toward the close of "the Doctor's War," a member of the hospital staff, Dr. Elmore C. Thrash, had publicly called for Emory to take over the entire institution.[72]

Millican's proposal in 1930 received support from an unlikely source. Dr. R. H. Fike alleged that patients in Black Grady received better care then those in White Grady. He based his claim on the single fact that Emory was responsible for Black Grady. The apparent freedom from politics in staff selections seemed to be the most important outcome of the arrangement Grady and Emory had worked out several years earlier. Dr. Fike claimed that political influence in making medical appointments had, in large measure, led to a relative neglect of Grady's white patients.[73] As might be expected, Dr. Fike's accusation outraged the medical staff supervising the white wards. Dr. Frank Eskridge, formerly the chairman of Grady's executive committee and then the Chief of OB-GYN, was especially upset at Dr. Fike's charge.[74]

While some sought to turn the hospital over to Emory in full, others took an opposite approach. Dr. L. Sage Hardin, an OB-GYN who had been an intern at Grady in the 1890s, believed Grady's status as a public institution meant it "should never be permitted to be controlled by any commercialized institution, or sect." Presenting what looked on the surface like a remarkably progressive proposal, Dr. Hardin offered a conservative solution to the governance of Grady. Following the logic of racial segregation and white paternalism to its conclusion, he proposed that African American physicians be in charge of Black Grady, "under the supervision of the white senior staff." In a letter to the editor of the *Constitution*, Dr. Hardin expressed confidence that "the negro doctor is competent." Yet, Dr. Hardin also recognized that physicians needed experience treating hospital patients in order to become more effective in their profession. He understood that excluding black physicians from practicing at Grady meant that they "had no clinical advantages as has been given the white physicians."[75]

A few months earlier the Atlanta Urban League had put the matter more plainly: "the average negro physician of Atlanta is less competent than the white to diagnose and treat many of the peculiar pathological conditions that they meet from day to day, because [t]hey are denied the opportunity of following their patients into the Gray clinic or the negro division of Grady hospital."[76] African American physicians had been lobbying for permission to see patients at Grady since 1910. Taking up the cause with a public letter in 1919, the National Association for the Advancement of Colored People (NAACP) noted the negative impact that blocking black physicians from Grady had on both physicians and patients. Unlike the NAACP, Dr. Hardin believed something else was at stake.

Dr. Hardin opposed having the city's taxpayers subsidize what he considered a "commercialized institution"—the Emory University School of Medicine. Reflecting the medical profession's longstanding opposition to (and fear of) the commercialization of medicine, Dr. Hardin urged divorcing Grady "entirely from outside influences." The way to do this, he suggested, was to return Grady to a board of outside trustees as it had at its founding. By separating Grady from Emory, medical treatment of patients would move from students to practicing physicians. That would give young physicians throughout the city valuable additional medical training. It would also be in the spirit of a resolution Grady's trustees passed in March 1914. In a bid to gain support from the city's physicians for a bond issue, the hospital's trustees pledged that as soon as facilities were available, any white physician in Atlanta would be able to send his patients to Grady and treat them there.

If that pledge were finally fulfilled, patients would be seen by licensed physicians rather than the medical students who, Dr. Hardin charged, "have no mature knowledge." Removing Emory from Grady would return the hospital to the city and its physicians. Dr. Hardin's proposal that Grady "should be open to the vast number of physicians, both colored and white, that they may better serve the community and the sick" would not carry the day, but it suggests that the continuing conflicts over politics, race, and professional control remained central for Grady.[77]

Other residents of Atlanta also opposed giving Emory control of medical care in Grady's white wards. For example, the Reverend Dr. Len Broughton, M.D., pastor of the Baptist Tabernacle (one of the largest churches in the Southern Baptist Convention) and founder of Georgia Baptist Hospital, strongly opposed allowing Emory to supervise all medical care at Grady.* While the Reverend Dr. Broughton publicly supported the passage of a $5 million dollar bond issue to finance a new structure for Grady, he firmly opposed giving Emory control over medical care at White Grady.[78]

It is possible the Reverend Dr. Broughton believed Emory's involvement in White Grady would lead patients to leave Georgia Baptist Hospital. That hospital already was a significant money-loser for its owner, The Georgia Baptist Convention. The loss of patients to a competitor could only make it weaker. While Southern Baptists in the state firmly supported Georgia Baptist Hospital and its mission, the hospital's leaders and supporters remained cautious. They knew some influential Baptists in Georgia wanted the state convention to support other projects rather than subsidize the hospital in Atlanta.[79] Therefore, the Reverend Dr. Broughton and other supporters of Georgia Baptist Hospital may have remained suspicious of anyone offering new or strengthened competition for white patients. The Reverend Dr. Broughton may also have based his objection on theological grounds.

From its start in 1845, the Southern Baptist Convention (SBC) kept out a keen eye for any possible state involvement in church affairs. The SBC continued its vigilance during the 1930s, alert to hints of tax dollars headed for sectarian religious causes. To them, a religiously grounded hospital (or school for

---

*The Reverend Broughton had received a medical degree from Kentucky School of Medicine and practiced for several years in North Carolina. After surviving typhoid fever, he entered the ministry.

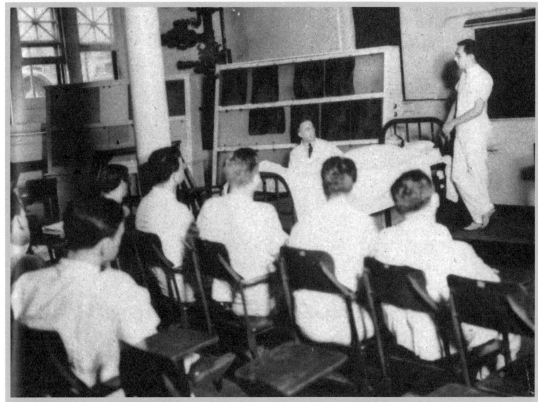
Student conference with a staff physician, patient, and fellow students (circa 1934).

that matter) by its very nature engaged in religious activity. Since Emory was founded by Southern Methodists and retained a strong sectarian identity into the 1930s, Southern Baptists would see it as a religious institution. Given Southern Baptists' traditionally strict understanding of the separation of church and state, any governmental financial connection with Methodists would start ringing Baptist alarm bells. In that context it would make sense for the Reverend Dr. Broughton to oppose turning over a public hospital's patient care to a Methodist medical school. From that perspective, transferring Grady's white wards to Emory would violate the separation of church and state. In a logic that might strike many Southern Baptists early in the twenty-first century as bizarre, the Reverend Dr. Broughton likely considered the use of public money to support Emory's work at Grady to be an unconstitutional government subsidy for Methodism. There was, however, more to Broughton's objection.

On Sunday evening, June 29, 1930, the Reverend Dr. Broughton preached his evening sermon at the Baptist Tabernacle on "The Exploitation of Atlanta's Negroes and Poor." In it he railed against placing all of Grady under the direction of Emory's medical school. The core of his objection, it turned out, hinged on the way medical research was being conducted. "Shall Grady hospital be made an experiment station with the poor blacks and whites as the victims while Atlanta's rich roll and fly in sumptuous luxury? I protest," he thundered.[80] Preaching on behalf of the poor, the Reverend Dr. Broughton blasted the city's wealthy for neglecting Grady's needs. "It is high time," he declared, "Atlanta's businessmen were heeding the hidden tears of her poor." The way things were at Grady, the city "cannot even provide the care due to a decent dog for our poor sick."[81] Indeed, the conditions at Black Grady were pitiful.

In his autobiography, Walter White, who later became the head of the NAACP, recalled the condition of Black Grady while his father was dying there in 1931. As he kept watch at night, Mr. White kept his feet off the floor; rats and cockroaches scurried incessantly across the floors of the hospital. Although nurses and orderlies cleaned constantly, Walter White believed that the building was too old for the staff to win that battle.[82] The age of the facility was not the only problem.

Six years earlier, physicians from Emory reported that rats had bitten several newborns at Black Grady. In addition, according to the hospital's medical board, "one premature child had apparently been killed by rats."[83] This horrifying incident would hardly provide favorable testimony for turning White Grady over to Emory's care. Although the physicians at Black Grady tried to have the rats eradicated, their efforts failed. It is unclear if different management could have fully solved Black Grady's serious problem with rodents. A change in leadership at White Grady, however, increasingly became a topic of conversation among physicians and politicians.

Alderman Millican's proposal in 1930 to turn White Grady over to Emory was joined with an attempt to divorce Grady from outside political interference. He believed, perhaps naively, that a transfer of control over patient care to the Emory University School of Medicine would eliminate politicians from insinuating themselves into the institution's operations. As might be expected, the president of Emory University, Harvey Cox, and Dr. Russell Oppenheimer, Dean of Emory's medical school, appreciated the proposal.

Supporting the transfer of responsibility for White Grady's medical care to Emory's school of medicine in 1930, Dean Oppenheimer reminded everyone of Emory's investment in Black Grady. In addition to donating the buildings, Emory contributed $30,000 toward the salaries of people working there. More than that, in the prior decade Emory purchased medical equipment for the hospital that the tight-fisted city government refused to fund.[84] In addition to asserting a kind of right resulting from Emory's existing association with Grady, Dean Oppenheimer saw the transfer of power to his institution as a progressive educational advancement. Grady's administration agreed that placing the white and black divisions under one group of physicians would benefit the hospital and its patients. Yet, important

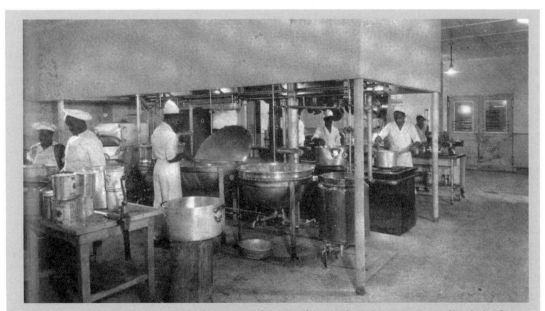

Grady Hospital kitchen (circa 1937) where more than one thousand meals were prepared each day for patients and employees.

developments at Grady would do more to change its medical service than any internal battle over which group of physicians would be in charge.

Investigating Grady

A major investigation of public corruption in Atlanta started in the fall of 1929 after accusations that the board of aldermen was paying $3,500 in bribes in order for a city building inspector to approve electrical wiring installed in the new Atlanta City Hall. The claim of a shakedown suggested blatant corruption in Atlanta. In the wake of the news, Clark Howell ran a blistering column in the *Constitution* urging the county grand jury to investigate "charges that certain influences have had to be bought in order to secure desired action on the part of council, or subsidiary branches of the city government."[85] On the same day, John A. Boykin, the county's solicitor-general (district attorney) began using the power of the grand jury to learn about corruption at city hall.[86]

At the time, Fulton County seated its grand jury for a two-month period. That meant that the panel of citizens installed at the beginning of November would be replaced by a new group of citizens at the start of January. The final report from the panel seated in November 1929 captured headlines when it was released at the start of January. The grand jury had found evidence of broad corruption. Indeed, corruption at city hall was so widespread that Solicitor-General Boykin likened it to the infamous Boss Tweed.[87] While the alderman's revelation had given the grand jury reason to investigate the city hall, several weeks later others provided Solicitor-General Boykin with allegations about Grady.

On March 20, 1930, Carl F. Hutcheson, an attorney in Atlanta, sent a lengthy letter asking the Fulton County grand jury to investigate Grady hospital.[88] Long involved in local politics, Hutcheson was someone with whom to reckon. He had a thriving legal practice, a close relationship with crucial political figures including Mayor Walter Sims, and had served on the Atlanta Board of Education. He also was associated with a politically influential organization in the city: the Ku Klux Klan.[89] Hutcheson's letter to the grand jury had credibility on arrival, and the jurors must have paid attention to Hutcheson's claim that people were using Grady "for private gain, which in the vernacular of current times is termed 'graft' and 'corruption.'" Most broadly, Hutcheson charged the hospital with discriminating against the poor in favor of the powerful and well-connected. His letter, however, was full of specific claims, especially about the illegal collection of fees. Hutcheson accused people at Grady of:

> extorting from patients illegal and excessive fees for making surgeon's reports of injured persons who carry indemnity insurance; of allowing internes to charge fees for blood transfusions, of conniving with a certain staff physician by allowing him to maintain beds in Grady where he sends his patients, allowing Atlanta to pay for their housing and hospital attention, while he charges said patients not only for his own services but for the services received by said patients in Grady hospital. Of knowing and willfully allowing internes to demand remunerations for appearing in the courts of Fulton county in behalf of plaintiffs who have damage suits for personal injuries, said plaintiffs having been carried to Grady when injured. Of referring charity patients who have gone to Steiner clinic for examination and treatment, to pay physicians, such practices smacking of suspicion and having earmarks of a 'cut' in fees between those in charge of Steiner clinic and those pay physicians not connected with said clinic.[90]

Hutcheson also accused the hospital of failing to keep records of what was done with the fees it collected.

Dr. Elmore C. Thrash, who chaired the medical committee at White Grady, labeled Hutcheson's accusations as false and malicious, and declared, "not a single charge can be substantiated."[91] The truth of that claim would be determined by the county grand jury's investigation into the hospital.

During several months of gathering testimony from hundreds of witnesses, successive panels of the Fulton County grand jury amassed substantial evidence of wrongdoing in city government. As for Grady, in October 1930 the grand jury reported that the hospital suffered from internal strife: "We regret to say that politics in the medical fraternity and politics in general, have played a large part in the management of the complex system that now composes this great hospital. The system is to blame, and no particular group can be singled out as being responsible for the lack of harmony among the various units."[92] Thus, infighting among doctors (which had continued in quieter form since the end of the "Doctors' War" three years earlier) and interference from politicians each contributed to the hospital's management woes. The problems at Grady were widespread and systemic.

The grand jury believed that creating a new board to run the hospital was the only solution. Optimistically, the grand jury expected that returning the hospital to the leadership of well-intentioned citizens would cure Grady's maladies. It reported, "we believe the only real and true way to eliminate the abuses and improve the general operation of the institution is to entirely change the political scheme of management to one based upon altruistic principles."[93] The grand jury recommended an independent board of trustees composed of five "competent, altruistic citizens" appointed by the mayor and confirmed by the council.[94] In addition, the board would include as ex officio members the mayor and the chair of the city council's Hospitals and Charities Committee. This would end the city council's direct control over Grady, leaving it only with approving mayoral appointments to the board.

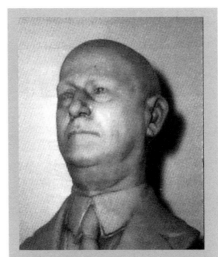

A bust of Dr. Elmore C. Thrash (1867-1931), president of the Fulton County Medical Society in 1919. He was the driving force behind the establishment of Georgia's Department of Health.

The grand jury had effectively endorsed a resolution that city councilman George Lyle had recently written. His proposal was popular in the city council and with James L. Key, the incoming mayor. (Some council members thought the city should solve all of its problems with Grady by turning the hospital over to the Emory University School of Medicine, lock, stock, and barrel.) In addition to endorsing Lyle's proposal to create a new board of trustees, the grand jury recommended that the city of Atlanta provide more money to Grady, which it expected would happen once Grady had been turned over to "capable trustees."[95]

The grand jury also urged Fulton County to increase financial support for the hospital. The grand jury suggested the county share equally in the hospital's costs, providing $300,000. The logic of the county paying up rested in the fact that the vast majority of patients treated at Grady were residents of Fulton County. The grand jury believed that the taxpayers of Fulton County could not object to bearing a higher share of the costs involved in running the hospital. Optimistically it supposed, "surely no taxpayer would begrudge funds properly

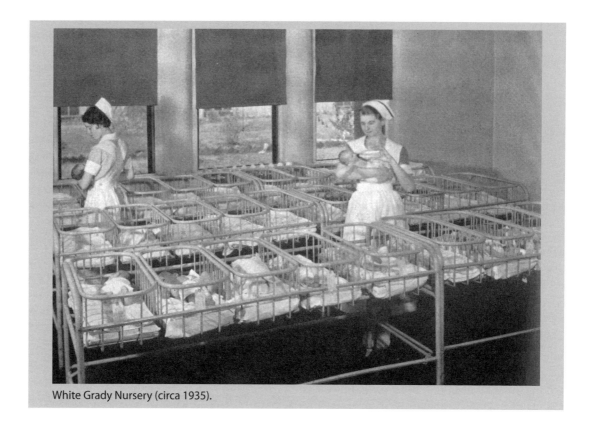
White Grady Nursery (circa 1935).

spent for the medical treatment of the poor, who are unable to get treatment elsewhere."[96]

The grand jury also recommended the hiring of a "national authority" to investigate and analyze the hospital's operations. This is among the earliest evidence of a recommendation that Grady hire outside consultants to provide advice on financing and operations. The grand jury even suggested the Rockefeller Foundation and the American Hospital Association as two possible consulting agencies. The input of the professionals, the grand jury indicated, would help the new board design an effective organizational system for the hospital.

The city's political leaders seem to have taken the grand jury's report seriously; in a few months the American Hospital Association would examine operations at Grady. The September-October sitting of the grand jury, however, did not have the last word. The corruption investigation continued for the next panel to consider.

While the November-December 1930 grand jury was impaneled, the city council committee overseeing Grady fired Dr. Julian H. Buff, head of the hospital's bronchoscopy and esophagoscopy departments, reportedly for talking to the grand jury. Dr. Buff, who had worked at Cincinnati General Hospital and had become chief of bronchoscopy and esophagoscopy for the United States government during World War I, was a distinguished expert in his field. In mid-November the city council committee, still functioning as the hospital's board of trustees, collapsed Dr. Buff's departments into the eye, ear, nose, and throat department and eliminated his job.[97] The council's shenanigans may have backfired; six weeks later the grand jury released an exceptionally critical report of the way Grady functioned.

The November-December 1930 grand jury traced the conditions at the hospital, ranging from corruption to low morale, to three causes. First, it blamed the city council's control over the hospital for favoritism in the appointment of physicians. While Emory had control over who saw patients at Black Grady, physician appointments at

White Grady could be directed by the city council. Council members took care of their physicians, friends, families, and themselves. Council members acted like they owned the place, using "the best rooms and facilities without charge." This practice, the grand jury maintained, lowered "the morale of the employees of the institution." Second, the grand jury claimed that some physicians at Grady, apparently members of the executive committee of the medical staff, had been abusing their positions, charging patients for services provided by the city. The grand jury asserted that this caused significant friction between members of the executive committee of the medical staff and other physicians in Atlanta. In addition, the grand jury found "staff doctors profiting from the conduct of the post-graduate school at Grady conducted at the expense of the city."[98]

Another major factor behind Grady's misery was "incompetent and inefficient management." Thanks to bad leadership in nearly every department, Grady suffered "unsanitary conditions, waste of supplies, excessive prices paid for drugs and foods, indifference to complaints, [the] disgraceful practice of disposing of bodies of charity patients dying in the hospital to such undertakers as are willing to pay internes and other employes [sic] for information of deaths, and lax methods of accounting for fees collected from patients in [outpatient] clinics."[99]

Like previous sittings of the grand jury, the November-December panel endorsed turning Grady over to an independent board of citizen trustees. It specifically endorsed the resolution Atlanta's city council passed on November 17, 1930, which was in essence Lyle's resolution giving a new citizen's board of trustees control over Grady. With the mayor nominating a board of five leading citizens, to be confirmed by the city council, the grand jury expected the problems with graft and corruption to dissipate. The measure to change the board of trustees alone, it expected, would largely "correct the evils of political control"— the primary aim of the grand jury's recommendations.

While it joined in the opinion of previous sittings of the grand jury, the November-December panel went further, recommending a new division of internal control of the hospital's operations. Instead of having one person be in charge of everything, the way it had been with superintendents Summerall and Johnston, the grand jury recommended dividing duties between a medical director who would be responsible for the care and treatment of patients and a business manager who would take care of administrative, operational, and financial issues. (The grand jury recommended appointing a practicing physician as medical director.) With both men reporting to the board of trustees, the grand jury expected that "the economy from efficient management of the hospital would more than cover any additional expense of such an organization."[100] The grand jury hoped a new management structure and a new board of trustees would solve Grady's problems. Yet, it did more than examine systemic issues; the November-December panel also blamed individuals for Grady's corruption and mismanagement. While it did not indict anyone, it recommended firing Grady's superintendent, Mr. Johnston, and an assistant superintendent, Mr. Lewis.

The Fulton County Medical Society endorsed the new board of trustees plan, as did both the outgoing and incoming mayors. At a meeting of the Fulton County Medical Society on November 6, 1930, Mayor-elect James L. Key declared, "no living doctor shall ever be appointed to that board if I have my way about it. Doctors generally can get along all right among themselves, but when you have a situation where one doctor begins telling other doctors what they should do, then you're headed straight for trouble and plenty of it."[101] In addition to depoliticizing medical care, Key hoped to remove Grady from the sphere of physician anxiety over their livelihood by abolishing the hospital's pay wards. Key declared he wanted "Grady hospital to be made into a strictly charitable institution and nothing else."[102]

Putting the issue of private-pay patients at the fore, Key echoed a long-standing complaint of many local physicians: Grady competed with private physicians and reduced their income. He also implied that many middle class people ineligible for charity assistance snuck into Grady for treatment. To the amusement of his audience, the mayor-elect declared, "why its gotten to be absolutely stylish to go to Grady hospital and have a baby." Key then made a pitch his audience of physicians was certain to like. "Doctors of Atlanta," he claimed, "are actually being shut out of a lot of practice they ordinarily would get. If a woman is threatened with having a baby let her make her application in advance for admission. In this way we can cut out two-thirds of Grady's obstetrical work and you doctors will get back your normal practice."[103] Playing to his audience, the mayor was both thanking supporters and solidifying their backing.

Soon after that meeting, the city council made a new citizens board of trustees responsible for Grady as of January 1931. Presenting his nominees for Grady's citizens board of trustees early in the new year, Mayor Key looked to an old hand from the city's corporate world to take charge. The mayor nominated Samuel Candler Dobbs, a highly experienced executive who had reached the pinnacle of corporate success in Atlanta, to be the chairman of the new board.

Emory and White Grady

At the same time that reformers repeatedly called for removing Grady from political control during the corruption probe of 1930, the Emory University School of Medicine continued to present itself as a potential source of physicians for White Grady. Gaining control over medical care at White Grady would let Emory keep fourth year medical students on the Grady campus instead of sending them to examine patients several miles away at the Wesley Memorial Hospital on Emory's campus in the Druid Hills neighborhood. In addition, it would reduce competition between the medical school and Wesley Memorial Hospital for funding from the university. (Dean Oppenheimer had been

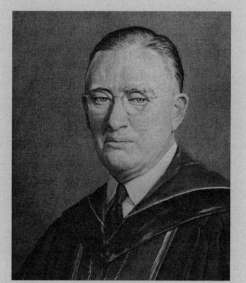

Dr. Dan C. Elkin was chair of the surgery department of the Emory University School of Medicine from 1930 to 1955.

begging the university's administration to provide greater funding to Wesley Memorial, in part because the institution was utterly inadequate for teaching medical students.) The prospects of gaining access to the patients of White Grady practically had Dean Oppenheimer salivating. In explaining his reasons for wanting control over White Grady, Dean Oppenheimer invoked racial stereotypes common among white physicians in Atlanta during the late 1920s.

Dean Oppenheimer explained in several annual reports to the president of Emory University that white patients offered important characteristics that black ones did not provide. While patients at Black Grady offered "excellent material for the students' study and instruction and for research work by members of the faculty," he believed they had innate limitations.[104] Dean Oppenheimer claimed one of the most important values in studying white patients was the chance "to study the relationship which exists between physical illness and the state of the patient's mind." According to the dean, "In the negro patient this relationship is manifested but little, if any."[105] That belief led Emory to send medical students to observe patients in a

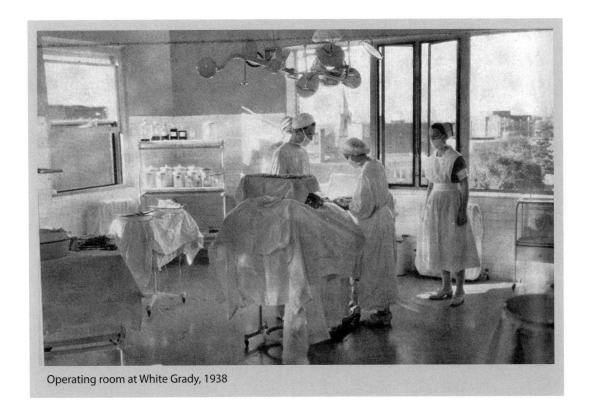

Operating room at White Grady, 1938

white hospital during their senior year. Dean Oppenheimer also believed working with white patients gave students experience in the different "manner of approach which must be used in dealing with the two races and in the differences that are found in the way in which the symptoms and signs of disease present themselves."[106]

By 1930 Dean Oppenheimer began moderating his tone about the differences between black and white patients. A report he gave that spring suggested it was not his personal or professional view that black and white patients were dramatically different. Instead, he faulted the professional accreditation agencies for insisting on the racial distinction. Dean Oppenheimer wrote that whether "accurate or not in their opinion, the Council on Medical Education feel that experience with white teaching material is essential for satisfactory student training."[107]

Significantly, at the same time Dean Oppenheimer was engaging in an experiment that was radical for Atlanta. In March 1930, at the instigation of Dr. Dan C. Elkin (a nephew of Emory's former dean), Dean Oppenheimer helped organize a teaching clinic at Black Grady for Atlanta's African American physicians.[108] This was a remarkable crossing of the educational and professional color line in the race-bound city. Only four years earlier, the physicians at Black Grady (which was run by Emory) opposed "the possibilities of holding a weekly clinic in the Grady Hospital for the colored doctors of the city."[109] At the time, Dr. Dan Elkin was chairman of the intern committee at Black Grady. His persistence led to the astonishing pioneering effort of 1930 that offered the city's black doctors an opportunity previously enjoyed only by white physicians.

For the first time, black physicians in Atlanta had a formal, sustainable opportunity to continue their medical education in the city. The teaching clinics for white physicians and membership in the Fulton County Medical Society, however, remained off-limits for black physicians. So too did actually practicing at Black Grady. African American physicians were well aware of the potential for the tax-supported Grady to "give far greater service and opportunities for the local Negro physicians."¹¹⁰ Thus, to help develop the teaching clinic that Drs. Elkin and Oppenheimer promoted, a group of black doctors created "their own organization, electing Dr. [Thomas] Slater as Chairman and Dr. [Homer E.] Nash as secretary."¹¹¹* African American physicians from throughout Georgia attended the meetings, including outstanding physicians like Dr. Relliford Stillmon Smith, a future president of the National Medical Association.¹¹²

Drs. Elkin and Oppenheimer facilitated access to Black Grady for the African American physicians; but they could not give them privileges to practice in the hospital. Distinguished black physicians like Dr. Slater and Dr. Nash were not allowed to admit patients to Grady. Any of their patients needing admission to the hospital had to be seen by a white physician first. Reflecting on the exclusion of African American physicians at Grady, Dr. Nash recalled years later, "I couldn't put anybody in Grady Hospital ... because of segregation. I couldn't even visit there as a doctor.... You lost your patient at the front door."¹¹³ Although he could come to the teaching clinics because he was a physician, when they were in session the white physicians presented the medical history, physical exam, and lab reports of the patients from Black Grady. The African American physicians, however, led the discussion of the information that the white physicians had presented. The group met bimonthly (on the second and fourth Wednesdays of each month during the academic year at 4 p.m.) "in the senior lecture room of [Black Grady]."¹¹⁴

Each of the first two meetings attracted about twenty African American physicians, with the topics split between medical and surgical areas of practice. Attendance at the clinics continued to be good through the following academic year. Dean Oppenheimer reported in April 1932 that the black physicians were "taking a larger part in the discussions of patients presented" and that he believed the black physicians appreciated the opportunity.¹¹⁵ Soon after helping to start the clinic for black physicians, Dean Oppenheimer and his colleagues from the Emory University School of Medicine began offering special lectures on clinical subjects to black graduate nurses—at the request of the nurses.

While Dean Oppenheimer and his faculty were becoming better acquainted with the city's black physicians, they also continued angling to become more involved with Grady's white patients. During 1930 and 1931, as the Fulton County grand jury uncovered shady practices at the hospital, Emory University continued selling itself as the answer to Grady's problems. After the new citizens board of trustees assumed control, Emory began serious negotiations to take control over medical care in the white wards. Recognizing the complexity of the issue, Grady's board of trustees created a liaison committee led by Mr. Arthur Harris, president of Atlanta Paper Company, to deal with Emory.¹¹⁶ Finally, in the summer of 1931 it was announced that Emory would control the white wards.¹¹⁷

Several significant provisions in the agreement with Emory would have especially great impact on Grady. First, Emory agreed to appoint sixteen of the staff physicians already serving the white unit to the Emory faculty. This meant that staff physicians would be affiliated with the medical school. Second, Dean Oppenheimer would decide which of the white wards to open to medical students. (He chose general medicine, surgery, obstetrics, and dermatology.) Therefore, Emory rather than the hospital exerted control over the relationship between patients and students. Third, Emory was "not to assume professional direction of the white hospital."¹¹⁸ This limitation, although worded vaguely, meant that the nature of Grady as

---

* These two men were among the most distinguished physicians in Atlanta. Dr. Thomas Slater (1865-1952) was a founder of the National Association of Colored Physicians, Dentists and Pharmacists, which later became the National Medical Association. He also co-founded with Dr. Henry Rutherford Butler (1860-1931) the first black owned and operated pharmacy in Atlanta. Dr. Homer E. Nash began his medical practice on Auburn Avenue in Atlanta in 1910 after graduating from Meharry Medical College and remained active into the 1970s.

a hospital would continue to be controlled by its owner, the city of Atlanta. Although the Emory University School of Medicine's responsibility for overseeing medical care in White Grady was announced in 1931, it did not become effective until the night of February 14, 1933.

A major event in Grady's history, the transition was well done and amicable. The closer ties between Grady and Emory offered important benefits to both institutions. Grady's patients continued receiving excellent care and access to top-flight physicians. The hospital's trustees and administrators believed the new arrangement greatly reduced the risk of turf wars among physicians. For its part, the Emory University School of Medicine gained the chance to give physicians, residents, and students more hands-on learning. Unfettered access to Grady became an integral and invaluable part of Emory's teaching program.

Samuel Candler Dobbs

Mayor Key made a wily choice in picking Samuel Candler Dobbs, formerly an executive with Coca-Cola, to head Grady's new board of trustees. Arriving in Atlanta in 1886 as a rural seventeen-year-old with little schooling, Samuel Candler Dobbs did two things quickly: developed a great appetite for the newly invented Coca-Cola soft drink and went to work for his uncle Asa Candler, founder of the Coca-Cola Company. Dobbs started out selling Coca-Cola to drug store fountains throughout the southeast. He rose through the company's ranks, and by 1906 he had become Coca-Cola's director of advertising. In that role Dobbs hired an outside advertising man who would place a significant stamp on the company, William D'Arcy of St. Louis (Coca-Cola was D'Arcy's second client). Together, they turned Coke's advertising in a new direction and made it central to Coca-Cola's legendary sales and marketing efforts. Dobbs became as responsible as anyone for Coca-Cola's success during the first two decades of the twentieth century. A key advisor to Asa Candler, Samuel Candler

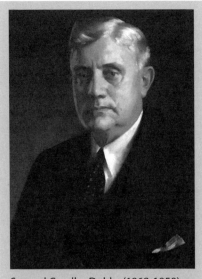

Samuel Candler Dobbs (1868-1950) Chairman of the Board of Trustees for Grady Memorial Hospital (1931-1937).

Dobbs seemed to have earned a secure place in his uncle's plans for the company.[119]

As the company prospered in the middle of the 1910s, the Methodist Asa Candler continued to examine the moral dimensions of the remarkable financial fortune Coca-Cola's success brought him.[120] By then Candler's brother had become president of Emory University and Asa Candler had become a generous benefactor of the school. Sounding like many Protestant moralists worried about the reported difficulties rich men encounter getting through the gates of heaven, Asa Candler had become convinced it was more important to make the world a better place than to amass a worldly fortune. Having struggled with the problem for some time, Asa Candler finally resolved what to do with the next phase of his life and also with his ownership of the company: divide his shares of the company's stock among his wife and children.

In what must have been a stunning blow to Samuel Candler Dobbs, Asa Candler did not include his nephew in the arrangement. Left out, Samuel Candler Dobbs would continue to own less than five percent of the company's stock. Despite close family and personal ties, and Dobbs' important contributions to the firm, his uncle did not give him additional stock. Following Candler's calculations, Dobbs did some reckoning of his own. Dobbs had felt slighted earlier when his uncle passed him over for the company's presidency. (Asa Candler gave the post to his son Howard instead.) The still nagging injury of not becoming company president combined with the insult of being left out of the stock distribution pushed Samuel Candler Dobbs to his next move.[121]

Quietly, daringly, without letting the Candler family suspect anything, Dobbs arranged to sell the Coca-Cola Company. It was especially audacious given Dobbs' small ownership of the firm's stock. The man he dealt with, the wheeler-dealer president of the Trust Company of Georgia, was a friend Dobbs had known and worked with for some years. In fact, Dobbs was a director of two companies that the Trust Company had organized, and in 1916 he joined the Trust Company's board of directors. The president of the bank, however, was someone Asa Candler despised and with whom he refused to deal. That must have made revenge seem all the sweeter to Dobbs. Stealthily he facilitated the sale of the Coca-Cola Company to a syndicate led by Ernest Woodruff. In the bargain, Dobbs became one of three members of a voting trust that effectively controlled the company. (The other two members were Ernest Woodruff and Eugene Stetson, a native Georgian turned New York banker.) Dobbs also became the new president of Coca-Cola, taking the job away from his cousin Howard, which caused significant discord between them.[122]

To mend fences with him, the triumvirate made Howard Candler chairman of the company's board of directors and also installed on Coca-Cola's board of directors someone Howard could consider a potential ally—his brother-in-law Thomas K. Glenn. The mending of the fences with his cousin would soon matter little to Samuel Candler Dobbs. Barely a year after those machinations, Samuel Candler Dobbs was no longer president of the company (although he remained on Coca-Cola's board of directors).

A decade later when Mayor Key chose Samuel Candler Dobbs to head Grady's new board of trustees, the decision depended on much more than Dobbs' experience at Coca-Cola. In addition to his background in sales, advertising, finance, and dealing with Ernest Woodruff, Dobbs also had been president of the Atlanta Chamber of Commerce. His close familiarity with the city's business leadership would prove useful in his role at Grady. Over the next six years the man with a wealth of senior level executive experience, and a full understanding of bare-knuckle business tactics, would guide Grady to a full recovery from its period of corruption and conflict—and do so in the midst of a national economic crisis. But it was not all smooth sailing for Dobbs.

A brief controversy erupted during his reappointment to the Grady board in 1934 when a few city council members tried to block Dobbs' confirmation. As it turned out, they were doing something far more radical than stopping an excellent board chairman from continuing his work. They were using the occasion (they later confessed) to abolish the citizen board of trustees. The architect

---

Minutes of the Medical Staff of Grady Hospital, October 9, 1934

"The meeting was on the whole most instructive and pleasant. After the first case was presented, however, there occurred the usual exitus of those of the staff who quietly leave the meeting in groups to attend the wrestling matches and other morbid entertainments, leaving a fairly representative group of physicians and surgeons present to continue their scientific efforts for the good of humanity.

The meeting was over at 8:45.
Respectfully submitted,
Jack C. Norris, Secty."[193]

of that failed effort, council member Joseph F. Berman, maintained that the board had accomplished its mission to "straighten out a badly disrupted organization."[123] Thanks to the new board, he argued disingenuously, it had become possible for the city council to reassert control over Grady. Berman was tipping his hand; for the next few years city council members would from time to time look for ways to return control over Grady to a city council committee. That effort shined forth again in 1937 when Samuel Candler Dobbs retired from chairing the board. He was sixty-eight years old and had successfully led a major turnaround at Grady.

Greater Grady, Again

In the mid-1930s Emory and Grady began reviving an old dream of the local medical community—turning Atlanta into a major center for medical care and research. In February 1936, in a speech to Grady's annual trustee-staff dinner, Dr. Harvey Cox, president of Emory University, articulated his vision for how Atlanta would become "the great medical center of the southeast." Those in attendance paid close attention as Cox proposed that Grady and Emory together form the core of a great medical center. Other hospitals in the city, he forecast, would join the effort. President Cox told his audience, "it would be fine if Grady hospital could be the center of a group of Atlanta hospitals grouped compactly and working in close co-operation." Perhaps, he suggested, local hospitals would move closer to Grady "so we can grow together."[124] Competing hospitals would, in his vision, turn into a federation.

President Cox asserted that concentration and cooperation were the keys to reducing costs. Among other benefits, locating all the hospitals in one part of the city would lessen the amount of time physicians spent traveling from one hospital to another. In his ideal world, visiting staffs from different hospitals could plan and work together. By purchasing goods collectively and sharing warehouses, hospitals would lower spending for supplies. In addition, physicians would enjoy better research facilities. Dr. Cox pledged Emory's support for making Atlanta the medical center for the region. A little more than a year later, as the dream of a Greater Grady seemed more plausible, internal battles at Grady threatened to undo President Cox's plans.

Infighting at the hospital, especially continued bickering between Superintendent John B. Franklin and Dr. Joseph Hines, the head of the medical board, looked like it could hurt Grady's chances of gaining the money it hoped to attract from foundations. The conflict also threatened to damage Grady's relationship with Emory. The problem was rooted in the Atlanta city council.

At its meeting on Monday, April 12, 1937, the council stripped the citizens board of its power over the hospital. In addition, it gave Superintendent Franklin complete executive and administrative authority. At the Grady board's monthly meeting two days later, Samuel Candler Dobbs announced he would not resign, despite the city council having taken away the board's power. Instead, Dobbs pledged to continue his effort to make Grady the heart of a great medical center

Uncle Jack

The following story was reported in the *Atlanta Constitution* on November 30, 1939.

"William 'Uncle Jack' Jackson, 99-year old negro who devoted a lifetime of service to Grady hospital, died there yesterday morning after a lingering illness. 'Uncle Jack' began his career as a laborer when the building site was being cleared and continued to serve in various capacities until he was retired on a pension a few years ago on account of his health. For many years he helped to take care of the horses which drew the first ambulances and when these were supplanted by automobiles he was employed as an elevator operator. He continued in that capacity until his retirement."

and graduate school. Dobbs was especially inclined to do so because the Rockefeller Foundation had shown some interest "in enlarging Grady." Although within days of its coup the council promised to restore some power to the board of trustees—the right to form policy and have final approval of hiring staff—its retreat did not go far enough to please Dobbs.

While Dobbs appreciated that the council was restoring some control to the board, he observed wryly, "You can not wipe out the tracks you make going down the hill even if you come back to the top."[125] The potential for political interference in the running of Grady continued to worry Dobbs. He warned, "there will never be any hope of obtaining help from the Rockefeller Foundation if council makes a political football of the city's charitable institution."[126] As Dobbs pointed out, and independent observers would attest, all hope of financial aid from the Rockefeller Foundation would vanish if "political chicanery or intrigue" reawakened around Grady.[127]

Noting that an official from the foundation had visited Grady recently, Dobbs said, "although we do not know what the foundation will finally do, we do know it is interested in enlarging Grady to the greatest medical center in the South, and it may mean that millions of dollars will be spent here to build this center."[128] While the foundation's rules prohibited it from donating to an individual hospital, they allowed it to grant money to universities. That made Grady's relationship with Emory its crucial conduit to the Rockefeller Foundation. (Dobbs hoped Grady would receive about eight million dollars from the Rockefeller Foundation.)

Three days after Dobbs spoke, *The New York Times* reported that the Rockefeller Foundation was negotiating to help fund a $10 million medical research center in Atlanta.[129] Emory would be asked to raise $2 million while the foundation would contribute $8 million. At the same time, the conflict between Superintendent Franklin and Dr. Hines remained on the edge of turning into a full-scale war.

There seemed to be little progress in furthering Greater Grady over the summer. On November 1, 1937, however, Emory announced it had purchased an additional five and a half acres of land near Black Grady. The land deal revived speculation that the

New Technology: EKG

When Dr. Carter Smith came from Boston to be a resident physician at Black Grady in 1929, he brought along what would become the hospital's first electrocardiogram (EKG) machine. The large apparatus was packaged in two cases. One of them held a camera and storage battery power source; the other had a string galvanometer.[191] The string, made of quartz, crossed between the poles of a magnet. A shadow of the elevation of the string, produced by a light behind the galvanometer, was projected into the camera box onto a moving roll of photographic paper. The measuring line on the paper came from the shadow of a small wheel with spokes that moved at a standard fixed rate.

The idea behind the new technology was that impulses from a normal heart would be recorded with specific shapes and sizes while in abnormal conditions the readings would show changes in the patterns. After performing the study, the camera box was taken to the X-Ray department for development. It usually took two hours to record a patient's heart.

The new machine was portable by moving the cases on a stretcher to any location in the hospital. After the machine was moved, however, technicians had to go through the time-consuming process of recalibrating the quartz string before an EKG could be taken. The introduction of the machine was a magnificent step forward for patient care at Grady Memorial Hospital. Four years later the hospital would open a heart clinic that featured a new Electro-Cardiograph donated by Jacob Elsas's heirs. After eight months, the clinic was credited with reducing the number of days heart patients spent at the hospital by thirty percent.[192]

Rockefeller Foundation would help fund the development of a medical campus near the hospital. President Cox of Emory admitted that the university bought the land just in case a major regional medical center would be formed, but he also indicated that creating the center would require a substantial increase in Emory's endowment.[130]

The possibility of a major medical research center in Atlanta was still alive in January 1939 when Emory University (then a school for men) and Agnes Scott College (a woman's college) received endowment grants from the General Education Board (a Rockefeller foundation) totaling $2,500,000. The money was to be spent on developing a university center in Atlanta, an idea initiated five years earlier by George A. Works, a professor of education in the University of Chicago. At the request of Emory University and Agnes Scott College, and with funding from the Lewis H. Beck Foundation of Atlanta, Mr. Works surveyed the state of education in the South.

Mr. Works' conclusions were simple. First, the South desperately needed strong universities. Second, Atlanta was the logical place to create the educational capital of the South. Third, with a moderate increase in financial strength, the private and public institutions of higher learning in Atlanta would be able to develop an outstanding university center. This certainly fit the bill for Emory. Dr. Cox, eager to form cooperative relationships among the schools of higher learning in the area, understood that the financial resources of private schools and public universities both needed to be enhanced. With more money in their endowments, and with a pledge to cooperate, the schools could collectively raise the region's relatively low educational standards. A university center would also involve the proposed medical center. At the announcement of the grant from the General Education Board in 1939, Thomas K. Glenn, a close associate of Ernest Woodruff and chair of Emory University's finance committee, noted that progress toward the development of the proposed medical center was continuing. He expected the medical center would become part of the university center.[131]

Continuing Medical Care and Innovation at Grady

Grady continued fostering medical innovations during the 1920s and 1930s. One of the more remarkable advances that changed medical practice in Atlanta and elsewhere in the American South took place on the night of February 12, 1923, when a resident surgeon, Dr. William Randolph Smith, carried out the first successful open heart surgery at Grady. He was able to repair damage done to a 22 year-old man who had been stabbed in the heart (literally, in the right ventricle). The wound to the heart was nearly three-quarters of an inch long. Because of Dr. Smith's success in the surgery, Grady organized members of its staff into a team that would be ready to care for similar cases.[132]

In 1931, Grady's Department of Surgery opened a surgical pathology laboratory for education and research. The hospital named Dr. John D. Martin, an Emory surgeon, as director of the lab. Surgical residents usually trained for one year on pathology of thyroid diseases, cancers, burns, and trauma. They also studied wound infections and tissue reactions to foreign bodies.

From the start, burn care was an area of particular interest to the staff in Grady's surgical pathology lab. In its early years, the hospital's attempts to treat burns centered on preventing infection and on physical therapy for the burn victim. Initially, the staff applied tannic acid to burns in the hope of creating a protective eschar (a dry scab) at the site of the wound. Grady quickly discontinued the therapy after autopsies of its deceased burn patients revealed liver necroses, possibly associated with the administration of the tannic acid. In 1935, several members of Grady's staff urged the hospital to establish a special burn unit. Unfortunately, in the difficult days of the Great Depression the funds for doing so were simply not available. Grady's dedicated burn unit would not be a reality for another 38 years. The pioneering surgical pathology laboratory at Grady continued until August 31, 1942, when a shortage of staff due to military enlistments pushed Grady to fold the lab into the hospital's general laboratory.

Despite continuing to suffer from inadequate financial resources, Grady persisted in providing superb medical care. During the Great Depression it opened a large number of clinics. By 1935, sixty-five clinics at the hospital were open at least one day per week. That year, almost 40,000 patients visited the clinics, averaging over five visits each.[133] Grady's clinics covered a wide spectrum of maladies. In addition to heart and diabetes clinics, Grady had a thyroid clinic, a post-partum clinic, and a children's venereal disease clinic.

Grady excelled in offering emergency care. The hospital's significant impact beyond metro-Atlanta was demonstrated clearly in the hours and days following a highly destructive tornado that swept through Gainesville, Georgia, in the early morning of April 6, 1936. Eight miles long and one mile wide, the tornado killed over 200 people and left approximately 1,200 injured. The scale of the disaster overwhelmed the area where the tornado hit. The small city, more than fifty miles northeast of Atlanta, was an hour away by automobile. Despite the distance, many of the most badly injured storm victims quickly were transferred to Grady. Mayor Key instructed Grady to send all possible aid to the stricken community. He even sent his personal car loaded with physicians, nurses, and supplies from Grady to help tornado victims in Gainesville.[134]

Hoping to address a major problem facing the hospital, in August 1937, Superintendent Franklin announced plans for Grady to establish the area's first blood bank.[135] The first blood bank in the United States had been established only months earlier, in March 1937, under the direction of Dr. Bernard Fantus at Cook County Hospital in Chicago. Planning for Grady's blood bank started only days after Dr. Fantus published a paper on his work in the *Journal of the American Medical Association*.[136] At the time, Grady frequently endured delays in obtaining the proper types of blood needed in emergencies. This was because patients who received blood at the hospital were responsible for finding donors who would replace a like amount. The patients could use a donor with any blood type, not just their own type, to replace the amount of blood they had received. Thanks to newly available technologies, hospitals could store greater amounts of blood. Obviously, keeping substantial quantities of all blood types made sense to Grady's administrators and physicians; thus they created the blood bank.

The story of Grady's blood bank points to the important role volunteers, women's societies, fraternal organizations, and other public groups played in the life of Grady over the years. On October 7, 1937, after the hospital finished buying and installing proper blood storage equipment, Mr. O. T. Smith, a printer for the *Atlanta Constitution*, became the blood bank's first donor. A few months earlier Mr. Smith set the type for the original newspaper story about Grady's need for a blood bank. Perhaps reading the story he helped cast in lead prompted Mr. Smith to volunteer to be the first donor. Three members of the Elks Club, L. P. Call, O. J. Stanley, and Ira Chance, also volunteered to be punctured by a needle on the blood bank's first day.[137]

One Grady physician's findings illustrate how medical breakthroughs often rely on an observant person noticing a medical development among a group of patients. During 1937, Dr. A. Park McGinty observed something about the impact of a new medication. Only a year earlier Bayer Corporation had released the first sulfa drug, sulfanilamide. Almost as soon as it became available, physicians in Europe and the United States started using sulfanilamide to treat bacterial infections like gonorrhea and urinary tract infections. Dr. McGinty observed that patients often experienced a sudden onset of fever and sore throat shortly after taking the medicine. With his curiosity about the connection quickened, Dr. McGinty looked for a cause. He diagnosed the patients who had taken the medicine as suffering from agranulocytosis (an acute, life-threatening lack of white blood cells). After looking into the problem more closely, Dr. McGinty presented a research paper, "A Review of the Complications of Sulfanilamides" to colleagues at Grady. *The Journal of the Medical Association of Georgia* subsequently published the results of his investigation.[138] Dr. McGinty won national recognition for his pioneering study of a previously unrecognized side effect of the new medicine.

In February 1939, Grady joined hospitals across the United States in investigating the effectiveness of sulfapyridine, an offspring of sulfanilamide, in fighting pneumonia. Their experimental use of the drug sought to confirm results scientists in England achieved— a reduction of up to 70% in the mortality rate for pneumonia. Grady's doctors hoped to reduce the hospital's mortality rate for pneumonia (35% in 1938) by two-thirds. Four months after they started prescribing the medicine, Grady's doctors confirmed that the hospital's mortality rate for pneumonia patients had fallen to 10%.[139] In addition to this significant impact, the drug was dramatically less expensive than the serum commonly used to treat pneumonia. The standard serum treatment cost from $50 to $90 per patient while the new drug cost about two dollars. Sulfapyridine also reduced the length

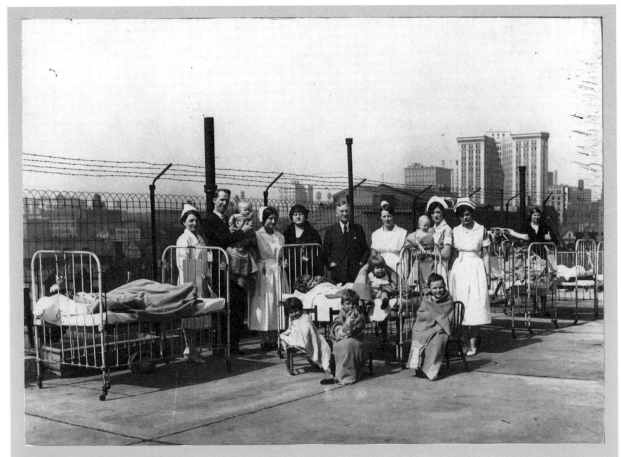

A Solarium for Children (1930)
Miss Durice Dickerson, R.N., supervisor of the children's ward at Grady and a graduate of the School of Nursing (Class of 1921), spearheaded the construction of the Solarium for the children. It was located on the roof and adjacent to the pediatric ward. The mayor urged Atlantans to mail a dollar bill to Miss Dickerson to support funding of the project.

> ### A False Alarm
>
> The Associated Press reported the following story on June 19, 1932 (published in *The Washington Post* the next day).
>
> "During a heavy downpour of rain that flooded numerous Atlanta streets last night, forcing water a foot deep into several stores, fire headquarters received an alarm from the box at Grady hospital. Five downtown fire companies fought through the pelting rain and vivid flashes of lightning to answer the call. Reaching the hospital they found a man, not later identified, who said he thought the box was used to summon taxicabs."[196]

of recovery by as much as two weeks, meaning patients spent less time in the hospital.

A milestone event quietly occurred at Grady in 1940 when a young black male, the son of a cook employed by a local white family, needed a blood transfusion. The child had a rare blood type; fortunately his mother's white employer carried the same blood type. Although the employer insisted that Grady use his blood for the transfusion, the hospital rejected his plea. It told him his blood could not be used—and the transfusion could not be done. The issue concerned race rather than the quality of his blood. Why the hospital's staff objected to mixing blood from two different races is hard to understand outside of racial prejudice. By 1940, long-standing racist assumptions about physiological differences among bloods from different races had been disproved. The transfusion could not have turned the child into a "white" since the legal definition of a "Negro" turned on a person having a small amount of "black blood." Having one great-grandparent of African descent (i.e., being 1/16 of African ancestry) qualified a person as "Negro." Yet, Grady's staff seemed to think that somehow the transfusion would mingle the races in an inappropriate way. The employer continued insisting his blood be used for the transfusion. After some time passed the hospital's staff finally relented; the black child and the white adult lay side by side in the hospital tunnel under Butler Street undergoing a person-to-person transfusion. The procedure succeeded and the young man survived.

The Great Depression

The Great Depression hit Atlanta and Grady hard. The hospital's finances reached a crisis-point in the autumn of 1930 when Mayor-elect James Key announced the city was facing a $1 million deficit for the following year. With the city trying to cut expenses and scratching for every dime, it looked to outside sources to help fund Grady Memorial Hospital. To Mayor-elect Key and other city officials it made sense to turn to Fulton County. At the time the county government paid only a fraction of Grady's $600,000 annual operating budget. Seeing a financial imbalance, Mayor-elect Key asked the county to significantly raise its contribution. He wanted it to pay one-third of Grady's operating costs. In making his request, the mayor-elect alleged that many people from Fulton County established a temporary residency in Atlanta in order to gain admission to Grady. They could do it easily because the city attorney had ruled that a person only had to live in Atlanta for one day to establish legal residency. Mr. Key promised to stop that practice once he was inaugurated.

At its meeting on April 14, 1931, the Grady board decided to ask Fulton County to appropriate $100,000 to support the hospital for the remainder of that year.[140] Shortly before the board meeting, Grady released a survey of admissions for the past five years. The data supported Mayor Key's contention that many of Grady's patients lived beyond Atlanta's city limit. Indeed, earlier estimates of non-resident use had been too low: It turned out that 23.5% of all of Grady's patients lived in areas of Fulton County outside Atlanta's city limits. In short, Fulton County's taxpayers were getting a great deal. Despite making up almost one-fourth of Grady's patients, Fulton County's taxpayers provided less than 2% of Grady's budget. The county's annual contribution of $10,000 to Grady stood in stark contrast to the hospital's cost of caring for patients from Fulton County—roughly $165,000. The county was paying for only six percent of the cost of care for patients from unincorporated areas of the county. Although non-Atlanta residents in Fulton were practically getting a free ride at Grady courtesy of Atlanta's citizens, Fulton County rejected the hospital's request that it pay for its patients on a per diem basis. The county did, however, give Grady $40,000 in 1931.[141]

In making its appeal for funding to the county government, Grady's board emphasized the hospital's desperate need for the money. Much of Grady's medical equipment was outdated because the hospital did not have the resources to buy the new devices that its physicians needed. Grady's fiscal situation was so dire that it could not even provide some basic needs. Indeed, visiting physicians often furnished their own supplies. At bottom, budget stringency prevented doctors from giving the level of care they would have liked and that their patients needed.[142]

By 1933, the average period of hospitalization at Grady dropped dramatically to just under nine days compared to an average of 13.6 days just five years earlier.[143] The shortened average length of stay in the hospital came as the number of patients more than doubled. The hospital served 41,149 patients in 1928; five years later the number had ballooned to 91,408.[144] With the onset of the Great Depression, an increasing number of people who once paid their own way turned to Grady for medical care. Although the rising demand for charity care added financial pressure, the public hospital impressively reduced expenses and improved operating efficiency. The cost per patient per day at Grady plummeted from $2.99 in 1930 to only $2.30

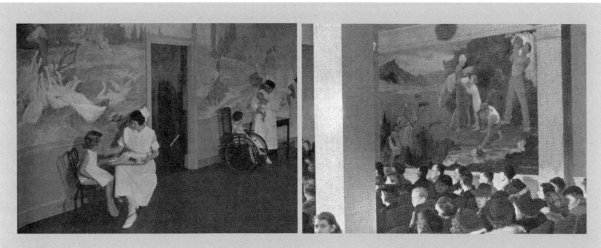

New Deal Murals Painted at Grady Memorial Hospital

In 1933 and 1934, James J. Haverty, the city's furniture tycoon and a great, informed patron of the arts, oversaw federal grants for a host of visual art projects in the southeastern United States.[194] Huddled in the state capitol, a small group of reviewers—led by the locally prominent painter Wilbur G. Kurtz—sifted through art proposals suitable for The Public Works of Art Projects. Like other New Deal art projects, this one attracted a number of proposals for the painting of murals in public buildings. One that won approval from Kurtz was the proposal from a local artist named A. Farnsworth Drew to create a mural for the newborns' area in White Grady's maternity ward. Later, in 1935, Ms. Drew developed a second mural for White Grady's children's ward. (She also crafted the mural that graced the Carnegie Library in downtown Atlanta.) Many hospitals in the United States obtained such murals during the New Deal. While some of the publicly funded murals proved controversial, notably those at Harlem Hospital in New York, Ms. Drew stuck to safe territory in her murals, illustrating children's nursery rhymes.[195] Sadly, Ms. Drew was murdered in her studio apartment in Atlanta in 1941.

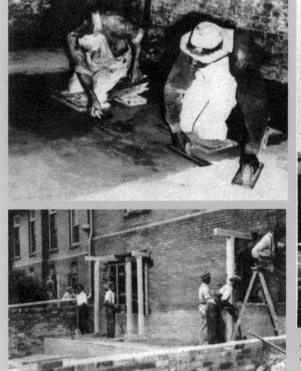
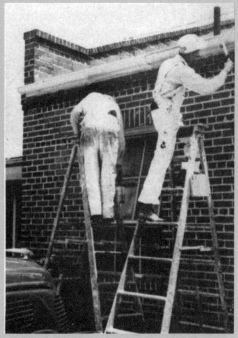

Aided by workers from the WPA, Grady built an Emergency Clinic in the basement of the old Clinic Building and remodeled the White Clinic Building in the late 1930s.

three years later.[145] It is likely that Grady's lower costs resulted from the savings found in its reformed, graft-free purchasing of food and other supplies. The falling expenditures also reflect the broader economic deflation gripping the United States.

Grady and the New Deal

Georgia's Governor, Eugene Talmadge, a Democrat and fiscal conservative, vigorously opposed President Franklin Roosevelt's New Deal. While he would not reject New Deal money, he responded to the economic crunch in Georgia by cutting state spending. Georgia's diminished budget during Governor Talmadge's reign reflected his priorities. In 1936, the fourth year of the New Deal, Georgia spent six dollars per resident for highways, but only a little more than one dollar per person to educate its citizens. Expenditure for public health programs and medical care was even smaller: three pennies per person in Georgia for the year.

In short, a gross lack of funding from the state blocked public health in Georgia from improving during the first years of the Great Depression.[146]

While Governor Talmadge opposed the New Deal, he could not block federal funds from entering Georgia to the benefit of public health projects and Grady. Indeed, when confronted with that reality, he tried to control the influx of New Deal dollars to benefit his political army. To his chagrin, officials in Washington bypassed Governor Talmadge and his cohort. Miss Gay B. Shepperson, a fine civil servant, effectively ran the New Deal in Georgia.[147] Under her leadership, federal dollars were used efficiently to improve public health.

In 1933 the Civil Works Administration (CWA) funded a program for southwest Georgia to combat typhus, employing 10,000 men to poison the rodents who hosted the lice that transmitted the disease. Late in 1933, Georgia's public health director, Dr. T. F. Abercrombie, working with the U.S. Public Health Service and CWA, developed projects to fight malaria (employing 2,995 workers) and hookworm (employing 1,453 laborers at the end of 1933). In addition, Georgia's state board of health worked with the Tennessee Valley Authority (TVA) to address health concerns in the seven counties in Georgia served by the TVA. That collaboration, employing 586 men at its launch early in 1934, built sanitary privies to control hookworm, engaged in malaria control through drainage programs, and conducted a sanitary survey of households in the area.[148] These public health programs reduced the incidence of typhoid fever, malaria, and hookworm. While the vast majority of these projects were undertaken many miles away from Grady, Atlanta's public hospital also benefited more directly in the early years of the New Deal. Indeed, the *Constitution* referred to Grady as "Atlanta's outstanding testimonial to the benefits of the national New Deal program."[149]

The CWA started $60,000 worth of improvements at Grady in mid-December of 1933. Federal funds paid for the construction and the repairs that held Grady's physical plant together. The projects included renovating the children's ward, building new sun porches, expanding the orthopedic outpatient department, and painting the building. The CWA paid for a variety of people to work at Grady, including nurses. Apparently this was too good to be true. Because of intervention by Georgia's Senator Richard Russell, the state's CWA commission cancelled the project nine days after it began, forcing Grady to fire 124 CWA workers, including 84 nurses. Senator Russell claimed that CWA workers were stealing jobs from other people. Even worse, CWA laborers were paid more than regular employees. CWA nurses at Grady earned $1 per hour (and worked five hours per day), earning twice as much as the regularly employed nurses.[150]

Over the next two and a half years Grady relied on the alphabet soup of New Deal programs for almost a half-million dollars of federal money. Grady profited from $110,000 spent on CWA projects, including improvements in building and grounds and a complete overhaul of the electrical system. The Federal Emergency Relief Administration (FERA) infused $235,000, including building additions to Black Grady and the Steiner Clinic, improvements to several wards in White Grady, remodeling of three clinics and the kitchen, and creation of a roof garden for the children's ward. The Works Progress Administration (WPA), which also administered some FERA money, contributed $87,000 during the spring of 1936. Ordinarily the WPA required matching funds be made available from local governments. Because it was owned by the city, however, Grady dealt directly with the WPA, providing the required matching funds itself rather than relying on a new grant from the financially ailing city.[151]

Spending for public health programs in Georgia increased soon after Eurith D. Rivers became Governor in 1937. In contrast to his predecessor, Governor Rivers strongly supported the New Deal. Soon after taking office, Governor Rivers pushed through the legislature a measure enabling the state of Georgia to receive more federal funding from New Deal programs. As a result, the state public health department's budget zoomed, growing by a multiple of ten in one year. It went from roughly $100,000 in 1936, the last year of Governor Talmadge's term, to one million dollars during Governor Rivers' first year in office. Although federal funding

Sending Fish to Grady

"Superintendent Steve R. Johnston, of Grady Hospital, has received a huge barrel of assorted varieties and sizes of salt-water fish from the Homosassa Fishing club, at Homosassa, Fla. The fish are being served to the patients at Grady Hospital. The Homosassa Fishing Club is composed of Atlanta men. Two of the members, H. Y. McCord and Charles T. Nunnally, are members of the Grady hospital board of trustees and they are responsible for the assortment of fish shipped to Mr. Johnston."[188]

played a big role in the jump, there is more to the story. The state legislature multiplied the public health budget six-fold in 1937, appropriating $600,000 for the department. The federal government, matching two-thirds of the state's spending, added another $400,000. With more money available, Georgia expanded the number of clinics for treating venereal diseases from 19 to 154.[152]

Like the state of Georgia, Grady benefited from increased federal funding during Governor Rivers' term. In 1937, the WPA erected a new obstetrics and gynecology clinic building at Grady. The hospital urgently needed the new facility since newborn deliveries at the hospital had risen rapidly during the Great Depression, reaching more than ten per day (nearly 4,000 per year) at the end of the 1930s.[153] The practice of having a white mother spend up to eight days in the hospital after giving birth—48 hour discharges were practically unthinkable then—makes Grady's urgent need for additional maternity beds even more understandable. (Black women stayed half as long as white women.)[154]

The WPA paid for $70,000 worth of other improvements to the hospital, including an updated Eye, Ear, Nose and Throat (EENT) clinic for black patients and a modernized pediatric clinic serving white children. The WPA also hired workers to organize the hospital's old records, creating a system out of a haphazard pile of materials. In addition, the WPA provided Grady with money to hire 150 other workers. This was not a "make-work" program. The hospital desperately needed dietitians, social workers, orderlies, and housekeepers. Because of stringent financial conditions, the hospital had been assigning its nurses to clean hallways, function as orderlies, and take on extra, non-nursing tasks.[155] With its new, federally funded employees in place, Grady's nurses enjoyed a rare reduction in their heavy workload. The added workers allowed Grady's nurses to spend significantly more time caring for patients.

In 1939, the WPA approved $81,528 to help pay for the creation of a Medical Social Service Department at Grady. (Grady's trustees contributed another $10,100 to the cause.)[156] The objective was to provide dozens of nurses who would offer a systematic follow-up for obstetrical, pediatric, diabetic, and cardiac cases treated in Grady's clinics. In addition, the social services department would teach dietetics to patients who needed help improving their nutrition. The program hired 126 people in its first year. With the WPA granting $154,844 the next year, hiring for the project increased to 223 people.[157] As the program expanded, more and more patients received badly needed follow-up care.

Throughout the Great Depression the South remained poorer and unhealthier than the rest of the nation. Widespread poverty contributed to poor health in the region. As late as 1940, per capita income in the Southeast was only slightly more than half of the national average. Even with the New Deal programs that were in place, a paucity of public health education and disease prevention played a major part in the citizenry's continued health-related problems. Separate city and county health departments contributed to the Atlanta area's comparative inefficiency in public health education. Important as it was for preventing the spread of venereal and other communicable diseases, health education had its limits.

Better public information might have helped reduce the dimensions of a malaria outbreak that struck in 1936. Publicizing information about eliminating mosquito-breeding areas, like pools of stagnant water, may have led to a reduction in the malaria-carrying insect's numbers. More than 11,000 Georgians contracted malaria that year, nearly 4,000 more than the prior year.[158] The number of malaria victims in Atlanta also rose in part because the city's sewage system was severely overloaded. Besides contributing to the outbreak, the system's problems enhanced the disease's unusual staying power. People continued contracting malaria well into the autumn. Atlanta reported two hundred cases of the disease during October and November of 1936, a remarkably high number for that time of year.

In addition to hosting a large number of malaria cases, Atlanta ranked among the top ten cities in the United States for outbreaks of diphtheria and typhoid. Together with the rest of Georgia, the city also suffered high rates of venereal disease.

Government interventions could have helped reduce the spread of several diseases plaguing the area. For example, the state of Georgia did not mandate immunizing school-age children for preventable diseases such as smallpox and diphtheria. Similarly, Georgia did not require premarital examinations. (In this era, many states required premarital blood tests to screen future spouses for syphilis.) The apparent apathy among many leaders in state and local government makes Grady's success in improving the public's health even more noteworthy.

Grady Superintendents Between the World Wars

Dr. Rudolph Bartholomew

Grady named Dr. Rudolph A. Bartholomew, a 32-year-old obstetrician on Emory's faculty, acting superintendent after Dr. W. B. Summerall resigned in 1918. At the time of his appointment Dr. Bartholomew already had impressed many of his colleagues with his initiative. With only one year of obstetrics practice under his belt, Dr. Bartholomew organized Grady's first prenatal clinic for indigent patients. His pioneering clinic set a high standard for future work in pediatric care at Grady. Dr. Bartholomew's tenure as acting superintendent was brief; his influence on Grady, however, lingered for decades. He played a vital role in training three generations of obstetricians who served Georgia and the southeast. Dr. Bartholomew's outstanding medical career brought him many local, state, and national honors. He resigned from the Emory medical faculty in 1955 but continued to be active in medicine, serving as chairman of Obstetrics

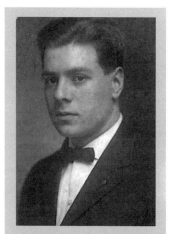

Dr. Rudolph Bartholomew (1886-1969)

and Gynecology at Georgia Baptist Hospital. In November 1966, nearly a half-century after Dr. Bartholomew joined the hospital's staff, Grady named the operating room in the obstetrical unit in his honor.

Mr. Steve Johnston

After the brief term of another chief, Lawrence Everhart,[159] Grady appointed Steve Johnston the hospital's new superintendent at the end of January 1919. Mr. Johnston was a successful business leader in Atlanta and one of the city's best-known citizens. At the time of his appointment, he served as alderman from Atlanta's fourth ward and as Mayor Pro Tem. He also served as chairman of two committees on the city council that had a major impact on Grady—the Hospital and Charities Committee and the Finance Committee. In addition, he was a founder and major benefactor of Battle Hill Sanitarium, a facility for treating tuberculosis patients. Long before becoming the hospital's superintendent, Johnston frequently appeared before the Fulton County Board of Commissioners to urge its increased financial support for Grady and Battle Hill. He resigned from all political offices after his appointment as Grady's superintendent.

Within two months of taking his new job, Johnston reported that the hospital was in chaos; he observed little discipline in the institution. For example, staff and patients alike smoked tobacco in the hospital's halls and wards. The situation prompted Johnston to institute important changes. First, he required the medical staff to visit each patient at least once per day. Second, he insisted the house staff and ambulance surgeons wear white uniforms. The quest for visual discipline went beyond clothing. Whether wanting to rid Grady of the smell of cigarette smoke or simply hoping to brighten up the place, Johnston also had the entire hospital cleaned and painted.[160]

Even with those simple reforms in place, Johnston remained dissatisfied with the way Grady operated. Looking for ideas, Johnston took a two-week leave of absence in order to visit two of Grady's peer institutions, Cook County Hospital in Chicago and Cincinnati General Hospital. Both had excellent reputations for the medical care given to patients. Like Grady, these prestigious (and publicly-owned) hospitals primarily cared for the indigent.

What Johnston found on his travels put Grady and Atlanta to shame. Atlanta city government allocated one-fifth as much money to its public hospital—$190,000 to Grady annually in 1919—as Cincinnati or Chicago. While serving half as many patients per day as Cincinnati General, Grady still received much less financial support on a per patient, per day basis, getting only two-fifths of the funding Cincinnati General enjoyed. To make matters worse, the city of Atlanta put all the money Grady collected from private pay patients into the city's general fund. By continuing to place Grady's revenue in the city's coffers rather than the hospital's treasury, Atlanta's government undercut an original purpose for Grady serving private pay patients. Instead of subsidizing charity care, private-pay patients were paying for such items as the paving of city streets. Looking for a way to strengthen Grady's finances, Johnston proposed blocking the admission of private-pay patients. Following Johnston's recommendation, Grady's board adopted that new policy at the start of October 1919.[161] It was later reversed.

On June 30, 1931, during a turbulent period in Grady's history, Superintendent Steve Johnston retired after leading the hospital for more than 12 years. During his tenure, Johnston oversaw the passage of several bond issues that provided Grady with money needed to expand facilities. He had also held the hospital together during "the Doctor's War."

Mr. John Franklin, Hospital Administrator

John Franklin became Grady's new superintendent on July 1, 1931.[162] Born in Mississippi in 1890, Franklin was a bookkeeper and schoolteacher early in his career. He entered the field of hospital administration serving as superintendent of Baylor University Hospital in Dallas, Texas, until 1925. During his time there, Franklin was First Vice President of the American Hospital Association for one year. He left Baylor to become superintendent of Hermann Hospital in Houston, Texas. The following year he accepted the same position at Georgia Baptist Hospital, a post he held for five years. Active in professional organizations, Franklin helped create the Georgia Hospital Association shortly after arriving in Atlanta. The year after Mr. Franklin became Grady's chief administrator, the hospital's board of trustees hired Dr. Joseph Hines, a practicing internist in Atlanta, as Grady's first medical director. At the same time, Dr. Hines also was appointed Assistant Superintendent. Thus, in theory at least, Dr. Hines reported to Mr. Franklin.

For the next six years Mr. Franklin repeatedly clashed with Dr. Hines over the hospital's administration. From Franklin's perspective, the division of authority between himself and the hospital's medical director did not work. On December 31, 1937, John Franklin announced his plan to resign effective March 31, 1938. Mayor William B. Hartsfield and the Fulton County Medical Society urged Franklin to stay, but he chose to leave, becoming director of John D.

Archbold Memorial Hospital in Thomasville, Georgia.¹⁶³

The Grady board of trustees would fire Dr. Joseph Hines effective March 1, 1938, and then eliminate the position of medical director in hopes of lessening friction among the medical staff. The board also named Dr. J. Moss Beeler as Grady's new superintendent.

Dr. J. Moss Beeler

Dr. Beeler was born in Clinton, Kentucky. He attended Clinton College and in 1918 graduated from the University of Louisville Medical College. He then worked for two years as an assistant physician at Connecticut's Middleton State Hospital. In 1920, he became director of the Department of Mental Hygiene in the South Carolina State Hospital in Columbia. Five years later he took charge of Spartanburg General Hospital. Seeing a close link between health and social problems, during his time there Dr. Beeler paid special attention to the hospital's role as a center for educating the general public.¹⁶⁴ He eventually also took on responsibility for the local county health department, holding the two positions until 1938 when he became Grady's new superintendent.¹⁶⁵ During his four years at Grady's helm he organized the hospital into various functioning administrative divisions. He also placed responsibility on the medical staff for all professional activities.

A New Chairman of the Board: Thomas K. Glenn

In early January 1938, just four days after John Franklin announced his resignation, Atlanta's city council once again abolished Grady's citizen board of trustees, returning control over the hospital to the city council's hospital's committee. Within several hours, soon after Mayor Hartsfield threatened a veto, the council rescinded its action. Rumors swirled about that the council wanted to create a new board of trustees in order to have the medical director, Dr. Hines, fired. Some council members, believing that the highly regarded Franklin

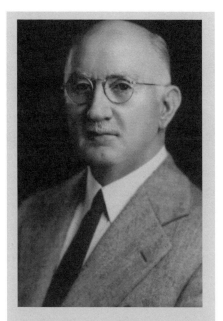

Thomas K. Glenn (1868-1946)
An outstanding businessman, banker, and philanthropist, Thomas Glenn established the framework that governed Grady hospital's second half century.

was leaving because of "political schisms" within the board of trustees, hoped that abolishing the board might help the hospital retain Franklin.¹⁶⁶ Still others believed infighting among physicians at Grady spawned the council's action. In introducing the ordinance to rescind the earlier action, however, councilman John White claimed Emory University, which was rumored to be planning a "hospital center" next to and in conjunction with Grady, preferred Grady be run by a citizen board of trustees rather than by the city council. (Rumors about the new medical facility centered on a group of financiers connected with the Trust Company of Georgia.)¹⁶⁷

The other main reason to rethink the abolition of the citizens board was a popular desire to keep politics out of the operation of Grady. Many council members feared the hospital would become a political football once more if control returned to a city council committee.

With the citizens board structure intact, Mayor Hartsfield promptly named Thomas

K. Glenn, then chairman of the board of directors of the Trust Company of Georgia, and three others—including Leon D. Wofford, vice-president of the Atlanta Federation of Trades—to the Grady board.[168] Thus, four of the six new board members were Hartsfield appointees.

A year later, in 1939, Mayor Hartsfield persuaded Thomas Glenn to become chairman of Grady's board. At the time, divisive city politics continued to bedevil the hospital. Labor unrest and disagreements between nurses and doctors also plagued Grady. To complicate matters further, the board of trustees was deeply divided. It took several months, but through a series of board meetings Glenn organized at his suburban Dunwoody home, Glenridge Hall, he managed to reunite the board.

As chairman, however, Glenn did far more than massage cranky board members into cooperating. A "hands-on" board chair, Glenn regularly looked into Grady's operations for himself. He frequently rode with Grady ambulance crews on Saturday nights to observe how effectively they and the rest of the institution worked. He also visited hospitalized patients to check on how they were doing and to solicit their suggestions for improving Grady's services. Looking back years later, Mayor William Hartsfield said, "the most fortunate appointment I ever made was naming T. K. Glenn chairman of the [Grady] board in the late 1930s."[169]

Thomas K. Glenn was born on January 21, 1868, in Vernon, Mississippi, and was the second of the family's ten children. His father, Wilbur F. Glenn, was a Methodist minister. The family moved to Georgia when Thomas was a small boy, and he was raised in the towns of Cave Spring and Marietta. Although his formal schooling ended after eighth grade, he continued educating himself for the rest of his life. By 1902, when he was thirty-four, Glenn had risen to vice-president of the Georgia Railway and Electric Company (descendent of Joel Hurt's streetcar company, run by Hurt's brother-in-law Ernest Woodruff, and forerunner of today's Georgia Power Company, the leading subsidiary of a huge electrical

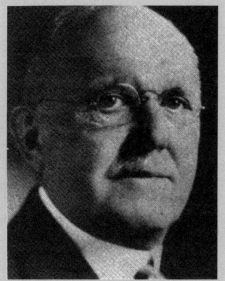

Dr. William S. Elkin (1858-1944) led three medical schools in Atlanta before becoming the first Dean of the Emory University School of Medicine.

utility, the Southern Company). Six years later Glenn became President of the Atlantic Steel Company and, in 1921, chairman of the Trust Company of Georgia. His accomplishments in business, however, may have been overshadowed by his strong contributions to Atlanta's civic welfare.

Thomas Glenn served Atlanta and its institutions in a variety of ways well before he became the chairman of Grady's board of trustees. He was actively involved in Emory University, La Grange College, Reinhardt College, Crawford Long Memorial Hospital (where his eldest son, Wadley R. Glenn, M.D. was a senior assistant to hospital founder Luther C. Fischer, M.D.), and the Scottish Rite Convalescent Hospital for Crippled Children. At the request of President Franklin D. Roosevelt, Glenn served as director of the Federal Reserve Bank of Atlanta from January 1, 1940, to January 31, 1945.

Thomas Glenn died on October 11, 1946, and is buried in Westview Cemetery; he left an enduring legacy as one of the most beloved and respected men in Atlanta's business and charitable history.

Three Important Physicians

Dr. William S. Elkin

A future giant of medical education in Atlanta was born in 1858 in the Commonwealth of Kentucky. He graduated from Centre College in 1879 and moved to Atlanta as a physician in 1882 after earning an M.D. from the University of Pennsylvania. Within two years he was appointed an anatomy professor in the Southern Medical College. In 1892, Dr. Elkin was named one of the original staff physicians of Grady Memorial Hospital. Five years later, together with Dr. Cooper, he opened the Elkin-Cooper Sanatorium. His professional stature increased when he became Dean of the Atlanta College of Physicians and Surgeons in 1905 and was heightened when he added a second role as its Dean of Pharmacy in 1910. A founder of the American College of Surgeons, he also served as president of the local medical society in 1884 and 1893. He became the dean when the Atlanta Medical College (AMC) formed in 1913. Two years later, approaching Asa Candler and others for support, he played an integral role in the transformation of the Atlanta Medical College into the Emory University School of Medicine. (He was its first dean and a professor of gynecology and clinical gynecology.) Although he resigned in

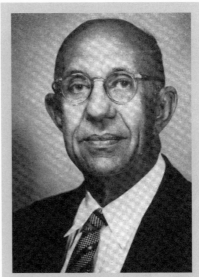

Dr. Russell Oppenheimer (1888-1971)

1925 after serving as a medical school dean for 20 years, he continued to actively advise and financially support the new school. He was frequently praised as the physician who had more effect on medical education in Atlanta than anyone else. Dr. Elkin died April 24, 1944.[170]

Dr. Russell Oppenheimer

In 1921, while practicing medicine in Detroit, Dr. Russell Oppenheimer saw an

Steiner Clinic Controversy

Steiner Clinic created controversy when it attempted to expand in 1938. More significantly, it also sought to make the institution independent of the city of Atlanta. In order to free the Steiner Clinic from city control, its board proposed to reorganize the clinic. Making the clinic a separate entity, unaffiliated with Grady, would free the clinic's board from dealing with public oversight. It assumed, perhaps naively, that separation from the city would ensure its survival and promote its prosperity.

The Fulton County Medical Society quickly opposed the proposed reorganization. It argued that the city could not legally give away the taxpayers' property. Initially the society's lawsuit designed to stop the Steiner Clinic's board from expanding failed. In 1939, a local magistrate ruled that the Steiner Clinic could proceed with its expansion plans. Later that year, the Georgia Supreme Court ruled that the city did not have the right to dispose of the property. The Steiner Clinic remained, for the time being, a part of Grady.

By city ordinance, control of the ward was transferred to the Trustees of Grady hospital In February 1941. Almost five years later, in December 1945, Grady paid the Steiner estate $15,000 for all of the contents of the Steiner building. In return, the trustees of Steiner's estate gave up all claims on $300,000 worth of real estate and equipment. Grady then made the Albert Steiner Clinic into a ward within Grady.[197]

advertisement in the *Journal of the American Medical Association* for a resident physician position at the Emory Division of Grady hospital. He contacted Dr. Lyle Robinson, a former roommate from the military, who then spoke on Dr. Oppenheimer's behalf to Emory's Dean Elkin. In August 1921, Dr. Oppenheimer became the first resident physician for Black Grady. Two years later the Emory Division promoted him to resident pathologist. Wesley Memorial Hospital (later Emory University Hospital) named him superintendent in 1924, a position he held until 1937 when he became the hospital's medical director. After Dr. Elkin retired in 1925, Dr. Oppenheimer also became Dean of the Emory University School of Medicine. Holding down both the deanship and the hospital superintendence made him the central figure in the development of Emory's medical school from the mid-1920s into the early 1940s. During his tenure he also served for a short period in 1938 as Grady's interim superintendent. Never married, he lived in the J. J. Gray Clinic building on the Grady campus until 1942 when he was persuaded to move to the Atlanta Athletic Club. He kept his office at Grady throughout his career. He was greatly responsible for the gradual change in medical education from a didactic approach to clinical teaching. Dr. Oppenheimer also played an integral part in Atlanta's development as a major medical center. After retiring as Dean of the Emory University School of Medicine, Dr. Oppenheimer moved to Jacksonville, Florida, to become director of medical education at Baptist Memorial Hospital. He died in Jacksonville at the age of 83.

Dr. James Edgar Paullin

James Edgar Paullin was born on November 3, 1881, in Fort Gaines, Georgia. He earned a B.A. from Mercer College in 1900, and, in 1905, The Johns Hopkins University School of Medicine awarded him an M.D. degree. He entered private practice in Atlanta in 1907 and two years later became a visiting professor at Grady. Dr. Paullin's private practice was thriving when he joined the

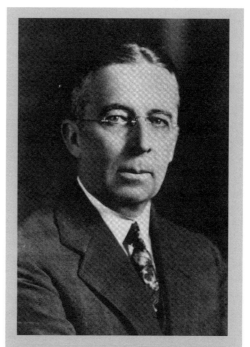

Dr. James Edgar Paullin (1881-1951) was the second president of the American Medical Association elected from Georgia.

military's medical service at the time the U.S. entered World War I.

He returned to Atlanta following his honorable discharge from the military and once again donated time to care for patients at Grady hospital, making rounds there twice each week. In addition to his other service, he also made significant contributions to educating medical students. He became the volunteer chairman of Black Grady in 1930, a position he held until 1942. Reportedly Dr. Paullin was the first physician in Atlanta to prescribe insulin for diabetes and to use the Wasserman test for detecting syphilis. During World War II he traveled throughout the Pacific Theater to study the medical care offered to civilians and soldiers. Dr. Paullin also served on the Procurement and Assignment Board, which recruited 65,000 physicians for the military during World War II. His service during the war won Dr. Paullin broad acclaim. Harry S. Truman awarded him the Presidential Medal of Merit, the highest civilian award for wartime service, in 1947. Five years earlier, in 1942, the American

Medical Association elected Dr. Paullin as its president.

Out of all of his many patients, President Franklin Roosevelt was the most famous. Dr. Paullin was in attendance when President Roosevelt died from a stroke at Warm Springs on April 12, 1945. In an attempt to save the president's life Dr. Paullin administered intra-cardiac adrenalin, but it had no effect. Dr. Paullin died in August 1951 at the age of 69.[171]

Fulton County Medical Society

The local medical society had a complicated relationship with Grady during the 1920s and 1930s. Its physicians played a major role at the hospital, provided countless hours of service to the institution, and treated its patients without charge. Many members of the society also served as clinical instructors to medical students at Grady. Their volunteer service provided an important benefit. Being elected to the hospital's visiting staff conferred prestige on physicians, giving them a seal of approval from the community they served. All this suggests physicians in the society had both a great deal of loyalty to the hospital and a vested interest in its success. Yet, by the 1930s the society's members were starting to see Grady as a competitor. During the Great Depression more and more women began giving birth at Grady instead of at home or in a private hospital. This further cut into physicians' already declining revenue. Similarly, more and more residents of Atlanta and Fulton County went to Grady's outpatient clinics for treatment instead of visiting a private physician. Again, Grady seemed to be taking bread out of the doctors' mouths. Even with economic concerns, the members of the Fulton County Medical Society remained staunch supporters of Grady Hospital and its mission. They consistently sought to make the best use of Grady.

In 1938, the Fulton County Medical Society seconded the recommendation of the Fulton County grand jury that patients with venereal disease receive their outpatient treatment at Grady instead of at the city's social diseases hospital.[172] The society's members believed patients with sexually transmitted diseases would be more likely to obtain treatment if they were advised to go to Grady. Being seen at Grady would lessen a patient's potential for public embarrassment since a patient there might be treated for almost anything, not only venereal disease. In addition, the patients would contribute to the training of medical residents and students. A year later, however, the Fulton County Medical Society changed its mind. It started urging Grady to refer patients with venereal diseases to private physicians. It claimed that visiting a private doctor would allow patients to avoid the long waits for treatment they endured at Grady. In addition, the society thought private physicians would provide superior education about sexually transmitted diseases. The medical society proposed that physicians charge a fee of only $1.00 for such visits in the hope that the low fee would help Atlanta's poor.

Public Health Reform and the Origins of the Fulton-DeKalb Hospital Authority

For six months in 1937 and 1938, Dr. Thomas Reed, an expert with the non-profit National Municipal League, conducted an exhaustive study of the Atlanta city and Fulton County health departments.[173] His highly critical report noted that the health departments operated in a difficult environment. Atlanta's infrastructure was in poor repair; its streets were dirty, garbage frequently went uncollected, and the city's equipment was old. According to Dr. Reed's report, the city's pitiful environmental health conditions led to about 1,000 needless deaths each year. To reduce that number, he recommended consolidating the city and county health departments. He rejected, however, leaving the resulting board in the hands of politicians and civic leaders alone. Among other ideas, Dr. Reed suggested placing at least six physicians on the consolidated agency's board. He also proposed big changes for Grady, an institution that continued to suffer serious maladies. Dr. Reed diagnosed Grady's facility as run-down, overcrowded, and fire-prone. He also observed inadequate living conditions for nurses and interns. Like others before him, Dr. Reed proposed a managerial solution for Grady's problems.[174]

Dr. Reed focused on the hospital's board of trustees. Despite reforms made after the city's corruption scandal, local politics (and politicians) continued to influence the hospital's operation. In the end, the city still set the budget and politicians still controlled who sat on the board. Dr. Reed believed Grady's management needed to become more fully insulated from local politics. That is why he suggested creating a new, permanent, non-political oversight body to replace Grady's board. Under his plan, Grady would still be a public hospital with public accountability; he did not envision a private group running the hospital outside the public eye. Dr. Reed hoped, however, that the proposed administrative structure would isolate the hospital's overseers from political interference.[175] Although the city did not immediately adopt his recommendations, eventually the seeds of the ideas Dr. Reed planted would germinate. As it turned out, the nurturing circumstance took a surprising form—a public bond referendum. It was an election on which Atlanta's civic leaders were pinning high hopes.

On September 4, 1940, the citizens of Atlanta voted on a $4 million bond issue, $2 million of which was earmarked for Grady. Half of the money from the bond would pay for a new hospital for whites at Grady; the other money would fund several public works projects. The Atlanta Chamber of Commerce and the city's newspapers led an all-out campaign to boost voter turnout. The Fulton County Medical Society strongly supported the measure.[176] Rich's Department store took out a full-page advertisement supporting the measure in the *Atlanta Constitution*.[177] The Atlanta Federation of Trades also lent its support to the effort.[178]

The bond campaign for Grady focused on the need to remedy the hospital's status as a firetrap and played on well-justified fears of fire in Atlanta. Burned down by Sherman, and having suffered a horrific fire in 1917, Atlanta had narrowly escaped disaster only two years before the bond referendum of 1940. On March 27, 1938, a fire started in an industrial building near Grady and quickly destroyed 25 nearby homes. As the flames threatened the Grady campus, firefighters gathered on the roof of the nurses' dormitory to blast water onto adjoining buildings in order to stop the blowing embers from igniting more buildings. The firefighters succeeded in saving the Grady complex, but the incident sounded a warning for the city.[179]

With this recent reminder of the threat that fire posed for Grady, Atlanta's civic leaders hoped the electorate would show up in the numbers needed to fund the hospital. Like a similar bond request in 1914, the proposal garnered overwhelming support from citizens who went to the polls (19,230 in favor to 1,807 against). Once again, however, the bond measure failed because of voter turnout. The proposal was left 161 votes short of the number of registered voters that it needed for passage.[180] The outcome prompted Grady's board chair, Thomas K. Glenn, to look for a way to get around the laws governing Atlanta's issuance of bonds.

Glenn's solution proved similar to Dr. Reed's proposal for de-politicizing Grady. Mr. Glenn called for changing state law in order to allow local governments to create a new kind of entity: a Metro Hospital Authority. He expected the new law would provide the City of Atlanta, DeKalb County, and Fulton County with the power to establish a hospital authority—a broad oversight body composed of local representatives. The authority would provide guidance and represent Grady's interests before the Atlanta City Council, the Fulton and DeKalb county commissions, the governor, and the legislature. Most significantly, the authority could float bond issues without a public referendum.[181] Creating the hospital authority system required a constitutional amendment and an act of the legislature. On June 3, 1941, the Georgia state legislature passed the "State Hospital Authority Bill" in order to allow such bodies to be created. The required referendum was passed a few weeks later. Governor Eugene Talmadge, having returned to office only a few months earlier, signed the measure into law. The ability to establish hospital authorities proved to be a lasting benefit for Grady and other public hospitals across the state. The Metro Hospital Authority (later the Fulton-DeKalb Hospital Authority) was established soon after the new law went into effect.

In August 1941, the newly established Metro Hospital Authority applied for $5 million from the federal government, half in the form of a grant and half as a loan. The authority planned to use the funds for a variety of projects. It proposed constructing a new White Grady (at a cost of $2,551,000), a new Battle Hill Sanitarium for tuberculosis patients ($1,250,000), and an additional nurses home for Grady ($175,000). It also would spend $150,000 for land acquisition, architect fees, and engineering costs. The rest of the money would be used to buy new equipment and furnishings.[182] The Fulton County Medical Society supported the plan but deplored its failure to address inadequate and deteriorating conditions in the hospital's black division. The society urged the hospital authority to include money for improving Black Grady.

The Japanese attack on Pearl Harbor put the hospital authority's expansion plans on hold. The attack also froze the Metro Hospital Authority's takeover of Grady from the city of Atlanta. Over the next four years the hospital's officials continued to develop their ideas, especially for improving the worn-out facilities. By the spring of 1945 it became clear that the authority planned to replace almost all of the existing physical plant. In its stead it would build a huge hospital with 1,000 beds. As World War II ended, the Metro Hospital Authority, under Mr. Glenn's direction, began final preparations for taking control of the hospital. On January 1, 1946, with the financial support of the two counties, the authority officially assumed control of Grady. The funding from county taxpayers in 1946 indicates the level of financial support required for Grady's operating budget; Fulton County paid $1,327,823 and DeKalb County spent $117,540 to support the hospital.[183]

Oglethorpe University Tries to Join Grady

The Medical College of Oglethorpe University, under Dean Frank Eskridge, welcomed its first class of 75 students in October 1941. With a shortage of physicians plaguing the South, it seemed reasonable for an ambitious university to create a medical school. Dr. Eskridge had previously served as Chief of OB-GYN at Grady and as an Associate Professor of Gynecology at Emory University. Dr. Joseph Hines, Grady's former medical director, served on Oglethorpe's faculty as Professor of Medicine. Recognizing that access to a good hospital was essential for the medical school's accreditation, the college's president, Dr. Thornwell Jacobs, asked Grady to host clinical training for Oglethorpe's medical school.

Emory University opposed the request, arguing that Oglethorpe's medical school should be refused access to Grady because it was not accredited. (This was years before the phrase "Catch-22" entered the lexicon.) Emory officials also claimed that giving the new school privileges to Grady would dilute scarce community resources. As their predecessors did when Emory sought to consolidate control over White Grady a decade earlier, university officials emphasized the school's investment of thousands of dollars in improving Grady's facilities. Supported by Drs. J. R. McCord, Eugene Stead, Russell Oppenheimer, and Mr. Preston Arkwright, Dr. James E. Paullin led the charge for Emory. The university's president, Dr. Goodrich C. White, also made his feelings known, arguing that bringing in a second medical school would sow confusion, lower the quality of care, and threaten the accreditation both of

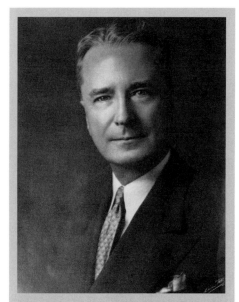

Dr. Thornwell Jacobs, a Presbyterian minister, was instrumental in starting a medical school on the Oglethorpe campus in 1941. The school first opened in 1836 in Midway, Georgia. It moved to Atlanta in 1870 but closed two years later. Through the energy of Dr. Jacobs, the Oglethorpe University reopened in Atlanta, beginning classes in the fall of 1916. Dr. Jacobs resigned as the school's president in 1943.

Emory's medical school and of Grady hospital. President White made it clear that Emory had no interest in relinquishing any control over its investment in Black Grady to another institution.[184]

In a desperate move, the Oglethorpe medical school's new dean, Herman D. Jones, appealed to Grady's trustees on racial grounds. Chicago's *Defender* newspaper reported Dean Jones had said the doctor shortage in Georgia was so dire that "veterinarians and Negro doctors" had been "delivering white babies and otherwise administering to the sick."[185] The appeal to racial fears, however, proved unsuccessful. Although Grady's trustees rejected Oglethorpe's request (by a single vote), they allowed that privileges at Grady could be granted to the students if Oglethorpe obtained the necessary accreditation. Inability to provide students clinical assignments at Grady led Oglethorpe University Medical School to close after three years.[186]

Dreams, Nightmares, and Hope

What once was the dream of a few of Henry Grady's friends and associates had become an integral part of the area's healthcare system, serving people from all walks of life. New facilities for black patients, a new cancer clinic, initiatives to treat the mentally ill, continued excellence in medical research, and a stronger affiliation with the Emory University School of Medicine all helped push Grady's growth in the years between the first and second World Wars. During that period, however, Grady's development continued to be hampered by an ongoing shortage of money. Its facilities, ceaselessly in need of patching up, fell into disrepair. Grady also suffered significant turmoil. Internal turf wars among physicians and political battles over institutional control battered the hospital as did corruption. Yet, despite these major hurdles, Grady Memorial Hospital significantly enhanced its reputation for excellence and solidified its place as an essential institution of medical care in the city. With a new governing structure for the hospital about to be implemented, supporters had every reason to hope that Grady would be freed from incessant political interference after the war.

Expansions
1942-1965

"To have a successful community you have to have well people. The function of this hospital is to keep people well or to care for them when they are ill and send them home."
—Hughes Spalding, Dedication Address, Grady Memorial Hospital, January 26, 1958

The Impact of World War II

During the first summer of American involvement in World War II, the United States Public Health Service asked Grady to train graduate nurses for the military. In order to comply with the request, Grady's nursing schools would need to accept more students; to do that the hospital needed additional housing—a nearly impossible task given Grady's tight budget. Under provisions of the Lanham Act of 1942, however, the federal government agreed to fund a new residence for Grady's nursing students. The building, designed by the architectural firm of Hentz, Adler, and Shutze, was intended to house 122 students. It took two years to complete and cost the federal government $174,763. The new building, later named Feebeck Hall in honor of Miss Annie Bess Feebeck, opened on August 5, 1944. Thus, Grady was unable to expand its nursing program until two months after the Allies' D-Day invasion of Normandy.

As part of the national mobilization for World War II, more than 200 graduates from Grady's nursing programs entered military service in 1942. Japanese soldiers captured two Grady graduates, Lieutenants Frances Nash and Mildred Dalton, at Santo Tomas in the Philippines. They were interred for three years before being released from captivity as the war was ending. Another graduate, Miss Louella White (class of 1943), lost her life on Saipan Island when she was murdered by three American sailors as she headed to a dance.[1]

Like physicians across the United States, doctors from Grady joined the military during World War II, a time when about forty percent of the nation's practicing physicians were brought into the army and the navy. As part of that call-up, the United States re-commissioned the moribund Emory Unit in September 1942. Deactivated after the First World War, the renewed Emory Unit attracted thirty-seven local physicians to its ranks. Among the doctors from Grady joining the corps, Dr. Ira Ferguson, who served as Chief of Surgery, and Dr. R. Hugh Wood, who oversaw the unit's medicine section, were two of the most prominent. After months of training at Camp Livingston, Louisiana, the Emory Unit went overseas in 1943. It staffed the 43rd General Hospital and served with distinction, first in North Africa and then, following the Normandy invasion, in southern France.

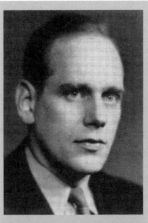

Eugene Stead, Jr., (1908-2005) was an outstanding teacher and researcher who helped make Grady Memorial Hospital a nationally recognized institution.

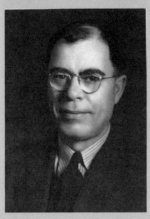

Dr. Stewart Roberts (1879-1941) was a highly respected teacher at Emory and president of the Fulton County Medical Society (1915), the Southern Medical Society (1925), and the American Heart Association (1933-34).

Medical Research at Grady Memorial Hospital

Dr. Eugene Stead, Jr.

Eugene Stead Jr., M.D., a native of Decatur, Georgia, joined the staff at Grady Memorial Hospital when he became a professor at the Emory University School of Medicine in 1942. Because of a severe shortage of offices, Grady remodeled an area in the basement of the black nurses dormitory to give him temporary work and laboratory space. It was the least they could do given Dr. Stead's status as the first full-time paid professor of medicine in Emory's history. Until he arrived, nearly every physician in the school's Department of Medicine was part-time. Dr. Stead recalled years later that when he arrived, "there was 1 full-time person in the clinical departments," an independently wealthy physician, Dr. Bert McCord.[2]

Dr. Stead earned his undergraduate degree at Emory University and then graduated from its school of medicine in 1932. During his time there Dr. Stead spent many hours at Grady. He also was a student of the famed Dr. Stewart R. Roberts, sometimes called the "Osler of the South"—a reference to Dr. William Osler, the Canadian-born physician who is known as the father of modern medicine. Dr. Roberts was the first heart specialist in Georgia, president of the American Heart Association, and had a profound influence on many students, including Eugene Stead.[3] After graduating from medical school, Dr. Stead held an internship at the Peter Bent Brigham Hospital in Boston and worked at the University of Cincinnati before engaging in medical research under the guidance of the legendary Dr. Soma Weiss at Boston City Hospital and then at the Peter Bent Brigham Hospital.[4]

In the 1940s, Dr. Stead developed a reputation as an exceptional teacher, researcher, and practitioner who enhanced the national standing of Grady and Emory, especially in cardiology. Dr. Stead's studies of shock, peripheral circulation, cardiac failure, and scleroderma (a disease in which the skin turns progressively harder and thicker) were published in many national peer-reviewed journals. Although his tenure at Grady and Emory lasted only five years (he became Chairman of Medicine at Duke University in 1947), Dr. Stead left a legacy of high standards for the quality of care, teaching, and medical research performed at Grady. He also set in motion far-reaching changes at the Emory University School of Medicine that would profoundly alter Emory University's campus, Grady Hospital, Piedmont Hospital (then located near Grady), and the delivery of medical care in the Atlanta area.

Dr. Stead's Associates at Grady Hospital

A remarkable group of physicians joined Dr. Stead at Grady. He lured them neither with large salaries nor by highlighting the potential excitement of medical work in Atlanta.

Indeed, he never even recruited them. They came to Grady hospital and Emory's medical school on their own. Dr. Stead recalled, "Jim Warren, Abner Golden, John Hickam, and Ed Miller were outstanding people on the Brigham house staff. They simply called and told me they were going to come to Emory the first of July and they thought it would be nice for me to know."[5]

Dr. James Warren

Dr. James Warren was at the center of the group of young and brilliant researchers who joined Dr. Stead in Atlanta. Dr. Warren graduated from Harvard University Medical School in 1939 and then served a residency at the Peter Bent Brigham Hospital before joining his friends in Atlanta. Working at Grady hospital with Drs. Arthur Merrill and Emmett Brannon, Dr. Warren focused his research on shock. At the time, the military's frontline physicians frequently needed to treat the wounded who suffered from this problem. Military doctors in the field, however, lacked a quick, effective way to treat the wounded that developed shock from the loss of blood. Through clinical research conducted at Grady, Drs. Warren, Merrill, and Brannon demonstrated that giving patients human serum albumin (a plasma protein) was an effective initial treatment for shock due to blood loss.[6]

This team also made significant contributions to the field of medicine through

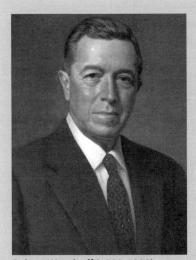

Robert Woodruff (1889-1985)

The Power of Robert Woodruff, Coca-Cola, and Philanthropy

Robert Woodruff and the Coca-Cola Company have had astonishingly great influence on nearly everything in Atlanta since the 1920s. Mr. Woodruff ran Coca-Cola, served on the Board of Directors for the General Electric Company and for the Southern Railway, and kept his hand on the Trust Company of Georgia; yet, Woodruff's leadership extended far beyond corporate boardrooms. Undoubtedly his vast wealth, close relationship with the city's leading banks and bankers, and role as a major employer in the city played a part in his being the prime mover among the city's elite. Woodruff actively served a variety of civic and cultural institutions and his was the vote that counted when those organizations made important decisions. (His also was the vote that counted for mundane matters.) Hughes Spalding, one of the city's most prominent attorneys, a member of the Coca-Cola Company's Board of Directors, and for many years a leader of Grady hospital, put it succinctly. Choosing his words carefully, Spalding told Floyd Hunter, a sociologist studying Atlanta's civic leadership, "When [Woodruff] gets an idea, you can depend on it, others will get the idea."

In a published interview with Dr. J. Willis Hurst, Dr. Eugene Stead recalled "Soma [Weiss] was the only person at Harvard who advised me to go to Emory. He thought that generous benefactors associated with the Coca-Cola Company were in the wings. ... It turned out that the reason I was able to be full time at Grady hospital was that Sam Mizell, in the development office of Emory, was able to get the money from the Coca-Cola Company. Robert Woodruff funded my department."

Mr. Woodruff's philanthropy did more than underwrite Emory medical school's Department of Medicine. His contributions to Atlanta, and specifically its medical community, have been nearly endless. Mr. Woodruff underwrote the creation of a new cancer center at Emory University in the late 1930s, would fund a new cardiac research station at Grady in the late 1950s, and do much more. Mr. Woodruff and Coca-Cola also wielded substantial power over Emory University and its School of Medicine's inner workings during the 1940s. A half-century after the fact, Dr. Stead told Dr. Hurst, "The administrative people close to the Woodruffs, who were financing the school with Coca-Cola money, thought it was time for Dean Oppenheimer to retire." They then asked Dr. Stead to become the medical school's dean, but Stead demurred until he was told, "If you want any financial support from the people who are now supporting the department, it's going to be withdrawn until you take the job." Dr. Stead accepted the appointment. [62]

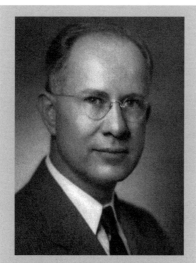

Dr. Joseph Massee (1899-1988) was an outstanding cardiologist. As President of the Fulton County Medical Society in 1945 he broke precedent by inviting black physicians to attend the society's scientific meetings.

research into the physiological causes of congestive heart failure. Taking advantage of the hospital's laboratory and the availability of technicians, Grady's doctors could study congestive heart failure when they didn't have a patient to treat for shock. They discovered that, in Dr. Stead's words, "the main difference in shock and severe congestive heart failure is that in one situation the blood vessels are empty and in the other, the blood vessels are full. A decrease in organ blood flow occurs in both conditions. The studies we made on heart failure led to the publication of many articles in which we tried to define the mechanisms involved in heart failure."[7] An article Drs. Warren and Stead published in 1944 in the *Archives of Internal Medicine* revolutionized physicians' thinking about edema in association with the heart.[8] The team also discovered the range of normal standards for cardiac output. In addition, they were able to determine the variations that different illnesses and physiological conditions caused.

In 1944, Dr. Joseph Massee, a prominent Atlanta physician, believed he had a patient with an atrial septal defect (a hole between the two upper chambers of the heart). Dr. James Warren suggested if that was true, then the patient should have an increase in oxygen saturation in the right atrium. This would happen as blood, fully oxygenated from the lungs, went into the left atrium and then was partially shunted through the defect into the right section of the heart. Dr. Heinz Weens (who in 1941 became the first radiology resident at Grady and soon became its Chairman of Radiology) and Dr. Emmett Brannon, along with Dr. Warren, performed a cardiac catheterization at Grady to verify the diagnosis. They reported their findings in the *American Journal of the Medical Sciences* in 1945.[9] Their pioneering article is among the earliest published reports of physicians using cardiac catheterization as a diagnostic tool for heart disease.

In 1946, Dr. Warren left Grady to teach at Yale University. He returned to Atlanta the next year and taught at Grady hospital and Emory for five more years before moving to Duke University in 1952. He later taught at the University of Texas Medical School before going to Ohio State University (where he had earned his bachelor's degree) to become professor and chairman of its department of medicine. He became professor emeritus in 1986. Dr. James Warren died in 1990 at the age of 74. Honored by the American Heart Association four times, his half-century of cardiovascular research and remarkable contributions to human understanding of sudden cardiac arrest (and its prevention) brought him global recognition.

Dr. Robert P. Grant

Dr. Robert Purves Grant was born in Ontario, Canada, in 1915 and graduated from Cornell University School of Medicine in 1940. After interning at the Peter Bent Brigham hospital, Dr. Grant served in the Medical Corps of the U.S. Army Air Corp during World War II. He joined Grady's Department of Medicine and Physiology in 1947. Dr. Grant established the Heart Station at Grady where he developed the concept and technique for spatial vector electrocardiography. His work helped explain why a particular pattern of electrocardiography (E.C.G.) occurred. His book *Spatial Vector Electrocardiography*, published in 1952, became a standard in its field.

A friend of Grace Towns Hamilton, who in the late 1940s would lead the efforts of the Atlanta Urban League to improve health care for Black Atlanta, Dr. Grant supported Emory's development of new teaching clinics for African American physicians. He also strongly favored Emory's involvement in creating a tax-supported teaching hospital for Black Atlanta. He would later prove instrumental in securing federal funding for training black physicians in Atlanta.[10]

In 1950, Dr. Grant took a position with the National Heart Institute. He eventually became the head of Training Grants and Fellowships for the institute, a position that led him to travel to cardiac research and teaching centers across the United States. He later became a representative in Europe of the National Institutes of Health. From his headquarters in Paris he traveled across the continent to extend collaboration between American and European scientists. He moved to Bethesda, Maryland, to become Director of the National Heart Institute in March 1966. Sadly, he suffered sudden cardiac death a few months later, in August 1966. His contributions to the field of cardiology and cardiovascular physiology are so significant that the International Society on Thrombosis and Haemostasis has named its highest award in his honor. The Robert P. Grant Medal is awarded biennially to an individual who has made an outstanding contribution to cardiology.[11]

Dr. Paul Beeson

In August 1942, Paul Beeson, M.D., joined Grady as director of its bacteriology lab. He would become one of the most influential physicians in the United States during the twentieth century. His reputation for outstanding ward rounds and clinical conferences was unsurpassed.

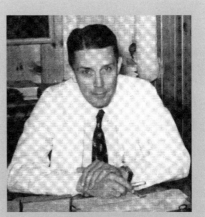

Dr. Paul Beeson (1908-2006) was one of the most remarkable physicians of the twentieth century. In 1943, Dr. Beeson became the first physician to use penicillin to treat a patient at Grady Hospital.

Born in 1908 in Livingston, Montana, Beeson grew up in Anchorage, Alaska, a town of 2,000 people where his father was the only physician. (At the same time, his father was also the physician for the Alaska Railroad being built from Seward to Fairbanks, Alaska.)[12] He attended the University of Washington and then earned an M.D. from the medical school at McGill University in Canada in 1933. After an internship at the University of Pennsylvania, Dr. Beeson spent two years as a general practitioner. A residency at the Rockefeller Institute Hospital followed by a second residency at the Peter Bent Brigham Hospital in Boston changed the course of his career. Where earlier he had hoped to enter into a general medical practice with his father and brother, the residency experience led him in a different direction. On the advice of Dr. Soma Weiss, Dr. Beeson went to Great Britain in 1940 as the Chief Physician of the Harvard Field Hospital Unit. During the two years he served in England, Dr. Beeson focused on infectious diseases including meningitis, hepatitis, and trichinosis. He found that treating meningitis early with sulfadiazine markedly decreased mortality. Returning to the United States, Dr. Beeson accepted Dr.

> **Margaret Mitchell**
> On August 11, 1949, at 8:00 p.m., Margaret Mitchell, author of the Pulitzer Prize-winning novel *Gone With the Wind*, was struck by a taxicab while crossing Peachtree Street at 13th Street. She was rushed to Grady but died five days later from her severe injuries. In her memory, Mitchell's friends raised $30,000 to be donated for improvements to Grady's emergency room. After the death of her husband, John Marsh, further money from his estate was left to the fund. The interest earned on income from this fund was designated toward purchase of equipment needed for the emergency room. Later, on November 16, 1965, the emergency clinic was officially renamed in her honor.

Stead's offer to become Assistant Professor at Emory and Director of the Bacteriology Laboratory at Grady hospital.

Soon after arriving in Atlanta, Dr. Beeson reported in the *Journal of the American Medical Association* on his observations that blood and blood plasma sometimes caused hepatitis in people who had undergone blood transfusions.[13] His research in this area of transfusion-transmitted hepatitis became national news for the medical community. Dr. Beeson also conducted research with his colleagues Drs. Brannon and Warren on bacterial endocarditis—a deadly infection of the heart's valves. Among their accomplishments, this group identified where to obtain a blood sample in the body to confirm the diagnosis of the disease. In 1943, Dr. Beeson became the first physician to use penicillin at Grady.[14] In other significant research he would show that a specific part of the body's immune system, the reticuloendothelial system (which is found in various parts of the body including the liver and spleen), removes bacteria from the blood stream. After World War II, Dr. Beeson joined a team of American physicians who traveled to Japan to help that devastated nation's medical schools reorganize and rebuild.

Dr. Beeson made a major contribution to science when he discovered a mechanism in the body that causes fever. He announced his discovery at the annual meeting of the American Society for Clinical Investigation in 1948. In an experiment using rabbits, Dr. Beeson learned that cells in the immune system secrete a certain type of molecule as part of the body's response to infection.[15] He was the earliest researcher to find this class of molecules—called cytokines—and their role in fever. More importantly, his discovery of the specific cytokine he found, now known as Interleukin-1, led to the creation of medicines used to treat hepatitis and cancer.

Dr. Beeson became the Chairman of the Department of Medicine after Dr. Stead left for Duke. During the five years that he served as chairman (1947-1952), the department continued to be dedicated both to the care of patients and to advancing the understanding of medicine. In 1951, for example, members of the department examined a broad range of medical problems. Dr. Arthur Merrill studied renal blood flow and heart failure; Dr. James Warren studied the dynamics of circulation; Dr. Phillip Body worked on adrenocortical hormones and the use of insulin; Drs. William Friedewald and David Ginder studied viruses in the production of tumors; and Dr. Belsam dedicated his time to studying the treatment of leptospiral meningitis. The following year, Dr. Merrill directed the use of an artificial kidney and offered the service to private patients in the community.[16]

In 1952, Dr. Beeson left Grady for Yale University where he served as Professor and Chairman in the Department of Medicine for thirteen years. In 1965, he became the Nuffield Professor of Clinical Medicine at Oxford University, one of the most prestigious medical positions in England. Upon returning to the United States in 1975 he became Professor of Medicine at his alma mater, the University of Washington. (He was also Distinguished Physician at the Veterans Administration in Seattle.) During his career, Dr. Beeson published an amazing 122 papers in peer-reviewed journals. He also edited two nationally recognized textbooks, including

Lucky in Funding, Happy in Research

The important clinical research that Grady's staff conducted during the 1940s on shock, blood loss, congestive heart failure, and cardiac catheterization grew out of relatively unusual circumstances. Practically the only ordinary thing about the genesis for Grady's research into these medical concerns is that the hospital needed more money for its clinical work. Even with Robert Woodruff's generous contributions, Dr. Stead believed he needed more money to run his department. Seeing no way to get what he needed from philanthropic foundations, he turned to the federal government. He was hardly alone. During World War II, America's universities and hospitals increasingly looked to the federal government to fund medical research. In the context of the war, the federal government was eager to oblige.

Looking for grant money where he could find it, Dr. Stead first wanted Grady to apply for federal grants that funded the study of venereal disease. That route made sense since a high percentage of Grady's patients were afflicted with the problem. By the 1940s, new methods to treat venereal disease had significantly reduced both the time and money needed for treatment. Patients and hospital administrators alike appreciated one of the new treatments' biggest highlights: a shorter stay in the hospital for patients. While Grady looked like a fine setting in which to study sexually transmitted diseases, the hospital's team of researchers faced a major hurdle: they knew relatively little about the subject. Their expertise lay elsewhere. Dr. James Warren raised this obvious issue, telling Dr. Stead, "[w]e certainly have plenty of venereal disease [among our patients] and the money is easy to get. But … maybe it would be more honest if we tried to get money for something we know something about."

At about the same time, Drs. Stead and Warren found out the United States military was eager to finance researchers examining shock and blood loss. Drs. Stead and Warren jumped at the opportunity to get funding for research in an area in which they had a background. According to Dr. Paul Beeson, James Warren went to visit Dr. André F. Cournand and Dr. Dickinson W. Richards, Jr., at Bellevue Hospital in New York to see how these pioneering investigators used a cardiac catheter to study shock.[63] (Dr. Cournand and Dr. Richards shared the Nobel Prize in Physiology or Medicine for 1956 with Dr. Werner Forssmann who, in 1929, performed the first cardiac catherization on a human.) Drs. Stead and Warren then submitted a grant proposal; it was the first time that they applied for a grant. As a crucial part of their application, the two physicians did their best to formulate a reasonably accurate budget for the proposed lab.

Luck rather than administrative acumen played a role in their getting enough money to develop a cardiac catheterization lab at Grady. As Dr. Stead later explained, "The grant was accepted, and when we looked at the money we found we had 10 times the amount of money we had applied for. My secretary had put the decimal point in the wrong place! It turned out that we could never have run the program on the amount of money we asked for. It took just about 10 times what we had asked for to do the work."[64] With the money in hand, they set up their laboratory at Grady Memorial Hospital, the fourth cardiac catheter laboratory in the world. According to Emory University records, the National Research Council supported the research with $44,500 for the year.[65] The articles the scholars published in medical journals meticulously noted (per their contract) the groups who funded their research.

With the lab in place they began studying shock in addition to "blood flow to the kidneys and to the brain as the result of severe hemorrhage." Grady had a very busy emergency room, especially on weekend nights. Stead recalled that he and Dr. Warren spent their weekends at the hospital, even sleeping there. With their laboratory conveniently located about fifty feet from the emergency room, and with technicians available on call, the researchers were in a good position to care for patients and, at the same time, make observations related to their medical research. Stead remembered that Grady's "population of patients were very fond of ice picks. They were used to stab the heart." While many patients had been assaulted with an ice pick, the majority of cases on which Dr. Stead and his colleagues reported involved knife wounds. The emergency room at Grady was so busy on weekend nights that some people in the community watched the scene unfold as a form of entertainment. For those bored on a Saturday night, and unwilling or unable to spend money to watch a movie, the reality show at the emergency entrance to Grady offered a parade of ambulances, cabs, and cars bringing in the wounded. Watching physicians care for the patients, however, remained out of sight.

As Dr. Stead recalled, "If the stab wound was in the ventricle, it usually just closed up, but if the stab wound was in the atrium and made a little tear in it, the patient could develop cardiac tamponade. The stabbed person would often make it to the hospital, so we studied cardiac tamponade."[66] In other words, they treated and studied the conditions that the patients developed as a result of injury and blood loss. According to Dr. Beeson, 1944 was the critical turning point for treating wounds to the heart at Grady. The research conducted at the cardiac catheter lab helped physicians understand that many patients would do well with more conservative treatment, an insight that led to fewer operations on emergency victims.

Harrison's Principles of Internal Medicine. Those who knew and worked with Dr. Paul Beeson will always recognize him as the ideal physician.[17]

Emory's Empire

Within a few years of gaining control over White Grady in 1933, Emory University officials began considering the medical school's long-term relationship with Grady in the context of the university's overall development. As early as 1937, the university's leaders began to consider putting "the major future developments of the [medical] school around the University Hospital on the campus" in the Druid Hills neighborhood several miles east of Grady.[18] The dean of the medical school, Dr. Russell Oppenheimer, resisted the idea. He preferred building future medical school facilities near Grady. If, however, Emory chose to move the bulk of the medical school to the university campus, he recommended that Emory retain a presence at Grady for undergraduate medical teaching and "our future program of graduate education."[19]

Two years later, in 1939, a planning committee on the future of the medical school sent a major report to the university's president. It allied itself with Dean Oppenheimer's viewpoint. The planning group recommended moving the medical school's basic science departments off of the main Emory campus and placing them close to Grady, home to the Emory University School of Medicine's clinical departments. In that way the medical school's two major research programs would be near each other.[20]

By 1941, Dean Oppenheimer understood that the planning committee had gotten it wrong—at least in the opinion of those who ran the university. Moving the science departments off campus was not what the university's leadership really wanted. The university, its board, and presumably its largest donors, apparently wanted to keep the medical school's science departments on the Druid Hills campus. More than that, as Dean Oppenheimer came to realize, the university's leaders hoped to consolidate the medical school in Druid Hills. In his annual report to the president of the university, Dean Oppenheimer wrote, "The faculty of the medical school definitely understand that it is the thought of the University Administration to fix the [medical] school on the campus…."[21] Although aware of that reality, the medical school faculty wanted to keep its teaching commitments to "other hospitals in the city." With that in mind, the dean lobbied for Emory to "maintain permanent affiliation with Grady Hospital."[22] Without Grady, Emory would lose access to the number and variety of patients it needed in order to give its medical students proper clinical training. Dean Oppenheimer firmly believed that Emory's medical and surgical teaching programs depended on Grady. At the same time that Emory was mulling over its option to continue working with Grady, the School of Medicine's effort to work with DeKalb County was in jeopardy.

For some time Emory's medical school had hoped to offer free medical care to all indigent residents of DeKalb County through Emory University Hospital (formerly known as Wesley Memorial Hospital). Emory was being more than munificent; it hoped to use the county's poor patients for "clinical material for the educational program of the medical school."[23] Because it lacked adequate facilities and staff, however, Emory could not treat all of DeKalb County's indigent at the Emory University Hospital. Given the size of its facility and the small number of paid physicians it could afford, Emory needed to make a decision: would it serve white or black indigent patients?

Since the Emory hospital on campus was for whites only, it seemed to make sense for the school to choose poor white patients. In short, there would be no "Black Emory" to serve the African American indigent of DeKalb County. Emory's inability to meet that need is one reason the DeKalb County Commission began working with Fulton County to jointly plan and erect a new Grady hospital. In the spring of 1941, with that plan far from being a reality, Dean Oppenheimer held out hope that "if the two counties are not able to complete these plans we may still be able to make acceptable arrangements with DeKalb County, either with or without including colored patients."[24] In any case, if the Emory campus were to become the center of the medical school, the Emory University Hospital would have to become much larger.

In the fall of 1941, the university created a committee to plan for the future of the hospital on Emory's campus. The new group met only twice before being replaced by an administrative committee that included the school's president, its treasurer, the dean of the medical school, the Emory hospital superintendent, and the director of university development, Robert C. Mizell—an advisor to Robert Woodruff. Shortly after it formed, Mrs. Robert W. Woodruff joined the committee. Two years later the school's president directed the medical school to create a separate planning committee to examine a broad range of concerns, including the place of the medical school in community life, how hospitals affiliated with the university fit in with the school's plans for education and service, the new departments the medical school needed, the pedagogical soundness of the medical school, the rules that would govern faculty appointments, and the school of medicine's budgetary needs. The school of medicine's new planning committee operated at the same time but separately from the Emory hospital's planning committee.[25]

After becoming dean of the medical school in 1945, Dr. Eugene Stead appointed yet another planning committee; it reported its recommendations the following year.* It hardly surprises that Dean Stead's committee came to a different conclusion from the planning committee that Dean Oppenheimer had led a few years earlier. Dr. Stead had convinced his committee that Emory's medical school should develop on the Druid Hills campus. Not only did he want to keep the basic science department on the Emory campus, he also wanted Emory to operate a private clinic and expand its own hospital. His reason for all this was simple: he wanted the school's administration to control the institution's future. He did not want Grady, or any other outside entity, to determine any part of what would happen to the Emory University School of Medicine.[26]

While Dean Stead resisted outside interference from anyone, Grady hospital was the institution at issue. Without owning Grady it would be difficult for Emory to control Grady—an institution that Dean Stead knew inside and out. Even with new management and a new board led by Thomas Glenn, the hospital seemed likely to continue to be a political football—if only because it remained publicly owned. In Dean Stead's view, to place the center of Emory's medical research and teaching at the public hospital would virtually cede control over a vital part of the Emory University School of Medicine to another entity.

Dean Stead argued that only by putting the center of medical research and teaching on the Emory campus could the medical school control its destiny and avoid political interference. Moving the center of teaching to the university campus would, however, do something else: cement Emory as the center for medical research and teaching in Atlanta. Grady and the city's other hospitals would continue to matter, but over time their power would lessen relative to that of Emory's medical school. It also meant that the long-standing dream of a Greater Grady would take shape as Emory's Empire.

If Atlanta were to develop into the major medical center for the southeast, Emory rather than Grady would be the hub. At the same time, money was becoming available for a new federal medical complex adjacent to the Emory Campus. The future headquarters for the Centers for Disease Control and Prevention (CDC) would soon be built on 15 acres of land literally up the street from the Emory University Hospital.[27]

---

* The committee's members included Drs. James Edgar Paullin, Phinizy Calhoun, Russell Oppenheimer, and Glenville Giddings.

It is probably no accident that Robert Woodruff's representatives had wanted Dean Oppenheimer to retire at about the time his planning group had recommended moving the medical school's science departments close to Grady. It is also unlikely that the politically astute Dean Stead would have pushed Emory to develop an independent medical center without a sense of Robert Woodruff's blessing.

What relationship, then, did Dean Stead envision Emory University School of Medicine would have with Grady hospital? More than once he noted, "the aims of the University and of a tax supported hospital are not always identical."[28] The medical school's desire to provide excellent patient care was part of its mission. Based on how public hospitals performed across the United States, Dean Stead believed that they were satisfied with providing only adequate care. While Grady hospital had high standards, Dean Stead worried that "political interference and budgeting considerations" could trump the desire of Grady's administrators to maintain these standards.[29] Dean Stead believed that

The Winecoff Hotel Fire

Grady hospital's ability to respond to a major disaster was put to the test on December 7, 1946, after a fire broke out at the Winecoff Hotel in downtown Atlanta. The blaze began at 3:00 in the morning and soon went out of control. (While the fire's cause remains unknown, evidence pointed to a cigarette burning on a mattress in the third floor hallway. Some investigators believed it was a case of arson.)

Built in 1913, the fifteen-story hotel with 200 rooms was supposed to be fireproof. Unfortunately, the facility had fatal flaws. The building had no exterior fire escapes and lacked a sprinkler system. The absence of fire doors allowed open stairwells to pull flames into the building's upper stories. The hotel's extensive woodwork and furnishings also fueled the fire. Tragically, because their ladders were too short, Atlanta firefighters were unable to reach the upper floors where many guests were trapped. A large number of the 280 guests were high school students attending a state YMCA Youth Congress. The devastating fire left 119 people dead. Of these, 41 died from burns, 32 from suffocation, and 26 from jumping or falling from the upper floors of the hotel. The cause of 20 other deaths was undetermined. The deadliest hotel fire in American history, it prompted the passage of new safety regulations.[67]

Nearly every victim of the Winecoff Hotel fire was taken to Grady. The hospital sent every ambulance available, each staffed with a doctor, to the scene to treat and transport victims. Hospital personnel worked nearly thirty hours straight to cope with the crisis. Grady's emergency department staff and many others—some were summoned, but many came on their own—treated the injured. They also arranged the bodies of the deceased for families to identify. The first bodies to arrive at Grady were taken to the bone clinic, an area near the emergency room. As that room filled quickly with victims, others were taken to a temporary morgue in the basement of a building across the street.

Blood donors began arriving at the hospital shortly after word of the tragedy was broadcast on the news. By 10:00 that morning, seven hours after the fire began, the hospital had more blood than was necessary to care for the victims. Two Grady interns, Dr. Bithel Wall and Dr. Joseph Hooper, were recognized for their heroic work in saving trapped hotel guests. Both doctors rushed to the roof of the Mortgage Guarantee Building from which they climbed a ladder to the hotel's upper level to rescue four guests. When acclaimed as a hero, Dr. Wall quietly demurred. He told an inquiring reporter that he was scared on the ladder and would rather have been home in Sylvester, Georgia, plowing fields with his mules.[68]

Grady's Superintendent, Frank Wilson, spent many hours comforting families and assisting them in the sad process of identifying deceased loved ones. Through the horror, Wilson noticed the heroism of Grady's workers and the remarkable response of Atlanta's citizens.[69] Grady's employees worked hard, but, Wilson noted, "Everybody helped. Salvation Army, Red Cross Nurse's Aides, Grey Ladies, the Motor Corps, volunteer technicians from other hospitals, doctor friends from all over Atlanta, and some from out-of-town."[70] Amidst the palpable horror and grief came a remarkable outpouring of kindness and generosity.

at their core the two sorts of institutions had different objectives. He also had other reservations concerning Grady.

Dean Stead hesitated "to continue development at Grady hospital" in part because of who the patients were. He doubted whether it was wise for Emory to expend its "highly skilled medical services" on the "section of our community which is socially and economically the least productive."[30] This is striking given that part of the original mission of the hospital was to restore people to economic productivity. It is difficult to know whether this concern about who was being cared for is something that Dr. Stead truly believed or whether he included these words in an official report because he thought it was something his boss wanted to hear. A university's administrative reports can be flavored by the author's ambition to get more money for his fiefdom within the school. Much in the way a job applicant will be tempted to shade his resume in an attempt to please a potential employer, university administrators may be tempted to take on a tone they believe will curry favor with their bosses. Whether it was Dean Stead's personal view or it represented a bias he believed others held, it is worth highlighting that his comments concerned social class rather than race. At the time Dean Stead wrote this report for Emory's president, Grady's patient load was almost evenly divided between white and black.

Dean Stead also worried about the financial side of Emory's relationship with Grady. He believed Emory needed to look out for its own interests first. As Dr. Stead saw it, this meant the university needed to invest in itself more than in the public hospital. As it stood, Grady generated absolutely no income for the Emory University School of Medicine—a fact that bothered the business-oriented and money-minded Stead. He believed the university should be paid handsomely for the service it provided to Grady's thousands of patients.[26] He knew, of course, that an army of volunteer doctors provided the bulk of physician services at the hospital. Even with that, however, Emory still incurred substantial costs for clinical work at Grady.

The prospect of the Fulton-DeKalb Hospital Authority dramatically expanding Grady with the erection of a 1,000-bed hospital—an idea that had been floated for several years by the time the war was ending in 1945—worried Dean Stead a great deal. He had no idea how Emory would be able to meet the challenges such a building implied. The size of the proposed structure suggested it would require far more physicians and medical staff than Emory needed to educate students, interns, and residents. If Grady built the new hospital, it was likely to ask Emory to provide more staff. To hire additional people would cost Emory more money—something continually in short supply at the school of medicine.[27]

Two recent phenomena made developing the medical school on the Emory campus plausible to Stead. The first of these was the rise of hospital insurance; the second was the growing acceptance of the group practice of medicine in the wake of the Great Depression and World War II.

With hospital insurance having become more widespread since the 1930s, hospitals with paying customers could be assured that the extensive costs of operating a hospital would be covered. "In former years," he wrote to the President of Emory University, "a school could not teach medicine satisfactorily in its own hospital because too much of the income of the school had to be directed to covering the basic cost of hospitalization. This difficulty has been removed by the rapid growth of hospital insurance. The expense of hospitalization for nearly all income groups will be covered by insurance either by voluntary payment, by industry, or by government."[33] In sum, the patient's hospital insurance would help finance the medical school's use of its own hospital.

The increasing acceptability of the group practice of medicine also helped make concentrating medical school education on campus more plausible. The group practice of medicine had drawn scowls from physicians and the public only a decade earlier. Physician experiences during World War II, however, when large numbers of physicians

Centers for Disease Control (CDC)

The CDC, a federal agency, grew out of the Office of Malaria Control in War Areas, which was organized as part of the U.S. Public Health Service in 1942 and headquartered in Atlanta. The malaria control agency's main domestic mission was to keep in check the South's substantial population of anopheline mosquitoes, the transmitter of malaria. Doing so would reduce the disease among soldiers training at bases in the South. Building on peacetime efforts by the WPA to rid the South of malaria (and using WPA workers until 1942), the malaria control agency found friends in Atlanta's business community.

Georgia Power, which ran hydroelectric plants that drew their water from man-made lakes, was an almost natural ally for the malaria control effort. Preston Arkwright, the company's president, turned over the firm's efforts to control malaria to his son-in-law, Dr. Glenville Giddings. The physician was a highly respected and influential member of Atlanta's medical community. He had served on Dr. Stead's planning committee for Emory's school of medicine and had been a strong advocate for improving public health. Dr. Giddings helped Georgia Power survey the incidence of mosquitoes and malaria in areas where the company generated hydroelectric power. Dr. Giddings also served as a medical advisor for Coca-Cola. It barely surprises, then, that Robert W. Woodruff would become a great ally of the public health service's malaria control board. According to historian Elizabeth W. Etheridge, it was Dr. Giddings who prompted Robert Woodruff's interest in bringing Emory and the CDC together.[71]

The chairman of Coca-Cola had a hunting lodge in southern Georgia located on an extensive estate he had named Ichauway Plantation.* Woodruff knew that mosquitoes and malaria bedeviled the area, and he wanted to do something about the problem. Indeed, a few years earlier Woodruff funded a research station near his plantation in Baker County that he staffed through Emory. Before long, a new, synthetic ally would transform the public health service's battle plan for fighting the malarial mosquito. The discovery in 1939 of the insecticidal properties of DDT meant that in the coming years victory over the anopheline mosquitoes would come more from spraying chemicals than draining stagnant water. Even after the arrival of DDT, however, malaria remained a problem across the South.

After World War II, the malaria control agency turned into the more broadly defined Communicable Disease Center. Under the command of the Surgeon General of the United States, it was to be headquartered in Atlanta. A general who directed much of the fight against malaria from his office in Washington, Dr. Joseph W. Mountin, took charge of the CDC when the new agency was organized in 1946. This was fair enough since, while he was working with the malaria control group during World War II, he had come up with the idea of creating a federal center that would improve public health by battling communicable diseases.

In 1947, the year after the CDC was formally organized as part of the U.S. Public Health Service, Robert Woodruff arranged for Emory to purchase 15 acres of adjacent land with the idea that the university would donate the land for the agency's future headquarters. Thus, the benefactor of Emory University became a patron saint for the new organization. In 1948 the land was officially turned over to the Surgeon General of the United States (the head of the public health service). While it held title to the land, the CDC needed funding from the U.S. Congress to begin building. The post-war ban on non-defense related funding meant that the CDC's fifteen acres would remain part of Atlanta's vaunted forest canopy well into the 1950s. Reportedly, it took a telephone call from a frustrated Robert W. Woodruff to President Eisenhower to prompt congressional funding for the CDC's new buildings. If such was the persuasive power of Robert Woodruff with the President of The United States of America, one can only surmise where he stood with administrators at Emory University.

---

*Ichauway is the Creek Indian expression for "where deer sleep."

in all specialties worked together successfully in the military, spurred the acceptance of group practice after the conflict ended. The changing attitude would help free the university to establish a clinic staffed by members of the faculty. Dean Stead envisioned Emory using its clinic for teaching. More importantly, by making a profit it would generate a significant source of income for the Emory University School of Medicine.[34]

It is hard to know where this idea originated. It appears to have started with Dean Stead, but there is some circumstantial evidence that points back to Robert W. Woodruff as the idea's incubator. Regardless of who first came up with the notion of the medical clinic funding the school of medicine instead of the other way around, the creation of a private clinic for Emory meant more construction on the Druid Hills campus. In order to concentrate medical education on campus, Emory would need to erect a clinic building. It also would gradually enlarge Emory University Hospital, turning over more of its beds to patients of staff members of the clinic.

Tellingly, Dr. Stead also indicated that concentrating "teaching facilities on campus" would require greater use of Crawford Long Hospital.[35] Deeded to Emory by its co-founder Dr. Luther Fischer in 1940, Crawford Long Hospital was located only about 1.3 miles northwest of Grady—and like Grady, it was about five miles west of Emory's Druid Hills campus. This suggests that the proposed consolidation of medical school facilities on campus was not about a spatial concentration. On the contrary, increasing use of Crawford Long would—in spatial terms—move medical school activity toward the center of Atlanta. Instead, by making more use of Crawford Long Hospital, Dean Stead would help Emory retain, indeed extend, firm control and authority over the medical school.

After Dean Stead left his post at Emory in 1947, his idea that Emory's medical school should exert full control over its own destiny, remained gospel for the university. The die determining Emory's dominance in Atlanta's medical community had been cast when Dean Stead's planning committee decided to concentrate the school's efforts at the Druid Hills campus and at Emory-controlled facilities.

Formalizing the Grady-Emory Relationship

Even after Emory decided to concentrate medical education on its own campus, it insisted that Grady would continue to "be of major importance in the teaching and research program" of the school of medicine. With this in mind, Emory tried to clarify its relationship with Grady. Since the primary issue concerned money, shortly after World War II, Grady and Emory began conducting accounting studies to determine the costs each institution should bear for the expenses incurred at Grady. Emory believed Grady should pay for "all costs of good patient care with adequate services" including the laboratory, pathology department, x-ray, pharmacy, and outpatient services.[36] The medical school, for its part, believed it should be responsible only for the costs of teaching and research. It took five years, but on September 1, 1951, the hospital authority and Emory's medical school presented a contract to formalize their relationship and, they hoped, settle what had become intense disputes over money, responsibilities, and lines of authority.

Dean R. Hugh Wood believed no contract could solve the problems between the hospital and school until Grady received adequate funding from the taxpayers. Even with Emory assuming responsibility for more of Grady's expenses, the hospital's annual operating budget remained inadequate. Grady served a rapidly growing number of people, yet the increase in its budget allocation from Fulton and DeKalb counties was barely keeping up with inflation. This led the medical school to complain that it was being "forced to supply certain services in order to maintain a minimum quality of patient care necessary for teaching."[37] Grady didn't have enough money to properly care for its patients. According to Robert Mizell, the close advisor to Robert

Woodruff and the director of development at Emory, people associated with Emory's medical school had long felt forced to spend money on things that were Grady's responsibility just to be sure patients had adequate care.

Writing in 1953, two years after the contract between Emory and Grady was signed and as Grady was about to enter into a new agreement with Fulton and DeKalb Counties, Mizell tried to assure Dean Wood that the days of Emory subsidizing Grady were over. The feeling of needing to provide what Grady lacked, Mizell indicated, had been a source of Emory's trouble with Grady. Trust was also a problem. Mizell did not believe that the "public authorities" were really short of money and he cautioned Dean Wood against being "pressured into doing what [Grady] ought to do" because, according to Mizell, "the public authorities have access to enough money to discharge their responsibilities."[38] Mizell, however, had a bigger concern than quibbles between administrators at Grady and Emory.

Mizell worried that donors would blame Emory for whatever sins Grady might commit. If donors got the impression that things were not being run properly at Grady, they might blame the school. More importantly, from Mizell's point of view, donors might begin to think Emory was being "careless in the expenditure of their funds, applying them to purposes never intended, and that the budget of the School is greater than necessary." Donors also might think Emory was paying for things that belonged in Grady's province. Writing to Dean Wood, Mizell concluded, "No donor, already a taxpayer, wants to subsidize a public agency."[39] Presumably Dean Wood understood from the note just

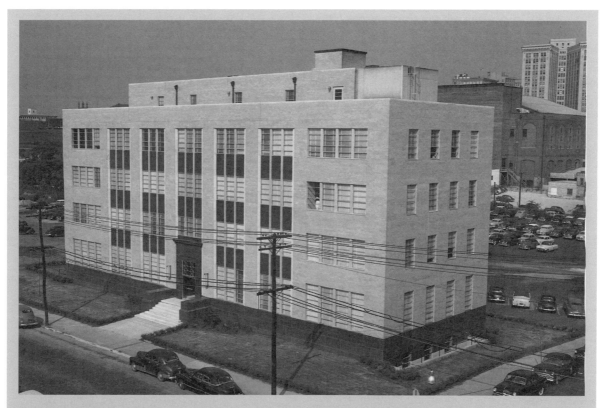

The Glenn Building at Grady Hospital
In 1949, the Wilbur Fisk Glenn Memorial Foundation made a generous gift to Grady to honor Thomas K. Glenn. The funds were used to build the Thomas K. Glenn Memorial Building, completed in 1953. Located across the street from the hospital, the facility provided offices for the medical staff and the medical school's administration, plus laboratories for the hospital's clinical faculty. The building cost $768,000 and was located on land purchased from Georgia Power at a cost of $175,000.

how Robert Woodruff felt. When the negotiations between Emory and Grady concluded, the funding issues were resolved in a way that Emory found congenial. Even having a contract in place, however, did not guarantee peace and harmony.

Dean Richardson and Medical Politics

Arthur Richardson, M.D., became Dean of the Emory University School of Medicine in 1956 when Dr. Wood decided to focus fully on his other position—director of the Emory Clinic. As word of Dr. Richardson's pending appointment leaked out, three department chairmen from Emory/Grady approached Boisfeuillet Jones, vice president of the university, asking that someone else be chosen. They claimed Dr. Richardson was unqualified because his scholarly focus was in one of the basic sciences, pharmacology, rather than patient care.[40] Soon after taking the post in September, Dr. Richardson found himself negotiating with the chairs who had resisted his appointment as dean. The discussion quickly moved from his scholarship to the substantial conflicts between Emory and Grady that began several years earlier, before Dr. Richardson became dean.

Emory physicians at Grady had been complaining that insufficient resources prevented them from properly caring for patients. Some Grady physicians became so frustrated with the way things were that they took out advertisements in the daily newspapers to publicize their dissatisfaction with Emory's handling of the problem. From the school's point of view, Emory couldn't privately fund the public hospital with money that donors intended for the university. The internal strife was related in part to the development of the Emory Clinic, a private clinic that was a partnership of physicians appointed to the medical school's clinical faculty.

Organized in 1952 and 1953, the Emory Clinic embodied what Dean Stead had envisioned for Emory's medical school. Although the group practice of medicine was becoming more acceptable within the profession, there was lingering resentment about it in the medical community. Physicians in private practice opposed the formation of the Emory Clinic because, in their view, it was the university's entrance into group medicine. In short, the university was competing directly with physicians in private practice. Indeed, some viewed the medical school as competing against its own graduates. While the university's attorneys had established a legal wall between the medical school and the Emory Clinic, the fact was that the partners in the clinic were members of Emory's medical faculty. In 1956, Dr. Eugene Ferris, the Chairman of the Department of Medicine at Emory and at Grady, laid out directives to clinical faculty working at the Emory Clinic. His action offended some of the physicians involved, but it also won the support of others.[41] (Dr. Ferris also had opposed centering medical school teaching on the Emory campus rather than at Grady.)[42]

To help resolve the issue, in November 1956 the Emory University Board of Trustees, at the recommendation of Dean Richardson, relieved Dr. Eugene Ferris of his post as Chairman of the Department of Medicine at Emory and, in effect, as chief of medicine at Grady Memorial Hospital. The board's action came only three days after the Chairman of the Fulton-DeKalb Hospital Authority, Hughes Spalding, had effusively praised Dr. Ferris and two other Emory faculty members—Dr. John Howard and Dr. William Caton—for their work at Grady.[43] Indignant at the removal of Dr. Ferris, twenty-nine members of the Grady staff signed a petition opposing the dean's decision. It is little wonder that shortly after firing Dr. Ferris Dean Richardson reported to the university's president that "the greatest problem facing us is the relationship between Grady Hospital and the School of Medicine."[44]

It was, in effect, a battle between the Emory Clinic and Emory faculty at Grady.[45] Certainly other elements were involved, including the authority of department chairmen within the school of medicine. Did their

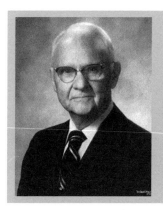

Dr. R. Hugh Wood (1896-1984) served as Dean of the Emory University School of Medicine from 1946 to 1956. During that time, Dr. Wood negotiated a 30-year contract between Emory University and the Fulton-DeKalb Hospital Authority. He was President of the Fulton County Medical Society in 1947.

authority extend to the activity of their faculty members at other clinical teaching sites, including Emory University Hospital and the Veterans Administration Hospital? What about the activity of clinical faculty, the part-time teachers who practiced at the Emory Clinic? The full-time Emory physicians at Grady were blocked from fully participating at the Emory Clinic and, thus, from sharing in its substantial profits. (Full-time teachers drew a salary from Emory, part-time teachers profited from their medical partnership.) With a partnership of thirty physicians who sent their patients to the Emory hospital, the clinic was a moneymaker for the doctors and the university. Whether it crossed the ethical boundary of being a "corporate practice of medicine" was up for debate. Apparently the three departmental chairs thought that the Emory Clinic had become focused on generating revenue rather than offering a way for part-time teachers to sustain themselves through private practice while being committed to clinical teaching and research. Although the complaining Emory physicians at Grady thought there was no way to separate clinical teaching from patient care, Emory insisted that it was being accomplished at the clinic.[46]

An important problem was that physicians in private practice resented being bossed by the chairmen of departments at the medical school. Dean Richardson claimed that the department chairmen wanted control over the faculty who spent 75% of their time at the Emory Clinic. Their doing so, he claimed, would itself amount to the corporate practice of medicine. While authority over faculty members was at stake, none of the department chairmen had claimed that they wanted to control what physicians did in the private practice of medicine.[47]

Many members of the Fulton County Medical Society who were not on Grady's staff also opposed Dean Richardson's removal of Dr. Ferris. They worried that the dismissal would generate morale problems among the hospital's house staff. Local physicians were concerned that the situation for doctors at Grady was becoming so toxic that the hospital might not be able to attract new physicians. Exasperated and concerned, Dr. Tully Blalock, a volunteer physician at Grady and a prominent member of Atlanta's medical community, asked the American Medical Association's Council on Medical Education to investigate the Emory University School of Medicine for its handling of staffing matters at Grady. Dr. Blalock believed that faculty members of a medical school who were also staff members of a public hospital should spend a majority of their time at the public hospital; customarily 80 percent of their time would be devoted to charity patient care with the remainder of their time allocated to private practice. Dr. Blalock saw the opposite happening with Emory physicians at Grady hospital. After consulting with other physicians, Dr. Blalock concluded that prolonging the conflict would hinder patient care and medical education at Grady. He then withdrew his request for an inquiry into the matter.

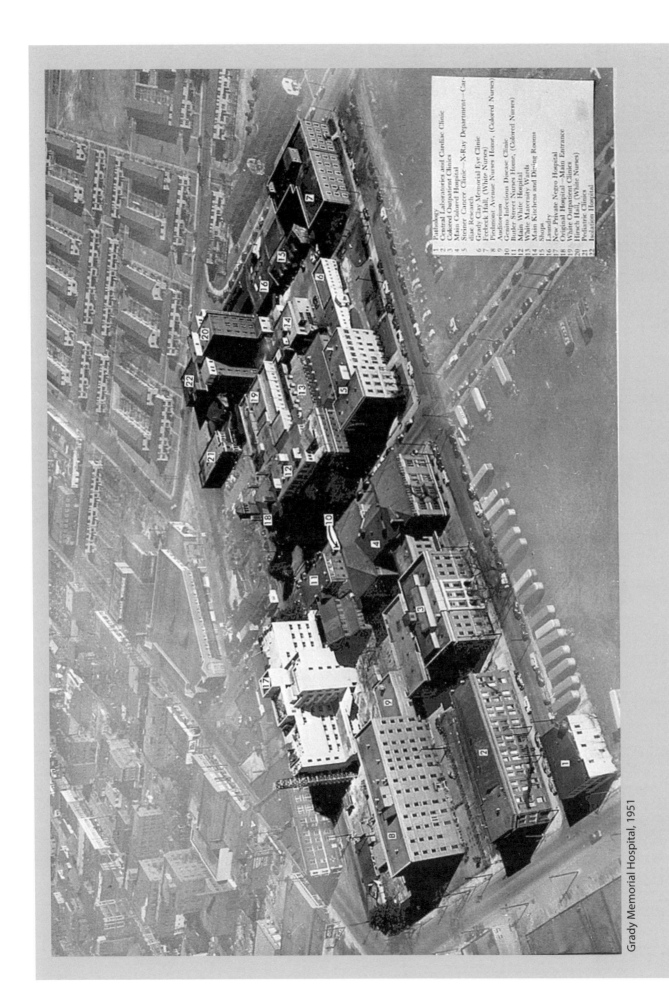

Grady Memorial Hospital, 1951

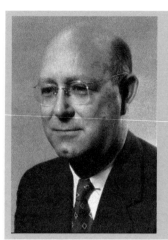

Dr. Arthur Richardson (1911-1993) was a forceful advocate for the growth and development of the Emory University School of Medicine. He was its dean from 1956 until 1979.

Appearing before the Fulton County Medical Society, Dr. Richardson claimed that the society's response to the conflict at Grady amounted to an attempt to interfere in the medical school's administrative decisions. He probably would not have viewed his comments as an effort to meddle in the society's affairs (he was a member). Still, he strongly objected to the society becoming involved in the conflict at Grady. He claimed the system through which Emory operated Grady would not work if he had to clear personnel and administrative decisions through the medical society.

The local physicians disagreed with Dr. Richardson. They claimed members of the Fulton and DeKalb county medical societies had a right to be involved in how Emory ran Grady's medical services. Among their reasons, the medical society's members noted that together they provided Grady with 350 volunteer attending physicians. This medical army provided much of the medical education and patient care at Grady for free. By doing so they had, in their view, earned the right to be involved in what took place at the public hospital. More than that, they insisted on holding Emory accountable to the local medical societies because those bodies represented physicians whose volunteer time at Grady benefited both the hospital and Emory's medical school. This position was hardly out of character for the local medical societies. Since Grady's founding, local physicians repeatedly asserted the right to have a say in what happened there. Not since the Steiner Clinic controversy of the 1930s, however, had the local physicians become so intensely upset over what were arguably administrative decisions made at Grady. Dr. Richardson thought the local medical society was unjustifiably angry. From his point of view, the society was living in the past.

Dean Richardson believed that the way medical schools in the United States operated had changed greatly in the decade since the end of World War II. Admittedly, they still relied on public hospitals to provide the "clinical material" used in teaching students. What was different, however, was the declining influence of local physicians on public hospitals. Their power waned in tandem with the rise of full-time faculty at medical schools. With increased federal funding after World War II, American medical schools began expanding residency programs and adding paid full-time faculty. Their need for volunteer teachers from local medical societies had diminished. The only problem Dean Richardson could see was that Atlanta's local medical society was having trouble hearing the news. It was not alone. Local medical societies across the United States didn't seem to understand that their army of volunteers no longer served as the soul of schools of medicine. Instead, medical schools increasingly relied on full-time faculty dedicated to the institution. Modern medical education, reflecting changes in the practice of medicine, demanded specialists who would teach first and practice medicine second.

To Dean Richardson's mind, the local medical society simply did not grasp the changing nature of medical education. Dean Richardson might have taken comfort in his knowledge that Emory was not alone in facing conflict with the local medical society. Similar "controversies" occurred in at least a half-dozen American medical schools at the same time. Summing up the dramatic revolution that had taken place in medical schools and teaching hospitals since the time of Abraham Flexner's exhaustive report nearly a half-century earlier, Dean Richardson succinctly noted,

"The volunteer faculty no longer has the time or background to dominate the medical educational program."[48] Where once the volunteer teacher could cover a broad range of material, increasing specialization and the accelerated growth of medical knowledge made it substantially more difficult for physicians in private practice to teach. The change in Emory's institutional character was remarkable, and the medical school's budgets provide one index of the shift's magnitude.

Research became a dramatically larger part of Emory's medical school budget between 1940 and 1958. In those eighteen years, research grew at an astonishing rate that rapidly outpaced inflation. Research funding rose from $5,000 to $1,000,000 during a period in which the school of medicine's total budget grew from $100,000 to $2.5 million. Put differently, research rose

County: Pay-Up Now!!

During 1957, Hughes Spalding threatened legal action against DeKalb County for failing to pay its financial obligations to the hospital for each of the preceding three years. Claude Blount, who became the new DeKalb County commission chairman in 1957, took these threats seriously and paid the obligations in full for 1954, 1955, and 1956.

from 5 percent to 40 percent of the school's budget. While the faculty had engaged in clinical research since the school's founding, basic scientific research was becoming more expensive. In addition, the school was hiring more full-time paid professors who were taking on much of the teaching responsibility that had earlier fallen on volunteer staff. Emory's spending at Grady increased from

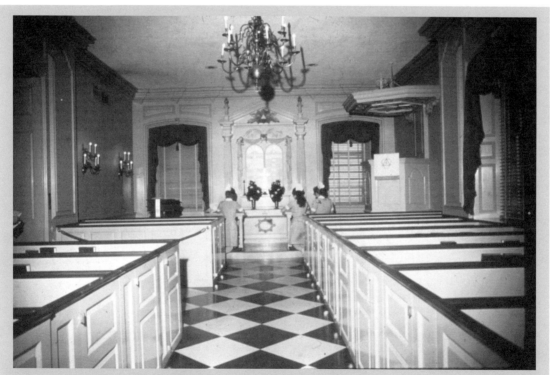

John Newton Goddard Memorial Chapel
The chapel, the first built in Grady hospital, was a memorial to John Goddard, a prominent philanthropist and successful businessman of Atlanta. It was funded by a $100,000 gift from Mrs. Goddard and her daughters, Mrs. Philip Alston and Mrs. Staunton Pickens. The chapel was designed by the classical architect Philip Shutze.

$65,000 to $356,000 from 1942 to 1957, excluding teaching and research grants of $350,000. Even with outside grants added to Emory's budget, its spending for Grady declined significantly in the decade after World War II, dropping from 65% to less than 30% of the medical school's budget.[49]

On January 5, 1957, Dr. Ferris appeared together with Dr. John Howard, the Chairman of the Department of Surgery, before the Fulton County Medical Society. Dr. Howard taught medical students, trained young surgeons, and researched clinical problems. He believed that the medical school's administration had given far too little support to its full-time physicians who both taught and conducted research at Grady. Instead, he claimed, Emory's medical school had focused its energy on supporting the Emory Clinic, which essentially had no direct involvement with academic research or teaching. Neither did the Emory Clinic provide medical support for Grady's indigent community. Dr. Howard said that he was resigning from Emory and Grady because he could no longer bring young doctors on to the staff in such an environment.

Dr. William Caton, Chief of Obstetrics, who opposed having Emory's medical faculty operate a private clinic, also resigned.[50] Like Dr. Howard, he claimed that Emory was evading its responsibilities for Grady. The argument was, in part, over Emory counting two physicians who worked part-time at Grady as being the equivalent of one full-time physician. In Dr. Caton's view, and that of others, the part-time physician would keep his first loyalty to his private practice.[51] While Dean Richardson admitted Grady was understaffed, he claimed that there were five full-time equivalents in medicine, five in surgery, two in obstetrics, and three in pediatrics. That was only true using full-time equivalents since only eight Emory faculty members worked full-time at Grady (out of fifteen "full-time" positions). Having been removed as chairman of the department of medicine, Dr. Ferris resigned from Emory and Grady's faculty effective February 1, 1957. (He became Medical Director of the American Heart

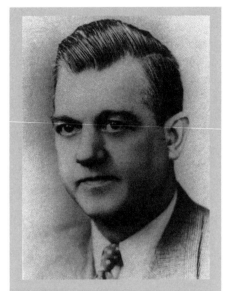

Dr. Eugene Ferris (1905-1957) had a distinguished career in teaching and research at the University of Cincinnati from 1936 to 1952 and at Emory University from 1952 to 1957. He was an authority on the pathological physiology of cardiovascular disease.

Association after leaving Emory, but shortly thereafter died of a heart attack at age 52 on September 26, 1957).

In the wake of Dr. Ferris' removal as a chairman, another member of the faculty, internist Walter Bloom, M.D., also left. In charge of the diabetes and endocrine clinic at Grady, he claimed Emory was "destroying the nucleus of the school's full-time faculty stationed at Grady" by accepting or asking for their resignations.[52] Given that the chairs of the departments of medicine, surgery, and obstetrics all would be gone from Emory by August 31, 1957, and would soon be out at Grady too, Dr. Bloom's assertion seemed reasonable. Dr. Bloom also indicated that Emory was no longer the place that he thought it had been regarding academic freedom and caring for the broader community. It didn't seem to him like an ideal place for a student to best learn how to become a physician.[53]

Dr. Bloom had conducted innovative research during World War II on high-altitude flying, protective masks for biological warfare, and the immunization and treatment of individuals exposed to anthrax. He had arrived at Emory and Grady in 1947 as an Associate Professor of Biochemistry and an Instructor in Medicine. At Grady his work included investigating Dextran, a volume expander used in emergency rooms to treat patients suffering shock. Dr. Bloom also established an endocrinology clinic at Grady. Prior to its opening, diabetes patients received care in the general medicine clinic. (The clinic that opened in the 1930s had closed during World War II.) Dr. Bloom became Director of Medical Education and Research for Piedmont Hospital in 1957, a move that was a substantial loss for Grady and Emory. After an outstanding ten-year career at Piedmont Hospital, Dr. Bloom spent sixteen years on the faculty of the Georgia Institute of Technology. The fallout from the firing of Dr. Ferris had been substantial, but the dean was ready to move on.

In January 1957, Dean Richardson named Dr. J. Willis Hurst to replace Dr. Ferris as Chairman of the Department of Medicine.[54] Several weeks after his appointment was announced, Dr. Hurst spoke to the Fulton County Medical Society (on March 21, 1957)—the same group that Dr. Richardson criticized for trying to "interfere" in Emory's internal affairs. Dr. Hurst's appearance before his friends and colleagues at the society's elegant building on West Peachtree Street proved effective. As the meeting ended on that spring day, optimism began to bloom among the society's physicians. Their interaction with Dr. Hurst led society members to anticipate a greater measure of cooperation between Emory and the society concerning medical service at Grady. A month later Dr. Richardson temporarily moved his office from the Emory campus to the Glenn Building at Grady to fulfill an agreement between the school and the hospital. The following year Grady appointed two members of the Emory medical faculty to administrative posts at the hospital. Dr. Bernard Hallman became Grady's Director of Professional Services and Dr. Charles LeMaistre became the Coordinator of Clinics for Grady. These steps helped lessen the tension that developed

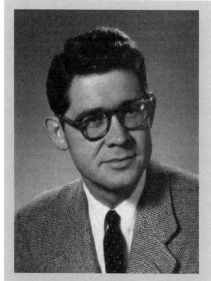

Dr. J. Willis Hurst (1920-2011), a widely honored and internationally recognized cardiologist, served for many years as Chairman of the Department of Medicine in the Emory University School of Medicine.

when Dean Richardson removed Dr. Ferris from his post as Grady's Chief of Medicine.

Dr. J. Willis Hurst

Born on October 21, 1920, in Cooper, Kentucky, J. Willis Hurst moved early in life to Carroll County in western Georgia. At the age of 16 he entered West Georgia College, where he stayed for two years before transferring to the University of Georgia. After earning his undergraduate degree he enrolled in the Medical College of Georgia. Having graduated at the top of his class in 1944, he completed an internship and residency in Augusta, which he followed with almost two years of military service (1946-1947). He then entered specialty training at Massachusetts General Hospital under Dr. Paul Dudley White, America's preeminent cardiologist at the time. In July 1949, Dr. Hurst returned to Georgia to enter private practice in Atlanta. One of a half-dozen cardiologists in the city, Dr. Hurst quickly volunteered to teach students at Grady Memorial Hospital.

In July 1950, Dr. Beeson offered Dr. Hurst a position at Emory that allowed him to work

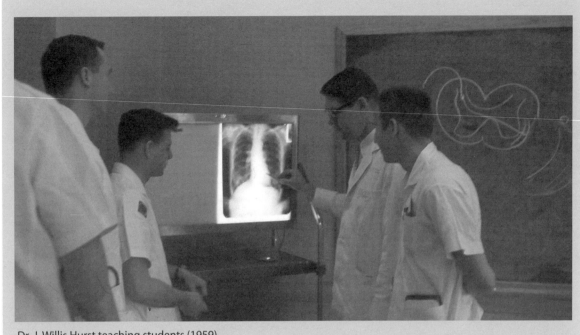
Dr. J. Willis Hurst teaching students (1959)

with Dr. R. Bruce Logue. Their work helped turn a private diagnostic clinic based at Emory into a major referral center for diagnosing heart disease. Recalled to military service in 1954, Dr. Hurst was assigned to Bethesda Naval Hospital. While there, he became the cardiologist for Senator Lyndon Johnson following Johnson's heart attack in 1955. After completing his second tour of duty as a military physician, Dr. Hurst returned to Grady and Emory. Several months after the resignation of Dr. Eugene Ferris as Chairman of the Department of Medicine, Dr. Hurst became the department's new chairman at the age of 36. He declined an offer to become White House physician after Lyndon Johnson became president, but Dr. Hurst remained his cardiologist for the rest of President Johnson's life.

Dr. Hurst retired as Chief of Medicine on September 1, 1986, after a thirty-year career. During his tenure he authored over 400 journal articles and edited or authored 74 books. He co-authored the definitive textbook, *The Heart*, with Dr. R. Bruce Logue and other leading cardiologists. (Now in its 11th edition, it has been renamed *Hurst's The Heart*). His leadership in numerous professional organizations included a term as president of the American Heart Association. He also received many major awards. His skill in teaching students, housestaff, and fellows became legendary, as did his deep concern for patients. A member of Grady's house staff echoed the feeling of generations of young physicians who learned from Dr. Hurst: "I practice as if Dr. Hurst is looking over my shoulder." His more than half-century of leadership in cardiology and medical education has left a mark on the medical community that may be impossible to duplicate.

A New Building For Grady

Grady's board members had been busy planning a new central hospital building ever since the failed bond referendum in 1940 and the resulting creation of the Fulton-DeKalb Hospital Authority. Before it even began formally functioning as an entity, the authority presented plans for a new building that would cost from $5,000,000 to $6,000,000. Viewed from overhead, the concept for the building, unveiled in mid-December 1945, took the shape of a capital

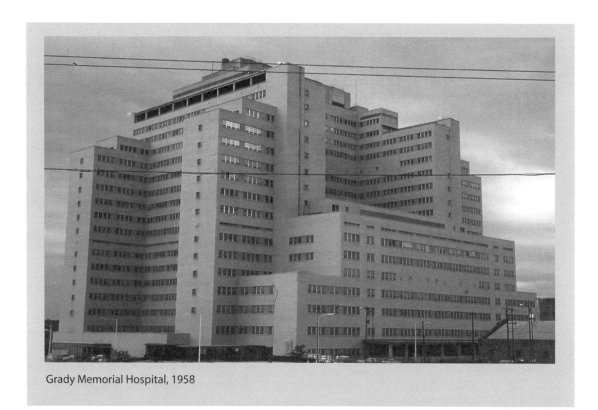
Grady Memorial Hospital, 1958

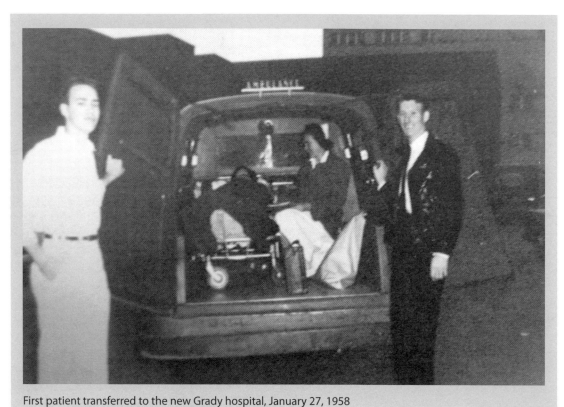
First patient transferred to the new Grady hospital, January 27, 1958

The Great "Fats" Hardy Bootleg Disaster

During a five-day period in late October 1951, 323 people who ingested bootleg whiskey tainted with methyl alcohol (it was 35% methyl alcohol) went to Grady for emergency treatment. Ranging in age from 10 to 78 years, almost all of the patients were African American; one-third of the victims were women.[72] Twenty-two victims were dead on arrival or died within thirty minutes after admission. More than a dozen other people treated in the emergency room for longer than 30 minutes or admitted to the hospital would die from the toxic whiskey. Many other victims permanently lost their sight. The mixture the patients drank contained corn whiskey, charcoal, stagnant well water, and the contents from a fifty-five gallon drum of methyl alcohol. Peach-flavored concentrate was added to the mix to disguise the undoubtedly putrid odor, although its affect on the whiskey's taste is unknown. The concoction had been mixed on a farm in Gwinnett County, near Duluth, Georgia. Ninety-nine gallons were brought to Atlanta and sold to a few individuals who then resold the mixture to the victims.

The police investigation revealed that John R. Hardy, a 44 year-old, 360-pound ex-convict with a fifth-grade education, also known as "Fats," made the whiskey. Hardy was arrested while hospitalized at Piedmont Hospital for injuries suffered in an automobile accident in Athens, Georgia. Hardy claimed he unintentionally added the methyl alcohol to the moonshine. Reportedly he knew nothing about a problem with the whiskey until notified by a distributor. Hardy assured his wholesale customer, "There ain't nothing wrong with that liquor. I drank me a half-pint and it tasted just fine." The distributor reportedly responded, "Mr. Fat, two of my people has died."[73]

Grady hospital responded remarkably well to the sudden influx of patients, and its staff put in many long hours to treat the afflicted. The most significant metabolic disturbance in humans with methyl alcohol poisoning is the development of severe acidosis; the most effective treatment is administration of sodium bicarbonate.[74] The Grady staff mixed baking soda from the hospital kitchen with a glucose and water solution and then administered it intravenously. During the five days of the crisis, 1,200 liters of the solution were given to the victims, most of who responded to the treatments with only minimal side effects.

The crisis offered substantial opportunities for Grady's staff members to collect and analyze data. Dr. Curtis Benton and Dr. Phinizy Calhoun of the Grady Eye Clinic studied and presented their findings of the ocular effects of methyl alcohol poisoning.[75] Drs. Ivan Bennett Jr., Freeman Cary, George Mitchell Jr., and Manuel Cooper later described their experiences in professional journals. Their valuable article in the *Journal of Medicine* reviewed the known literature on the subject and included the laboratory findings and autopsy reports from The Great "Fats" Hardy Bootleg Disaster.[76]

Dr. John Powell, from the University of Maryland, worked with the Social Service Department of Grady hospital to collect data that would provide a basis for predicting mass behavior in a time of crisis.[77] Among Dr. Powell's other interesting findings, he learned several patients denied drinking the alcohol even though they became severely ill. Perhaps more oddly, the emergency room saw about 100 patients with symptoms of methyl alcohol poisoning but who had never drank any of the contaminated whiskey. Apparently these patients began feeling ill after hearing about the outbreak. Less surprising, but still notable, a large number of spectators gathered outside the emergency room to watch the incoming patients. This was fairly commonplace on weekend nights when small groups of people gathered to watch emergency cases being brought into the hospital. This macabre form of entertainment drew a larger than usual crowd during the alcohol poisoning crisis, but it was unusually sedate.

A jury tried and convicted Hardy of killing John Blount, one of the African American whiskey victims. He was also found guilty of murder in four other cases, including John Blount's wife, Annie. He was sentenced to life imprisonment on the first murder, with consecutive five-year sentences for each of the other deaths. Fats won parole in 1967 after the judge who tried the case, Judge E. E. (Shorty) Andrews, testified before the parole board on Hardy's behalf. Judge Andrews said that without the case's widespread publicity, Fats Hardy would not have been convicted of a charge more serious than manslaughter. Fats Hardy died in 1970 at Grady from a heart ailment.[78]

H. Designed fully for the segregated world of separate but equal facilities, the proposed scheme reserved one side of the building for white patients and another side for everyone else. A corridor would connect the two sides of the facility. The building would stand as a testament to separate but equal medical care. Because of material and labor shortages after the war, the board understood it would have to wait before proceeding. Originally the authority planned to build a twelve to fifteen story building that would accommodate up to 1,000 patients. Over the years, as their plans matured, the building became taller and provided more room for clinics and services.

It took nearly a decade for the Fulton-DeKalb Hospital Authority to break ground for the new hospital; it finally did so on March 18, 1954. Grady completed its new building four years later, in January 1958 (months behind schedule thanks to labor disputes and shortages of material). When it was finally completed, the New Grady was a veritable Noah's Ark of hospitals, containing two of everything—one for black patients and one for white patients. Although it was designed to suit modern theories of medical

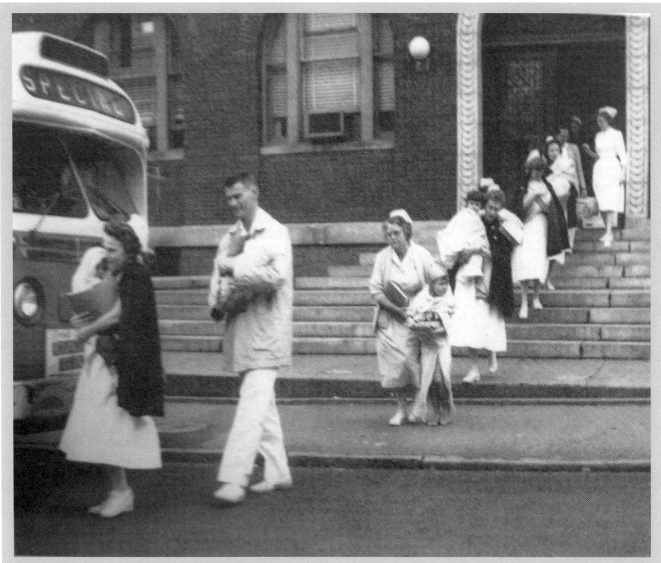

The transfer of pediatric patients to the new Grady hospital

practice and hospitalization, the overwhelming message was segregated medical care. The new hospital building stood 21 floors tall and covered 27.6 acres. It contained 1,100 beds, 17 operating rooms, 19 elevators, 10 delivery rooms, and 12 x-ray rooms. The construction cost 26 million dollars. (The original estimated price of construction of the new hospital was $20,523,000. Rising costs for labor and material helped push up the price and accounted in part for the cost overruns.)

Thousands of Atlanta's residents attended open houses at Grady on January 24 and 25, 1958. On January 26, the hospital dedicated the white section of the hospital with a ceremony held in the auditorium at 3:00 p.m. The Black Grady section was dedicated later that evening, at 7:30 p.m. Hughes Spalding, the hospital authority's chairman, delivered the dedication address on both occasions. Members of the hospital's board of trustees, local clergy, political leaders including Governor Marvin Griffin and Mayor William B. Hartsfield, together with several members of the Emory faculty and administration joined Hughes Spalding in the festivities.[55]

In his remarks, the ever-upbeat Mayor Hartsfield described the new hospital as "a fruition of a great dream of our community."[56] Governor Griffin, a committed segregationist, followed the mayor, invoking the New South theme of economic development. He exulted, "this magnificent structure is symbolic of the extremely rapid growth that we are enjoying in all fields of endeavor in our great state."[57] The Reverend Stuart R. Oglesby, pastor of Central Presbyterian Church, offered a dedicatory prayer asking for the Almighty's blessings on all who would enter through the hospital's doors. The core of Hughes Spalding's remarks focused on Grady's mission. Echoing the sentiment of the New South boosters who founded the hospital three generations earlier, Spalding said, "to have a successful community you have to have well people. The function of this hospital is to keep people well, or to care for them when they are ill and send them home."[58] It was, Spalding noted, not just the destitute who showed up at Grady. Its patients, he said, "are those of moderate incomes who can't raise a family and go to a private hospital."[59]

The hospital's philanthropic mission continued to mesh with the founders' aim to keep their community economically fruitful. In addition to the humanitarian hope to bring healing, the hospital would make Atlanta better by restoring patients to economic productivity. At the same time, the community continued its fundamental moral commitment to treat all who showed up at the hospital, regardless of their ability to pay for services. With the new hospital, the larger community reiterated its mission that no one should die from neglect of medical attention. The new Grady truly would make Atlanta a better place.

By noon on January 28, 1958, all patients had been transferred from the old Grady to the new facility. The first child to be born at the new hospital arrived that afternoon at 4:47 p.m. The baby, a boy weighing 7.5 pounds, was born to Mr. and Mrs. James Miller, the first of 7,713 newborns delivered at the new Grady that year.

The hospital had 160 doctors on its house staff. Another 500 physicians from the community volunteered their time and expertise to teach students and care for patients. Over 550 other volunteers who helped out on a regular basis joined the hospital's 1,217 employees. The campus housed three professional schools: the Grady School of Nursing (divided into black and white divisions), the School of Radiologic Technology, and the School of Medical Technology.

Staffing Up at Grady and Emory

With the coming of the new building, Grady had room for the first time in thirty years to substantially expand its staff and services. Since Emory's medical school ran the medical staff, Dean Richardson was responsible for making sure the departments had first-rate doctors. Although Emory began expanding its staff at Grady in the early 1950s, there were still only a few full-time Grady-based staff members when Dean

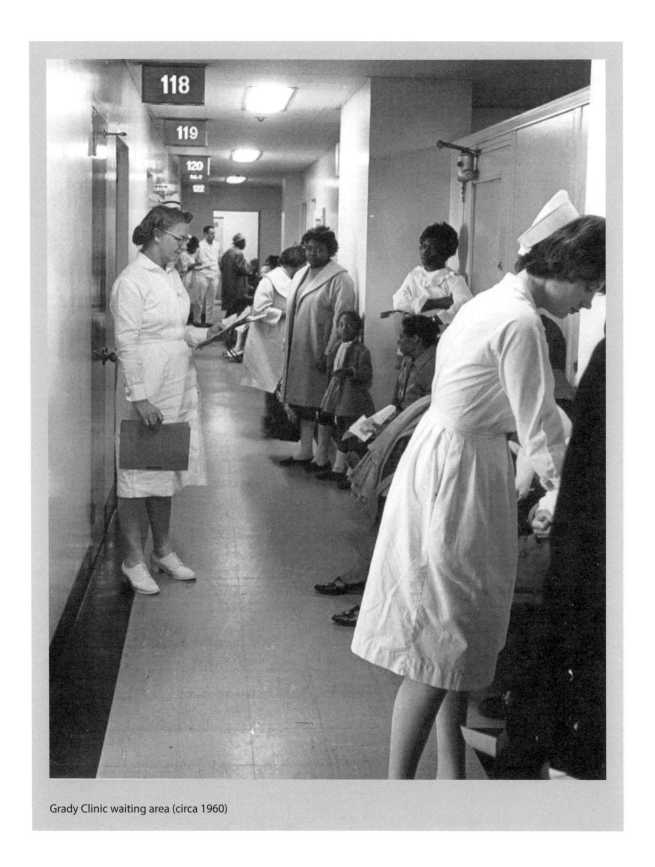
Grady Clinic waiting area (circa 1960)

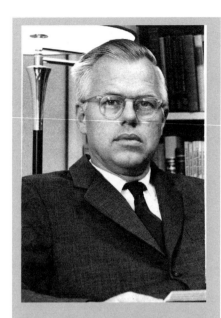

Dr. Bernard Holland (1916-2008) was an outstanding teacher and a forward-thinking leader of efforts to improve mental health care in Georgia.

Richardson took the medical school's helm in 1956. In particular, the departments of obstetrics-gynecology, radiology, and anesthesiology were severely understaffed, especially in light of the 350 additional beds that would come with the new facility. The departments of hematology, neurology, psychiatry, and gastroenterology also lacked the full-time faculty needed to broaden research, teaching, and patient care. In 1960, Emory and Grady agreed that at the rate of one department per year, control over radiology, pathology, and anesthesiology would be turned over to Emory. In January 1961, Dean Richardson reported to the president of Emory that "the pathology service under the supervision of the Hospital Authority deteriorated to such an extent that it threatened the accreditation of the hospital. The medical school was, therefore, asked to take over this service twelve months ahead of schedule and under rather difficult circumstances."[60]

New leadership made a noticeable difference in several important departments. The appointments of Dr. John D. "Dan" Thompson to head gynecology-obstetrics and of Dr. Bernard Holland to head psychiatry radically altered those departments at Grady. Under the leadership of Dr. Thompson, in the first years of the 1960s Grady's gynecology-obstetrics program developed significant major programs, including the Maternal and Infant Care Project, the Gynecological Cancer Program, and the Family Planning Project. Under the guidance of Dr. Holland, Grady's psychiatry program was dramatically improved.

Together with Drs. Richard S. Ward, H. Lee Hall, and C. Downing Tait, Jr., Dr. Holland

How to use an elevator

On January 24, 1958, a memorandum that Mrs. R. F. Schrader, the hospital's personnel director, sent to all employees gave seemingly remedial instruction in proper elevator etiquette and usage. This was necessary because the hospital would not be employing elevator operators in the new building.

She informed Grady's employees, "The passenger elevators are completely automatic, set on a pre-arranged time cycle, and they are equipped with a light and bell signal to indicate in which direction each elevator is traveling." She then reassured them, "The doors will not close while any passenger is entering or leaving, and you need only to press the button indicator for the floor you wish."[79]

Mrs. Schrader then let the hospital's workforce know what would happen on their elevator ride. "After you have entered, the door will close, and the elevator will leave the floor and discharge any other passengers en route who may have pressed indicators for floors between your point of departure and your destination."

Finally, to leave nothing out, she let it be known, "It is expected that Negro employees will use the elevators on the Pratt Street side of the building, and that white employees will use those on the Butler Street side."[80]

More than a few employees later recalled that the request for self-segregation was routinely ignored without penalty, even when the new building first opened at the start of 1958.

led Grady's psychiatry department into an affiliation with Columbia University. Appointed as training analysts on the faculty of Columbia Psychoanalytic Clinic, they commuted to New York to participate in faculty meetings, executive committee meetings, select students, and supervise candidates in psychoanalytic training. This relationship led to the development of a psychoanalytic institute in Atlanta which would dramatically improve the quality of care in the area. The institute also significantly enhanced the training of residents in psychiatry at Grady and improved the psychiatric care afforded to the hospital's patients. By the mid-1960s, Grady's psychiatry department was providing the core leadership for the development of mental health care in the Atlanta area. Indeed, Grady's department became the center of gravity for mental health treatment in Georgia.

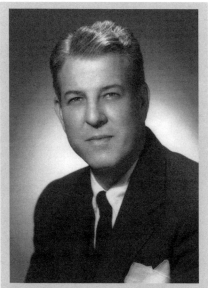

Frank Wilson, Sr., (1902-1964) was the administrator of Grady Memorial Hospital for 22 years. He oversaw the development of the new hospital building completed in 1958.

Grady's Superintendent Mr. Frank Wilson, Sr.

Following the resignation of Dr. James Moss Beeler in May 1942, Grady's trustees chose one of their own, Mr. Frank Wilson, as his replacement. Mr. Wilson agreed to serve as acting superintendent only until the hospital found someone to fill the vacancy. Late in 1942, at the urging of the board's chairman, Thomas Glenn, Mr. Wilson agreed to take the job permanently.

Frank Wilson was born in Atlanta on February 1, 1902, and educated in the Atlanta public schools and the University of Georgia. His successful business career and his service on the Atlanta City Council from 1933 to 1943 helped prepare him for the paths he would follow (and sometimes blaze) as Grady's superintendent during the next twenty-one years. Under his leadership, Hughes Spalding Pavilion and the new $26 million dollar Grady hospital were both erected. Mr. Wilson died on February 19, 1964, compiling a record as one of Grady hospital's longest-lasting and most effective chief administrators. After he died, the Atlanta Association of Independent Insurance Agents donated two heart machines to Grady in his honor. One, a "Scopette," allowed physicians to view a heart's electrical impulses on a monitor. The other was a pacemaker.[61]

The Fulton-DeKalb Hospital Authority

Mr. Hughes Spalding, Board Chairman

Mr. Hughes Spalding, an Atlanta business leader, succeeded Thomas K. Glenn as the chairman of the Fulton-DeKalb Hospital Authority. Mr. Glenn had been the driving force in making Grady hospital financially independent of voter-approved bond issues and in modernizing and reforming its administrative practices. Hughes Spalding would prove to be equally committed to Grady's mission of providing care to the area's neediest patients and of offering an unsurpassed facility for medical education and research.

Hughes Spalding was born on August 10, 1886, and raised on a small farm on Peachtree Road north of Atlanta, near the present site of Piedmont Hospital. (His

Consulting Report, 1960

The growth of the patient population and increasing costs to care for the indigent led Grady to hire a consulting firm to examine hospital operations and make recommendations for improving care. The consultant's report, issued in February 1960 but not released publicly until August, stated that Grady was one of the finest institutions of its kind in the United States; but the report also subtly criticized the organization and administration of the hospital. The consultants suggested changing the agreement between Emory and Grady Memorial Hospital to better define the role of department heads. Among other things, they hoped to improve morale among physicians. The report also urged an increase in nursing staff—especially in the clinics—and suggested improvements in intensive care nursing. Finally, the consultants also recommended Grady increase its fees. The chairman of the hospital authority, Fred Turner, rejected that suggestion on the grounds that the hospital's mission to serve those unable to pay meant it must limit charges for people without funds.

Superintendent Wilson was disappointed because the report provided few suggestions for how the hospital could save money. On the contrary, to Mr. Wilson's dismay, if all of the recommendations were put into place, the hospital would spend almost a quarter-million additional dollars during the next fiscal year. For example, the report recommended splitting the operations of the Hughes Spalding Pavilion from Grady Memorial Hospital. In order to implement that suggestion, Hughes Spalding Pavilion would need more staff, including a Director of Internal Medicine, a pathologist, and an anesthesiologist. Those three positions combined would cost the Grady system an extra $100,000 per year.

father, an extremely successful attorney, had moved the family two miles north from 14th and Peachtree streets.) He graduated from Atlanta's Marist College (later Marist High School) in 1903, earned a bachelor's degree from Georgetown University in 1908, and completed studies at the University of Georgia Law School in 1910. During World War I, he served as a First Lieutenant with the field artillery. After the war, he reentered the private practice of law with the firm Spalding, McDougald, and Sibley (later restored to its original name of King and Spalding).

In 1932, Governor Richard B. Russell appointed Spalding to the State Board of Regents, which oversaw the state's public universities; he served as its chairman in 1933 and 1934. His selection sparked controversy in rural Georgia where newspapers criticized the appointment because Mr. Spalding was a Roman Catholic. Anxious editorial writers claimed that the Pope would soon take over Georgia's public school system. When Governor Russell selected another Catholic to supervise the state banking system, equally gifted seers in the opinion columns predicted with astonishing certainty that the Vatican would soon control all of Georgia's banks in addition to its schools. Other newspapers praised the governor for selecting the most capable individuals without considering their religious beliefs. Hughes Spalding served a second term as chairman of the board of regents from 1949 to 1951, during the administration of Governor Herman Talmadge. While on the board of regents, Spalding oversaw the merger of several separate state schools and abolished many outdated agriculture and mechanical schools. He was also instrumental in establishing the University of Georgia Foundation. In addition, Mr. Spalding served as a director of the Coca-Cola Company and as a director of the Trust Company of Georgia. He was a skilled attorney and an insider among the insiders of Atlanta's business establishment. The Trust Company was Coca-Cola's bank of choice, and executives from the bank and the soft drink giant held seats on each other's boards of directors. In short, there was only the slightest degree of separation between Mr. Spalding and Robert Woodruff.

When Hughes Spalding stepped down from the hospital authority one year after the new Grady facility opened, Superintendent Frank Wilson correctly commented, "There would have been no Grady hospital, as we know it today, without Hughes Spalding." Mr. Spalding died at St. Joseph's Hospital on March 30, 1969, at the age of 82.

Fred J. Turner, the president of Southern Bell Telephone and Telegraph, was appointed in January 1959 to succeed Spalding as board chairman. Health concerns forced him to resign three years later. W. O. Duvall, president of Atlanta Federal Savings & Loan Association, was elected board chair in March 1962 but would serve for less than two years.

Mr. Clayton Yates

On January 22, 1964, the Fulton County Commission integrated the Fulton-DeKalb Hospital Authority by appointing Clayton R. Yates to the board. Sixty-seven years old at the time, Mr. Yates had a remarkable career building businesses in Black Atlanta. At the time of his appointment he was chairman of the board of trustees of the Citizens Bank Company, president of South-View Cemetery Association, and president of Southeastern Fire Insurance Company. A trustee of Morehouse College, he also served on the board of First Congregational Church and the Hunter Street YMCA.

After graduating from Morehouse College in 1918, Mr. Yates became a teller at Citizen's Trust Bank. Three years later, together with Lorimer D. Milton, Yates bought the Gate City Drugstore (at the corner of Auburn Avenue and Butler Street) from Herman Perry, a legendary business leader in Black Atlanta. Reopened as the Yates and Milton Drug Store, it became a neighborhood center as people flocked to its elegant soda fountain. It also had a substation of the U.S. Post Office. Over time, Yates and Milton added four drug stores to their holdings. In addition, each pursued more business ventures.

Volunteers

Ever since the idea of building a public hospital moved forward in 1888 and took shape from 1890 to 1892, volunteers played a major role at Grady hospital. It is difficult to imagine the hospital fulfilling its mission to care for its patients without the untold numbers from the community donating their time and money to ensure that Grady provided the best care possible. The year 1961 typifies the importance of physician volunteers for Grady when almost 600 doctors in the community, representing all specialties, gave time to help educate students, treat patients, and conduct research.[81]

Non-physician volunteers also continued to be crucial for the hospital. On any given day, thirty or more people helped out at Grady. The 509 volunteers from the community who served in 1965 logged 33,666 hours at the hospital. These included members of the Service Guild. Founded in 1936, the guild ran the hospital's gift shop and each year donated its net proceeds ($5,000 in 1965) to the hospital. In 1971 it would donate $10,000 to buy incubators for the Premature High Risk Nursery.[82] Other volunteers came in for special occasions. The Council of Jewish Women generously gave parties on Christmas, Halloween, and Thanksgiving for the children hospitalized on those days.

Two notable volunteers during the 1960s include Harry Sunshine and Officer Don (Don Kennedy). Starting out with a horse-drawn peddler's wagon, Harry Sunshine developed a chain of department stores in Atlanta. He convinced manufacturers to donate clothes and shoes for patients at Grady who needed them. A sweet man, he made certain that every child who visited the pediatric outpatient clinic received a lollipop. Officer Don, the much loved star of a local children's television program, "The Popeye Club," visited the pediatric outpatient clinic each Christmas.

Garden clubs were especially active with the Pine Center Garden Club beautifying the Spalding Pavilion, the Mayflower Garden Club enhancing the children's play area on the 16th floor of Grady, and the Castlewood Garden Club placing plants and planters at Hirsch Hall for the benefit of the student nurses.

Building on its contributions from the previous year when it donated rocking chairs for the pediatric areas and equipment for operating rooms, in 1965 the Junior League, with Mrs. Allen S. Hardin as its president, brought in provisional members to volunteer for three months. It also provided courses for nursing students, including a class in "grooming and slimnastics" that Mrs. J. P. Garlington, Jr., and Mrs. Frank Kelsey III taught for two hours twice each month during the autumn.[83]

During the 1940s and 1950s Clayton Yates played a significant role in supporting the development of Hughes Spalding Pavilion and served as a member of its advisory board. The appointment of Mr. Yates to the Fulton-DeKalb Hospital Authority was a major breakthrough for the county commission and for Grady. At last, someone from Black Atlanta had a voice in the hospital's oversight.

Edgar J. Forio

Edgar J. Forio was appointed to the Fulton-DeKalb Hospital Authority on January 22, 1964. A native of New Orleans and a 44-year veteran of Coca-Cola, Forio had been a senior vice-president of Coca-Cola since 1956. He was elected the authority's chairman less than a year after being named to its board. Unfortunately, he was forced to resign from the authority a little more than four years later (on April 1, 1969) because of health concerns. During his years as chairman, Mr. Forio oversaw the hospital's adaptation to Medicare and Medicaid. He also helped it prepare for an expected decline in patients because of the new insurance programs. In addition, he guided the board toward longer-range planning.

Desegregating the Gradys After World War II

The Stealth Strategy

The Atlanta Urban League (AUL) provided the leadership to improve health care for Black Atlanta in the years immediately after World War II.[1] Affiliated with the National Urban League since 1920, the AUL took a scientific approach to studying problems in the community. With the facts in hand, it moved to improve the way things stood. In the segregated city, access to jobs, housing, schooling, and health care stood out as big problems for African Americans in the 1920s and 1930s. These hardly lessened after the United States entered World War II.

In 1944, the AUL formed a Citizens Committee on Public Education to address racial inequities in local planning for postwar school construction. A proposed bond referendum from the Atlanta Board of Education would provide one million dollars for building public schools for black students. While substantial, the amount was merely one-tenth of what white schools would receive. After carefully analyzing the needs of Atlanta's black schools, the league published a report that deftly argued for more funding.[2] Based on hard-nosed statistical evidence, and publicized with assistance by executives from the J. Walter Thompson advertising agency, the AUL's report helped push the Atlanta Board of Education to dramatically increase funding for black schools. In the revised proposal, $4 million of a $9 million bond referendum would go to black schools. While funding for black students continued to lag behind the appropriation for white students for the rest of the 1940s, the shift by the school board marked a significant victory for the league and its new executive secretary, Grace Towns Hamilton.[3]

In December 1947, the AUL finished a path-breaking report about health care in Black Atlanta. The account of how things were attracted serious attention among African Americans and liberal white leaders when it came off of the press in January 1948.[4] "A Report on Hospital Care of the Negro Population of Atlanta, Georgia" surveyed hospital facilities for Black Atlanta and raised a series of big issues about health care for the city's African American communities.

The questions could hardly have been more basic: What were the basic health care problems? Did blacks get "adequate and competent care?" What hospital services were available to them? Could black physicians serve on the medical staff of approved hospitals? To what extent were black nurses used? What opportunities for continuing education were available to black physicians in Atlanta? Could the health needs of Black Atlanta, constituting one-third of the city's population, be met "by having one-third of the public health facilities?"[5] The survey data indicated disturbing answers to those questions.

Presented in a matter of fact style, the report revealed a dismal state of affairs. The basic health care problems for blacks in Atlanta were legion. With access to only a small number of hospital beds, black citizens were far from having anything close to adequate hospital care. The prohibition of black physicians from practicing in most of the city's hospitals, including its public charity hospital, also limited health care for Black Atlanta. For one thing, it meant that it was hard to attract black physicians to the city. Barred from residency training in hospitals in Atlanta, black physicians went elsewhere for postgraduate training and were unlikely to have a reason to come south to Atlanta afterwards. Black doctors also were excluded from the local white medical societies whose membership was a prerequisite for gaining privileges in hospitals. The number of physicians, dentists, and nurses in Atlanta's black communities was beyond inadequate. The evidence damning the state of health care in Black Atlanta led to a central theme: the health and well-being of black residents suffered directly from Jim Crow.

Racial discrimination was a central cause for the poor health conditions in Black Atlanta. The data showed that "the health of Atlanta's Negro population compares unfavorably with that of the white population of the city."[6] Indeed, the racial contrasts told the story of two cities. Atlanta's black citizens had significantly higher mortality rates than did whites, especially for infants and among women giving birth. The infant death rate for African Americans in 1946 was double that of whites. The death rate in giving birth showed the biggest difference. In 1946 the maternal death rate was almost five times greater for black women than for white women: 2.11 per 1,000 live births among black women; only 0.43 for white women in Atlanta. The overall death rate also had a clear racial disparity: 13.02 per 1,000 people for blacks compared to 7.48 for whites. (The overall death rates for blacks in Atlanta had dropped sharply since 1938, when it was 22.7 per 1,000 for blacks and 9.48 for whites.)[7] Blacks in Atlanta had higher mortality rates than did whites for each of the seven leading causes of death except cancer. Black Atlanta also had proportionally far fewer physicians. There were 37 black physicians in the city, twenty of which were over 55 years old. There were even fewer black dentists—nine. Remarkably, Atlanta had only 98 active black registered nurses. (The report claimed another 13 black registered nurses were "inactive.") Written largely by Grace Towns Hamilton, the AUL's report justifiably claimed, "Hardly a single phase of hospitalization in the city is unrelated to the racial nexus."[8]

When the AUL published its report, racism restricted the number of private hospital beds available to blacks. Emory University Hospital, Crawford Long Hospital, Georgia Baptist Hospital, and Piedmont Hospital each refused to admit black patients. The vast majority of hospital beds in Atlanta that were open to blacks, 300 out of 391, were at Grady. More than half of Black Atlanta, however, couldn't go there; their family incomes were too high for them to qualify for treatment at the charity hospital. That effectively left Atlanta's more than 70,000 middle class blacks access to 91 general hospital beds. Of these, 87 beds were at three black-owned proprietary hospitals.[9]

The report put health care for Black Atlanta in the context of a recently enacted federal law. The Hospital Survey and Construction Act, which Harry S. Truman signed into law in 1946, provided for the federal government to pay up to one-third of the cost of erecting a new hospital. Known as the Hill-Burton Act, the law required states to formulate a statewide plan for hospital capacity. The law's goal aimed for each state to have 4.5 hospital beds per 1,000 residents. No state would receive federal funding for hospital construction unless the Surgeon General of the United States approved its plan.

Georgia's State Hospital Plan, approved by the Surgeon General in November 1947, indicated a need for 6,992 additional hospital beds in the state for people of all races. Black Atlanta alone needed access to about

250 more hospital beds, the vast majority (approximately 220) for its middle class.[10] Significantly, the federal law prohibited state agencies from providing funding to hospitals that discriminated against people "on account of race, creed, or color." A loophole in the law, however, allowed states to bypass the anti-discrimination clause if plans for a new hospital "otherwise made equitable provision on the basis of need...."[11] In essence, any hospital could freely discriminate on the basis of race, creed, or color and still be eligible for federal construction money.

In measured tones, the AUL showed that Atlanta's health care system needed major improvements. Black Atlanta was underserved in every category imaginable. Although Black Atlanta's health had improved in the preceding decade, the statistics showed it was far behind White Atlanta.[12] In addition to a higher mortality rate, fewer hospital beds, and a lower number of physicians, dentists, and nurses, there was also remarkable inequality in the opportunities for professional development in medicine. This was largely because such opportunities did not exist in Atlanta for black health care professionals.

The AUL indicated practical, seemingly simple ways to give Black Atlanta better access to medical treatment. While the report was more suggestive than polemical, its underlying message was hard to miss. Overall, the report was a brief in support of a new hospital for Atlanta's black middle class. (It was an old cause that the AUL and others had been pushing for years.)[13]

Leaders in White Atlanta recognized the reports' compelling argument that Atlanta's black middle class needed access to more hospital beds. Among these white leaders, none was more significant for the AUL's chances of achieving success than Hughes Spalding, the recently appointed chairman of the Fulton-DeKalb Hospital Authority. Possibly the second most powerful man in the city after Robert W. Woodruff, Hughes Spalding was an accomplished attorney and a devout Roman Catholic whose firm ideas of Christian morality

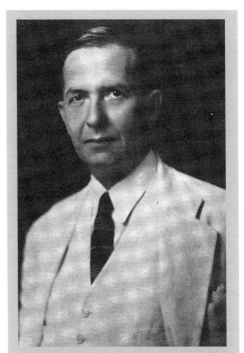

Hughes Spalding (1886-1969) was a prominent attorney, philanthropist, and civic leader who oversaw the Fulton-DeKalb Hospital Authority from 1946 to 1958.

had been sharpened by the Jesuit fathers during his college years at Georgetown University. (He would later indicate that the history of American anti-Catholicism and his own Catholic identity made him "more sympathetic" toward the Civil Rights movement.)[14]

Spalding sought support for a new pay hospital for black patients from other white civic leaders. He invited G. Arthur Howell, Jr., who together with his brother-in-law F. M. "Buster" Bird had founded Bird and Howell, one of the city's more powerful law firms, to join him for a meeting about the hospital project. This was no accident since Howell and his firm, which later became Jones, Bird & Howell after merging with the golfer Bobby Jones's law firm (and through a later merger became Alston & Bird), represented the agency. Writing to Howell, Spalding suggested that White Atlanta had a responsibility to improve conditions in Black Atlanta. "Unfortunately," he wrote, "so many of us are full of platitudes about helping the negroes and do nothing."¹⁵ Hughes Spalding had decided to do something about the health and welfare of Black Atlanta.

White advocates for a new hospital for the black middle class offered several arguments in support of the proposal. Some, like Spalding, believed it was simply the right thing to do on moral grounds. There was, to them, no question that the current state of health care in Black Atlanta was morally indefensible; they thought it self-evident that the black middle class deserved better access to hospitalization. A new institution would remedy the embarrassing and critical shortage of hospital beds for the city's black middle class and dramatically improve the community's health and welfare. While some leaders in White Atlanta believed the way things were was morally wrong, they had other reasons to support creating a hospital for the black middle class.

As he tried to persuade whites leaders of the virtue in creating the new hospital, Frank Wilson, the superintendent of Grady, appealed to their economic interests. The desire to return citizens to productive labor as soon as possible had been central in the logic behind creating Grady in the first place. After World War II, leaders in White Atlanta applied the same argument to erecting a new hospital for the black middle class. In recommending white candidates for an advisory board for the new hospital, Wilson—who would be instrumental in cultivating White Atlanta's support for the hospital—named people he believed were interested in the problems of Black Atlanta, men for whom "it would certainly mean money in their pockets to return Negroes to an employable status as promptly as possible."¹⁶ White Atlanta's arguments, however, went beyond morality and money.

Much of Atlanta's white leadership hoped building a hospital for the black middle class would block efforts to desegregate the local white hospitals. When the time came to sell the idea to White Atlanta, the all-white hospital authority claimed that unless a hospital was built for the black middle class, the area's white hospitals would be forced to accept black patients. The hospital authority seems to have floated this idea as a way to build support for a black middle class hospital among white taxpayers. (Surely, any official arguments directed to Black Atlanta would have been different.) While white leaders argued that the new hospital would keep medical care racially segregated for all of Atlanta, the goal of keeping Jim Crow in his place was anything but the aim of leading figures in Black Atlanta. Grace Towns Hamilton and her cohort at the Atlanta Urban League hoped to achieve something quite different.

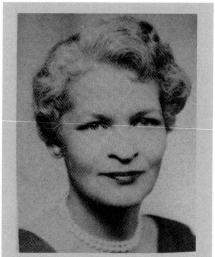

Grace T. Hamilton (1907-1992) was the first African American woman elected to a state legislature in the Deep South. Her pioneering efforts paved the way for many future black women to achieve public elected office.

At first glance, the AUL's call for a segregated "private-pay" hospital seems remarkably cautious. While it would lead to better health care for Black Atlanta, it would also reinforce the power of Jim Crow. The meekness of this approach bothered a number of national African American leaders, including Dr. Louis T. Wright of Harlem Hospital.¹⁷ According to historians Lorraine Nelson Spritzer and Jean B. Bergmark, the timid request masked a remarkably audacious plan. Indeed, the AUL hardly could have set its sights higher. It reasoned that putting the new hospital under the control of Grady's board would, by extension, link it to the Emory University School of Medicine. They hoped the connection between the new publicly owned black middle class hospital and Emory University (via Grady) would eventually force the university to desegregate its medical school.

Grace Towns Hamilton recalled years after the fact, "our hidden agenda was to provide a means of cracking the door at Grady-Emory."[18] As Spritzer and Bergmark suggest, however, the real objective was hidden better in memory than in fact. At the time, Mrs. Hamilton, Mr. Spalding, and others—including leaders at Emory's School of Medicine like Drs. R. Hugh Wood and James P. Grant—were aware that using the new hospital to train black physicians and surgeons would involve Emory. Indirectly, at least, it would force the university's medical school to desegregate.[19]

Leaders in Black Atlanta were especially eager to foster educational opportunities in medicine for blacks. That is why they urged Grady to admit black students to the hospital's x-ray and medical technology schools.

This seemingly innocent proposal was also part of a broader agenda. African American leaders reasoned that if Grady allowed black people to study in those schools, then the hospital would be forced to train them in other areas. In addition, since Emory's faculty trained students admitted to the x-ray and technology schools, having them teach black students at Grady would serve as another step toward desegregating the university's medical school. Black leaders, however, publicly masked the larger aims behind their proposals for medical education. Instead, they emphasized the need to attract more black physicians to Atlanta.

Black Atlanta's civic leaders put their point simply: opening Atlanta's hospital doors to black medical residents and interns would help attract a new generation of black physicians to Atlanta. Almost a year before the AUL's report on health care in Black Atlanta was finished, black physicians in Atlanta resumed their drive to open Grady hospital to African American interns and

Hospital Beds

According to figures published by the American Medical Association in 1948 and from local hospital records in 1947, there were 1,850 general hospital beds available in the Atlanta area as follows:

HOSPITAL BEDS	White	Black
Public		
Grady Hospital	322	300
Private		
Catholic Colored Clinic	0	4
Crawford W. Long Hospital	324	0
Dwelle's Infirmary	0	18
Emory University Hospital	231	0
Georgia Baptist Hospital	194	0
Henrietta Egleston Hospital (Children)	44	0
McLendon's Medical Clinic	0	34
Piedmont Hospital	132	0
St. Joseph's Infirmary	148	0
Scottish Rite	64	0
Wm. A. Harris Hospital	0	35
TOTALS	1,459	391

physicians. (Atlanta's black physicians had pushed for the admission of black physicians to practice in Grady's wards as far back as 1910.)[20] In their argument for opening Grady to black residents, they noted that many physicians who trained at Grady (including those from foreign lands) had made Atlanta their home after their residency ended. Allowing black medical school graduates to train in Black Grady would lead to alleviating the city's shortage of black physicians.

On February 19, 1947, Dr. Roderick L. Chamberlain, President of the Atlanta Medical Association, the city's professional society for African American physicians, requested that the Fulton County Medical Society support allowing black physicians to have staff privileges at Grady Hospital and permit black interns to train there. His timing could not have been better. Not long before Dr. Chamberlain made his appeal, a white physician, Dr. Paul Beeson, had asked the medical director of the Homer G. Philips Hospital in St. Louis how they had organized their training for African American physicians.[21] Whether or not he had heard about Dr. Beeson's query, Dr. Chamberlain certainly knew that Black Atlanta needed new physicians to replace the aging African American physician population; more than three-quarters of the Atlanta's African American physicians had over 25 years of experience practicing medicine. Dr. Chamberlain hoped the white physicians would agree to his proposal. While the white medical association accepted Dr. Chamberlain's opinion about the need to attract young black physicians, its leadership claimed the society had no right to determine policy for Grady hospital (a position it had rarely followed before and would reverse within a decade).[22]

A year after rejecting the call to press Grady to accept African American physicians, the all-white Fulton County Medical Society endorsed the concept (on December 2, 1948) of building a separate hospital for middle class black patients.[23] Although they favored creating such a hospital, several medical society members opposed building it on public land. Hughes Spalding, however, responded that it should be on public land because taxpayers would control the institution through the Fulton-DeKalb Hospital Authority.

Some doctors in the medical society worried that public ownership of the hospital could limit a patient's choice of physicians. (This was a real concern for them since a large number of middle class blacks saw white physicians.) Hughes Spalding quickly moved to dispel their anxiety. He told the society's members that while the authority would govern the hospital, patients could still freely choose their doctor. Although this removed one potential problem, many society members stayed wary of placing a private-pay hospital on public land. Disagreements arose within the society about where to put the new institution. The medical society suggested two potential sites for the new facility: one on the Grady campus, and another on the city's west side near the Atlanta University Center complex of historically black institutions of higher education. Emory University ended the debate by donating land for the new hospital directly across the street from Grady hospital.

To oversee the construction and operation of the new hospital, Hughes Spalding appointed a special joint committee composed of both white and black citizens. As fit Atlanta at the time, everyone involved understood that the committee's black members would play only an advisory role. In short, they would not have a vote. The biracial committee included Dr. R. Hugh Wood, the dean of the Emory University School of Medicine, Dr. Benjamin E. Mays, President of Morehouse College, and Dr. Rufus Clement, President of Atlanta University.[24] After the committee formed, Hughes Spalding regularly met with Grace Towns Hamilton and other leaders in the Atlanta Urban League, keeping them apprised of his careful effort to cultivate support for the proposal among the city's white leadership. It didn't take long for more and more white civic and business leaders to come aboard.[25] While white and black leaders worked together on a common cause, the underlying racial tensions were evident in symbolic decisions.

Hughes Spalding scrapped gently with black leaders over naming the hospital. Initially Spalding proposed calling the new institution Margaret Mitchell Hospital. Naming a hospital designed to serve the black middle class in honor of a white author who had glorified the Old South of slavery and secession must have seemed, at best, like a clumsy idea to Atlanta's black leaders. Hughes Spalding, however, had good reasons to honor her.

Almost two years before the Atlanta Urban League's report was completed, Margaret Mitchell had persuaded Spalding that Atlanta needed "a negro hospital of this nature." She became very interested in the cause in part because of what had happened to a black woman who had worked for her for twenty years. As her laundress was dying from cancer, Margaret Mitchell, the most famous and culturally powerful woman in the city, could not find a hospital bed where the woman "could die more comfortably than at home." Mitchell wrote to Spalding in 1946, "I do not think people who have not experienced so heartbreaking a time can realize the need for more beds for our colored population who are able to pay something for medical and hospital care…. Most people are unaware of the Negro problem and are apt to dismiss it by saying 'why don't they go to Grady.'" Through conversations with Margaret Mitchell in the wake of that letter, Hughes Spalding came to believe that a pay hospital for Black Atlanta "was a step that could be successfully taken."[26]

While Mrs. Mitchell had inspired Hughes Spalding, the leaders of Black Atlanta were not convinced the hospital should be named for her. They countered by suggesting the hospital be named for the late Dr. Charles Drew, an eminent black physician and medical researcher. In pleading the case, Dr. Asa Yancey, an African American who was born and raised in Atlanta, and was then the chief of surgery at Tuskegee Veterans Administration Hospital, told Hughes Spalding that no one had done more "toward the training of the Negro physicians in Georgia" than Dr. Drew.[27] Spalding rejected that argument because, while a heroic figure in the American medical community, Dr. Drew had no direct ties to either Atlanta or Georgia.[28]

With the naming of the hospital unresolved, Mr. Spalding might have come to prefer naming the hospital for an outstanding black leader. If so, he did not press the case. Perhaps the influence of Grace Towns Hamilton led other black members of the hospital advisory committee to suggest naming the hospital in honor of Hughes Spalding. With their having done so, there was little Spalding could do to refuse the honor. The black hospital was named for the white Fulton-DeKalb Hospital Authority Chairman who skillfully navigated its creation through the complicated politics of White Atlanta.

At a ceremony on Sunday, June 22, 1952, Governor Herman Talmadge presented the new hospital for African Americans to the City of Atlanta—and stood before a racially mixed crowd. Officially, Dr. Benjamin Mays, one of the most remarkable leaders in Atlanta's history, was supposed to accept the hospital on behalf of Black Atlanta. Dr. Mays, the great educator who had earned his Ph.D. at the University of Chicago, seemed to see his role differently. Standing at the podium, he took advantage of what a later generation would call "a teachable moment." While calling the event "a majestic step forward in Negro higher education," Dr. Mays saw the hospital as signaling something more significant: a major step forward in race relations. He declared that the project's significance rested in the process more than product. Optimistically, he suggested that the completion of the building marked a new beginning. For the first time in Atlanta, the segregationist reality that "Negroes are planned for rather than planned with" was turned on its head. "As a rule," President Mays observed from the podium—likely to the discomfort of Governor Talmadge—"we live on the periphery of American life, on the edge of the ragged edge. We are not part and parcel of the commissions, committees and boards that make up and shape the policies that govern our destiny." But this project was different. President Mays noted, "this hospital has culminated in a happy situation

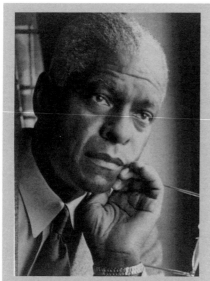

Dr. Benjamin Elijah Mays (1894-1984) was a remarkable teacher, preacher, scholar, mentor, and activist. He was President of Morehouse College (from 1940 to 1967) and, in retirement, President of the Atlanta Board of Education (from 1970 to 1981). He was awarded 56 honorary degrees.

because Negroes were not planned for. They were planned with. Step by step, in every detail.... As a result, interracial goodwill has been generated, interracial respect has been increased, interracial confidence has been strengthened, brotherhood has been furthered, and everybody feels better in his heart."[29]

Atlanta could finally boast of having an institution dedicated to training black interns and residents. Certainly the city's civic and medical leaders of both races hoped the young physicians would make Atlanta their permanent home after finishing medical training at the Spalding Pavilion. In addition, the new facility meant that black physicians finally had a modern hospital in which to care for their private-pay patients. Certainly it was a first-rate facility, as well-equipped and modern as any hospital in the South. The first and fifth floors, which housed administrative offices and modern surgical suites, respectively, were fully air-conditioned (as were the "pink" and "blue" nurseries on the fourth floor). With icemakers on every floor, oxygen piped into every patient's room, marble walls, and terrazzo floors, the new hospital was meant not only to be separate, but to be truly equal in the quality of construction and furnishing.[30] Dr. Mays noted that segregation generally meant "inferior services and inferior goods" for blacks. The Pavilion was different, he said, comparing "favorably with the best hospitals in the land."[31] The hospital opened its doors for patients on July 7, 1952, two weeks after the dedication ceremony. (The first person admitted, Miss Ruby Mae Miles, a patient of Dr. James B. Harris, president of the Atlanta Medical Association, came for a tonsillectomy.)[30]

Spalding Pavilion owed its existence to the reign of Jim Crow. To White Atlanta the hospital proved that Jim Crow worked and should be left in place. From their perspective, they could be proud that the new hospital remedied the racial imbalance in access to health care in the city. White Atlanta viewed the new hospital as a bulwark supporting segregation during a period of intensifying uncertainty about the future status of "separate but equal" treatment under the law. Without the new hospital, whites had feared, federal courts might force the integration of every white hospital in Atlanta. With the new black hospital, they hoped, separate medical treatment might be sustained. Black Atlanta took a nearly opposite approach.

Leaders in Black Atlanta celebrated the opening of the new hospital with a very different spirit. Instead of symbolizing the success of Jim Crow, they saw the Pavilion's creation as a sign that the noxious system of racial apartheid could be dismantled. For people who died disproportionately early because of medical segregation, the death and burial of Jim Crow could not come fast enough. At a time when the federal courts remained a promising but still uncertain route to killing off the existing system, the hospital represented the promise of negotiating toward freedom through the Atlanta way. Not only did the new facility give the black middle class access to modern hospital facilities, it also promised to attract more African

American medical professionals to the city. Because the hospital was also dedicated to the training of black physicians and surgeons, leaders in Black Atlanta expected the new hospital would lead to the desegregation of the Emory University School of Medicine.

Still, not everyone was so sanguine about that result. The Pittsburgh *Courier*, for which Dr. Mays served as a columnist, was succinct: "Disturbing to many observers was the revelation that the $1,850,000 structure will play a role in perpetuating the institution of segregation even unto death."[33] A number of black physicians had expressed similar fears early in the planning stages for the new hospital. Grace Towns Hamilton, Clayton R. Yates, and other leaders in Black Atlanta understood the anxiety. But they were not about to fail.

The not-for-profit Spalding Pavilion's early years involved a series of challenges. They differed, however, from those that plagued Grady hospital in its early years. Where Grady experienced management conflict and turnover during its first few months, Spalding enjoyed administrative consistency. While Grady endured labor strife as its outset, Spalding's workers seemed relatively satisfied, even with the adjustments people have to make when a new institution opens. While leadership and labor proved stable enough, the finances quickly became alarming. The hospital lost $37,000 in its first six months. This was in part because of surprisingly low occupancy rates. In its first three months the hospital averaged only 27 patients per day—less than 25% of capacity.

One reason for the low occupancy rate was simple: The black middle class was excluded from Blue Cross hospital insurance. The companies that did offer hospital insurance to blacks provided only a few dollars a day in benefits—not enough to cover the $9 to $15 per day cost of staying at Spalding Pavilion. The hospital's Advisory Board recognized that helping Atlanta's black middle class gain access to hospital insurance would be critically important for improving the pavilion's finances.[34] Taking their advice, Hughes Spalding argued the case with Blue Cross officials in Atlanta, and before long the company began making its hospital insurance available to blacks. While other firms were slower in writing policies for African Americans, the number of patients at Spalding Pavilion rose as hospital insurance became increasingly accessible to African Americans. Over the next two years the average daily number of patients stood at about forty. By July 1954, Blue Cross and Blue Shield had accepted the Pavilion and two private black institutions—Harris Memorial Hospital and McLendon Medical Clinic—as member hospitals.

The Pavilion's occupancy rate rose slowly because white physicians sent few patients there. They kept their patients away from Spalding in part because the hospital's services seemed inadequate—a direct result of not having a teaching program and therefore no interns. (While the hospital was supposed to become a training center, it struggled to get one off the ground.) In addition, Atlanta's two other private black hospitals kept their operating rooms open 24 hours per day. In order to comply with American Medical Association rules, however, Spalding Pavilion only conducted surgery during the day.

Although a large number of African Americans saw white physicians (in part because of the shortage of black doctors in Atlanta), they did so with the understanding that many white doctors treated African Americans as a sideline. White physicians would operate on white patients during the day. Since they couldn't use Spalding Pavilion for surgery at night, they had an incentive to place patients with the other black hospitals—facilities that continued to be crowded in the first years after the Pavilion opened.[35] While physicians tended to choose the hospital for their patients, the cost of being treated at Spalding also affected occupancy. With rates 30% above competing private black hospitals, Spalding was relatively expensive. In addition, the wealthiest members of Black Atlanta continued to go to northern cities for specialty treatment.

As Spalding Pavilion's deficit continued to mount, the county grand jury looked into the finances and questioned the rationale for keeping the hospital open. In response, the FDHA moved patients from Black Grady's obstetrics department to Spalding Pavilion in the summer of 1953. Dedicating forty beds to Grady's obstetrics program would double the occupancy and generate income for the Pavilion. Grady's move also meant that more nurses and support staff were available to help private obstetrics patients at Spalding Pavilion.[36] Still, even with more patients through insurance and from Grady's overflow, Hughes Spalding Pavilion ran an annual deficit of nearly $100,000 by its third year of operation. Facing such losses, the FDHA was straining to keep the pavilion open.

As the 1950s ended, the hospital authority appeared increasingly uncomfortable with managing Hughes Spalding Pavilion. Part of this was because Hughes Spalding himself had retired from the FDHA. He had proved to be a steadying hand for the Pavilion during its first few years. With Spalding's absence, however, the authority became increasingly concerned about the Pavilion being a private hospital. By 1960, the authority had trouble reconciling governing Spalding Pavilion with its responsibility to warden Grady's mission to care for the poor. The basic conflict between Grady's purpose and that of the Hughes Spalding Pavilion was only part of the problem. Varying accountings for the cost of operating Hughes Spalding Pavilion led to intense arguments between administrators and trustees. Grady's administration claimed Spalding was losing money; Superintendent Wilson putting the operating deficit at $50,000 for the first 6 months of 1960. In contrast, the Spalding Pavilion's board claimed the hospital enjoyed a net operating surplus of $89,585 during the same period.[37]

While finances grabbed headlines, the biggest problem lay elsewhere: the educational program that was to be at the core of Spalding Pavilion had been going nowhere. While the Pavilion was established in part to be a training ground for recently graduated African American physicians, it would take over five years to get a program up and running in just one department. Almost as soon as it got off of the ground, however, the training program for black physicians and surgeons began drawing attention from critics. After holding their fire for a brief period, in 1960, eight years after the hospital opened but only two years after the training program was launched, critics declared that it was a failure. They hammered home the fact that only three interns had received any meaningful experience in the hospital.

The failure to develop a significant teaching program may have rested even more heavily upon the Emory University School of Medicine than on the Fulton-DeKalb Hospital Authority. At first the medical school showed significant signs of interest. By 1947, Dr. Paul Beeson had been corresponding with Dr. Charles R. Drew and other outstanding African American physicians about how to improve training for African American physicians in Atlanta. That year Dean Wood met with Dr. Drew and with Dr. Murray Brown of Meharry Medical College, and by that December plans for "a Negro hospital which would accommodate the Negro physicians" was already in the planning stages. As early as 1948, Dean Wood had said that Emory would be willing to train black physicians at the new hospital. As if to seal the promise, in the summer of 1948 Emory and Grady put together post-graduate clinical seminars for African American physicians, restarting the program that had been held for a few years in the early 1930s. Widely publicized, and praised in an editorial in the *Atlanta Journal*, the seminars suggested Emory's openness to offering post-graduate training to African American physicians. Clearly, Dean Wood was trying to improve health care in Black Atlanta.[38] While there were no legal contracts in place, officials at Emory had indicated their support for the African American physicians training program at Spalding.[39] Indeed, the dean of Emory's medical school helped oversee Spalding Pavilion's planning and construction.

While officials from Emory had made it clear in the spring of 1948 that they would "train Negro physicians and surgeons" at the new hospital, for more than a decade Emory made little effort to begin full-scale training programs for physicians and surgeons at Hughes Spalding Pavilion.[40] Through the 1950s Emory offered the same reason time and again: It lacked the personnel to take on the responsibility for teaching at Hughes Spalding. It also worried that additional students would reduce the "clinical material" available to students from Emory.

Were these just excuses? Some physicians with close ties to Emory thought so. For example, in a long letter to Dr. Beeson, Dr. Robert Grant accused Emory of evading its promise to establish the training program.[42] Yet, adequate funding was a real concern—one that black physicians like Dr. W. Montague Cobb recognized and hoped to resolve through funding from foundations. Grace Towns Hamilton did too, and sought help from people associated with the Rockefeller and other foundations.[41]

When federal funds for such training programs became available later in the 1950s, it was Spalding Pavilion's advisory board that pursued the opportunity. With crucial support from Dr. Grant, by then at the National Heart Institute, the FDHA won a grant from the U.S. Department of Public Health to fund Dr. Yancey's position at Spalding Pavilion. Emory University, in contrast, did little if anything to pursue similar opportunities for developing the teaching program at Spalding Pavilion. When pressed in 1959 to make the inpatients at Black Grady available to black residents being trained in surgery at Spalding, Emory found "it would not be practical … to modify the existing teaching and service programs" at Grady. More plainly, it rejected doing what Dean Wood said was necessary five years earlier. To get the training program off the ground, he had argued, required the hospital authority and Emory to make a decision: one of them would have to take the lead in integration.[43] Instead, Emory suggested turning Spalding Pavilion into a training site for fourth-year residents in surgery at the Veterans Administration Hospital in Tuskegee, Alabama.[44] Frustrated leaders in Black Atlanta privately faulted Emory University for the sluggish development of the Pavilion's training program.

By the end of 1961, with the new Grady building long since opened, Spalding Pavilion was running far over its full capacity of 125 patients. The apparent success was rooted mostly in the continuing shortage of hospital beds for Black Atlanta. The black population of Atlanta had risen by 50% between 1950 and 1960, from 121,285 to 186,464 residents.[45] The crushing need for more hospital beds that the AUL documented in 1947 had only intensified by 1960. Even with the 125 beds that Hughes Spalding supplied to Black Atlanta, the number was inadequate for a population that had grown by slightly more than 65,000 since the planning for Spalding Pavilion began.

Even as the demand for its services increased, and its wards became as overcrowded as those of Black Grady, Spalding Pavilion continued to be the hospital authority's poor stepchild, underfunded and understaffed.[46] Circumstances were so difficult by the end of 1961 that the hospital's nurses threatened "direct action" unless hospital administrators increased their pay and lightened the work load. The size of the nursing staff simply had not kept pace with the growing number of patients. "Every nurse at Hughes Spalding can tell you we've been overworked, underpaid and treated like anything but professionals for years," an exasperated nurse exclaimed as she reported that the nurses had circulated a petition to let hospital administrators know that the workload was leading to substandard patient care.[47]

With too little money, inadequate equipment and facilities, and a training program barely begun and hardly used, even the pragmatic leaders in Black Atlanta were reconsidering their strategy. In 1952, the opening of the new hospital for the black middle class had seemed to validate the negotiating strategy of Dr. Mays and Mrs. Hamilton. Less than ten years later, their faith in the Atlanta way seemed to have been mocked more than rewarded. The strategic resistance of Emory University, Grady hospital, and the Fulton-

DeKalb Hospital Authority had delayed the start of Spalding's teaching program, prevented the desegregation of the x-ray and medical technology schools at Grady, and left the Pavilion under severe financial pressure. By 1961, Grady's wards were still segregated by race, still closed to black physicians. The problems that leaders in Black Atlanta had hoped to solve through the new hospital remained. A younger generation, one that would begin direct action through sit-ins and protests at lunch counters in 1960, was starting to ask follow-up questions to those Mrs. Hamilton and the AUL had raised more than a decade before.

The Direct Approach

When the new Grady hospital building opened in 1958, it provided separate spaces for the care of premature newborns: one for blacks and one for whites. That isn't too surprising given the hospital's desire to maintain Jim Crow in architecture as much as in patient services. What is remarkable is that the hospital's physicians, all of whom were white, protested the re-segregation of a previously (if unofficially) integrated section of the hospital. In 1945, Dr. M. Hines Roberts and his associate Dr. Elsworth Cale opened a nursery for premature infants near the obstetrical unit in White Grady. This highly specialized nursery accepted both white and black newborns and remained "unofficially" desegregated into the 1950s. At first blush, it seems that the physicians might have spoken up about keeping their arrangement in the new building before the hospital authority built a segregated unit. Because their desegregation was "unofficial," they may have been in no position to make waves before the building was designed, much less before construction was finished.

Once the building was in place, however, the physicians advised Grady's administrators that the Neonatology Service barely had enough staff for one premature baby unit, much less two. Hospital administrators might have hired additional staff and provided more money to keep the premature babies segregated from each other. Instead, Frank Wilson and his assistant Bill Pinkston decided to keep the Neonatology Service desegregated. As a practical (and cost-saving) matter, the administrators provided a single unit to care for premature newborns of both races. This small episode is the first official desegregation of patients at Grady. As the 1950s drew to an end, another small step in Grady's official desegregation came when Dr. John B. Holton, a black physician from Nashville, was hired as a full-time radiologist at Hughes Spalding Pavilion; he was the first black physician that the Grady system employed. These small steps added up for Grady, but they were barely noticeable on the outside. The Fulton-DeKalb Hospital Authority's movement toward desegregation was far from what Mrs. Hamilton, the AUL, and other black leaders were trying to achieve.

The city's established black leaders believed in using their limited political leverage with care; this helps explain their patient and cautious push for desegregation. The circumspect strategy that Grace Towns Hamilton and the AUL used to create a separate middle class black hospital and a training facility for black medical professionals typified their approach.

For those pragmatists of the older generation the central issue was how best to get from Jim Crow to desegregation without sparking a riot. They had grown up with stories about the race riot of 1906. Neither the "old guard" leaders of Black Atlanta nor the white power structure wanted to see anything like a repeat of that disaster. They were intent on not provoking the kind of inflammatory rhetoric that had led to a terrible, deadly race riot. In the decades since the riot, what was at first an uneasy truce arranged by the leaders of White Atlanta and Black Atlanta settled into a pattern of negotiation. By the start of the 1960s, the leaders of the two Atlantas had managed to keep racial peace (if not complete harmony) for more than fifty years. That way of avoiding civil strife, the backroom alliance between the leaders of Black Atlanta and White Atlanta, seemed to take on even greater urgency after the U.S. Supreme Court ruled against Jim Crow in *Brown v. Board of Education* (May 17, 1954). The *Brown* case and subsequent decisions led to intensified negotiations between Atlanta's black and white civic leaders.

One of the Supreme Court's decisions following *Brown* concerned Atlanta's policies about public space. In 1951, the municipally-owned Bobby Jones Golf Course summarily refused to allow a black foursome—an elderly physician, Hamilton M. Holmes, two of his sons, Alfred ("Tup") and Oliver, and a friend, Charles Bell—to play on the links.* Located at the southern edge of the solidly white Buckhead community, and named for the hometown golf icon, the course did not permit black patrons. Two years after the incident, when the usual negotiations had produced no movement, the physician and his two sons sued the city.

The case, *Holmes v. Atlanta*, eventually found its way to the U.S. Supreme Court where, in November 1955, eighteen months after the *Brown* decision, the court ruled that the city's golf courses had to be open to members of every race. *Holmes v. Atlanta* brought the *Brown* decision home to Atlanta. In the wake of the *Holmes* ruling, Mayor Hartsfield proved ready to guide the city to peaceful (if languid) desegregation. Eager to avoid the violence of a half-century before, he worked with leaders in Black Atlanta to see that the desegregation of the city's public golf courses went smoothly. The black leadership, also eager to avoid racial violence in the city, agreed to work with the mayor.

Following *Holmes v. Atlanta*, the leaders of Black Atlanta and White Atlanta would collude in staging integration events. For example, the arrest of black protestors on a bus was staged to begin a legal process that would quietly and peacefully integrate the transit system. (Such events were routinely arranged with cooperation from Atlanta's chief of police). Through this system, public officials hoped to sidestep some of the political consequences of integration—especially the substantial loss of white votes—by blaming the judiciary. Progress in ending segregation was deliberately slow but usually steady. (The city's stalling maneuvers, which it regularly employed, seemed to become an almost scripted part of the process.)

Although Atlanta haltingly moved toward desegregating municipal golf courses and parks during the later 1950s, the city's public school system moved with less alacrity. It only began to desegregate in the early 1960s when it ran out of ways to stall implementation of the Supreme Court's decision in *Brown*. Although Atlanta's white flight had been underway for some time, the coming of public school desegregation intensely accelerated the migration of middle and lower income white residents to the suburbs.

Their move away from the city had significant consequences for Grady. It meant that one of the white constituencies that had long used and supported Grady lived farther away from the hospital and, in many cases, became ineligible to be treated there.

Whites who moved north into Cobb and Gwinnett counties could no longer use Grady since those areas were outside of the hospital's zone of service. Citizens in these counties neither paid taxes to support Grady nor were they represented on the Fulton-DeKalb Hospital Authority. (While they were technically excluded from being seen at Grady, patients from those counties were admitted as emergency cases, to the burn unit, and to other services that only Grady offered to the metro area.) As a result, the ratio of black to white patients at Grady steadily rose.

The white movement away from the city, and the accompanying racial re-segregation, would hinder political support for Grady in the coming decades. While that was still in the future, the immediate issue of desegregating public space drew attention within

---

*Alfred "Tup" Holmes was the father of Hamilton E. Holmes. The young Hamilton became the first black male to integrate the University of Georgia (1961) and the first of his race to attend and graduate from the Emory University School of Medicine (1967).

and to the city. While some whites fled, others stood their ground in the fight over desegregation.

Rather than simply opposing civil rights, Georgia's segregationists saw themselves in positive terms.[48] In particular, they viewed the defense of segregation as protecting American liberty. They believed they were guarding against an assault from civil rights agitators against a supposed basic American right to "freedom of association" in public space—an assault that helped fuel a backlash in Atlanta against the city's "progress."

Many whites disdained the "race improvements" Atlanta's civic leaders promoted in large part because they believed that they paid more taxes than did blacks. The historian Kevin Kruse notes that the "supposed disparity between the tax burdens of whites and blacks took on a strongly racist tone."[49] Atlanta's whites increasingly asserted that their tax dollars were subsidizing the welfare of black communities when public spaces became desegregated. In the voting booth white Atlantans opposed a bond initiative city leaders presented in 1962 to fund public works projects. (The next year a revised, "stripped-down" version of the bond—one that removed the most obvious benefits for black communities—narrowly passed.) As Kruse shows, the bond proposal's white opponents saw the public programs it funded as unfair; they believed that the tax burden fell more heavily on whites while, in their view, black residents won benefits at the expense of white pocketbooks.[50]

In contrast to the city's leadership, working class and middle class whites came to equate what civic leaders saw as the public good with benefits for black neighborhoods. It became nearly impossible for city leaders to win white support for public works spending. Whites came to believe their hard-earned tax dollars would only benefit others—people newly free to use parks, swimming pools, and other public facilities that once were designated to benefit only whites.[51]

Although whites failed to block integration of public tennis courts and golf courses, wealthier participants in those sports retreated into de facto segregation in the safety of private clubs that quietly excluded blacks from membership. (The most elite private clubs in Atlanta, the Piedmont Driving Club and Peachtree Golf Club, would not have black members until the 1990s.) White Atlanta had resisted the desegregation of public parks. Whites found the prospect of "race mixing" at swimming pools especially vexing. As with a hospital room, using a swimming pool involved in its very nature a form of physical closeness that gave rise to concerns about whom one associated with. Given white stereotyping of blacks as carriers of contagious disease—particularly syphilis—their intense desire to keep public swimming pools segregated barely surprises. As they had with tennis and golf, wealthier white residents would retreat to private clubs. Desegregating public swimming pools would also lead to a boom in personal swimming pool construction. For the majority of white residents, however, retreating into private recreational space was financially impossible. They could not afford to replace lost public space with equally segregated private space in the way wealthier Atlantans did.[52]

The antipathy of some whites toward desegregation of public spaces and to having the government take their hard-earned money away only to turn it over to the welfare of the black community gives context to the Fulton-DeKalb Hospital Authority's anxiety about desegregating Grady hospital.

Early in 1960 a group of younger blacks began to challenge Atlanta's system of backroom negotiation between black and white leaders. Born more than a generation after the race riot of 1906, these young people were in a hurry, impatient with the way things were done, and more than ready to claim their inalienable right to full participation in American life.

Idealists on the move, they proved to have little patience for their elders like Morehouse College's President Mays. Like so many others across the South, they were inspired by the sit-in that began on February 1, 1960, at the Woolworth lunch counter

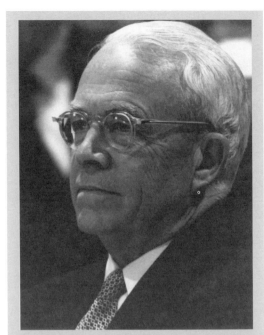

Ivan Allen, Jr., (1911-2003) photographed shortly before his testimony to the U.S. Senate Commerce Committee.

in Greensboro, North Carolina. Although they were ready to mimic the action of the students at North Carolina A&T University (as students were doing across the South) Atlanta's black students held off for several weeks. They followed the advice of their teachers, especially Dr. Rufus E. Clement, the President of Atlanta University, who urged them to write out and publicize their goals before taking direct action. In a full-page advertisement (paid for by the presidents of Atlanta's black colleges) in the city's newspapers on March 9, 1960, the students presented an articulate and passionate manifesto, an "Appeal for Human Rights." The student leaders who drafted and signed the document were direct: They were not going to wait for their rights—or for a redress of the glaring inequities in education, housing, and services blacks suffered in Atlanta and across the nation. They declared themselves ready to take legal, non-violent action to up-end the racial system. Except for a small protest at governmental buildings, however, they would wait for more than six months before beginning massive sit-ins in Atlanta.[53]

With their own organization, the Committee on Appeal for Human Rights (CO-AHR), and leadership, students in Atlanta's black colleges took to the streets, sat-in, got kicked out, and arrested in the pursuit of equal citizenship. Even before they began protesting, the gulf between the students and the city's black power structure seemed so deep and wide that the two groups formed a liaison committee in the spring of 1960. (Yet, student activists received strong support from the older generation, especially the Reverend William Holmes Borders, the dynamic and eloquent pastor of Wheat Street Baptist Church, and his congregation.)[54] The student activists and others outside the city's established black leadership, however, pressed more publicly for desegregation than did their elders.

Starting in the fall of 1960 with sit-ins at lunch counters in downtown Atlanta, including the restaurants at the city's most luxurious department store, Rich's, the students—allied with other organizations—led the fight for access to public accommodations. A settlement that Ivan Allen, Jr., the head of the Atlanta Chamber of Commerce, brokered in March 1961 helped halt sit-ins and boycotts for several months. (Later that year Allen defeated the segregationist Lester Maddox in a bitterly contested mayoral election.) To break down Jim Crow in Atlanta would require pressure from the city's black leaders and student activists, but also commercial pragmatism among the city's white leaders. In short, the profit-motive would help shape the response of Atlanta's white civic and commercial elite to race relations.

Lunch counters, stores, churches, and public schools were the public spaces first subject to negotiation, but medical services soon followed.

The effort to desegregate hospital care in Atlanta gained momentum in May 1961 when Georgia Baptist Hospital, a whites-only hospital owned by the Georgia Baptist Convention, refused to give emergency treatment to an eight-year-old child who had been hit

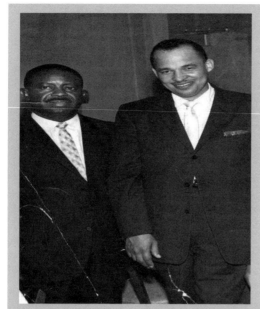
Rev. Ralph David Abernathy (1926-1990) on the left with Dr. Roy C. Bell (1927-2011) on right.

by an automobile.⁵⁵ The driver of the car had taken the bleeding child to Georgia Baptist for treatment. While he knew that the hospital did not accept black inpatients, he was astounded that they refused to give a child first aid. He didn't think they would do that to a dog.⁵⁶ Nurses at Georgia Baptist told him to head for Grady. It was there that the child was treated for lacerations to the face, two broken ribs, and a "large knot on the head." Having made sure that the child was cared for at Grady, the automobile's driver, a white man named Harold Ross, indignantly returned to Georgia Baptist to ask why the hospital refused to treat the child. The answer was supposed to have been obvious—Georgia Baptist had no facilities for black people.

Within days the board of *The Atlanta Inquirer* newspaper took up a new cause: outlawing the refusal of emergency treatment by any hospital in Atlanta.⁵⁷ Under the signature of its president, Jesse Hill, Jr., the newspaper's board of directors sent a letter to Alderman G. Everett Millican. Eloquently echoing President Kennedy's inaugural address, the company's board claimed it was willing "to bear every burden, pay whatever price, and extend ourselves as necessary to the end of protecting human rights, health and welfare of all citizens regardless of race."⁵⁸ In the effort to prevent hospitals in Atlanta from refusing emergency care on the basis of race, the newspaper turned for assistance to the black and white medical societies and nursing societies, the Atlanta Christian Council, several ministerial groups, and the Atlanta Committee For Cooperative Action (ACCA).⁵⁸ It quickly became a cause for the Atlanta Medical Society (whose president, Dr. Clinton E. Warner, also was vice president of *The Atlanta Inquirer's* board).⁵⁹

As a result of the effort, Georgia Baptist Hospital soon apologized for the incident and promised that it would give emergency treatment to blacks. Dr. Warner responded prophetically, saying, "the fight against racial bias in the broad area of health care in a sense is just beginning."⁶¹ At that point, the North Georgia Dental Association and the ACCA showed support for a movement to end discrimination in all areas of health care.⁶⁰ Within weeks the Butler Street YMCA would name Dr. Warner its "Man of the Year" for his leadership in "crusades such as the current effort to secure equal and unsegregated hospital care for all Atlantans."⁶³ The *Inquirer* continued its campaign to desegregate health care with a front-page story at the end of July. It noted that Grady continued to prevent black physicians from serving there even though two-thirds of Grady's patients were black. In obstetrics, blacks had an even larger majority—5,580 of the 6,883 babies born at Grady in 1960 were black.⁶⁴

The push to desegregate Grady won significant publicity thanks to the effort of Dr. Roy C. Bell.⁶⁵ A dentist who was married to Clarice Marijetta Wyatt, a cousin of Dr. Martin Luther King, Jr., Dr. Bell led public discussions in Black Atlanta about segregated health care in the city. In the summer of 1961 he appeared on radio station WERD with Dr. Warner. Together they raised follow-up questions to those Grace Towns Hamilton and the AUL had asked more than a decade earlier. Were the black and white taxpayers being cheated by having to pay more because health services were segregated? Did being cut off from access to proper hospital facilities limit the quality of care black physicians and dentists could offer? What had Emory and the hospital authority done to give a "fair shake" to black physicians and patients at Hughes Spalding Pavilion and Grady hospital?[66] Dr. Bell was certain that the answers would be obvious to any disinterested observer. The solution, Dr. Bell insisted, was for Grady to end its segregation and racial discrimination.

Dr. Bell asked the Fulton County Commission to end racial segregation of patients at the public hospital. Dr. Bell also wanted Grady hospital to open membership in its medical staff to qualified Negro physicians and dentists. In addition, he pressed the Fulton-DeKalb Hospital Authority to appoint blacks to its board and urged the authority to make improvements to Hughes Spalding Pavilion. He pointed out that the hospital dedicated to Atlanta's black middle class lacked an emergency room, a 24-hour doctor on duty in the hospital, and a sufficient number of nurses.

Carlyle Fraser, Chairman of the Fulton County Commission (and the founder and Chairman of Genuine Parts Company), responded to Dr. Bell's appeal in simple terms: the Fulton County Commission did not control Grady. The commission only appointed seven FDHA board members. Chairman Fraser also allowed that the commission did not name people to the board in order to accommodate or represent a certain group. In addition to not having a black member, the hospital authority's board also lacked a physician, a representative of the labor movement, and a Roman Catholic. (Hughes Spalding, an active Roman Catholic, was no longer a member of the authority.) Chairman Fraser's response to Dr. Bell did not end there. Regarding the Pavilion's lack of emergency facilities, Chairman Fraser noted that with Grady hospital standing across the street, emergency facilities were but a few heartbeats away from the Spalding Pavilion. The county board chair also defended staffing practices at Spalding, emphasizing that many hospitals in Atlanta lacked in-house staff physicians 24-hours-per-day.

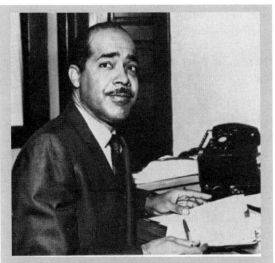

Dr. Clinton E. Warner, Jr., was a World War II veteran, Morehouse College (1948) and Meharry Medical College graduate (1951), civil rights leader, and co-plaintiff in the federal suit to desegregate Grady.

By the middle of August, Dr. Bell had won support for his demands from three prominent national organizations—the National Association for the Advancement of Colored People (NAACP), the National Medical Association, and the National Dental Association. In addition, he was working with the ACCA, the Atlanta Medical Society, The Empire Real Estate Board, The Interdenominational Ministerial Alliance, and local fraternities, sororities, and civic clubs to map out a larger strategy for desegregating all of Grady—including its schools and staff.[67] A new committee, co-chaired by Drs. C. Miles Smith and Clinton Warner, sought meetings with the federal Department of Health, Education, and Welfare, and the U.S. Commission on Civil Rights. It also won backing from Roy Wilkins and Jack Greenberg at the NAACP.[68]

Dr. Bell noted that in order to practice at Grady, a physician needed to be a member of the local medical society affiliated with the American Medical Association. The relevant group, the Fulton County Medical Society, however, did not accept black members. He also noted that "White doctors practice on Negroes to get their training and later do not want to touch them; or have Negroes coming through the back door or after his white patients leave."⁶⁹ The calls for desegregating Grady and the admission of black physicians to practice on its wards won the black activists a rebuke from the *Atlanta Constitution* editorial page, which warned that violence might follow.

In response, Margaret Long, a liberal columnist for the *Atlanta Journal*, wrote, "I'm sure I can't remember how long the idiotic situation at Grady has prevailed so that Negro physicians, in a giant hospital hard put for doctors, can't work in Negro wards of this tax-supported wonder."⁷⁰ Wondering just when the *Constitution* thought it would be the right time for blacks to seek their rights, she mockingly wondered if "the disapproval and possible violence of this illiterate, lawless and emotionally sick native fringe and their imported cohorts" served as a good reason "to delay the simplest rights of respectable Atlantans or to improve operations at Grady Hospital?" Did the city's tranquility really depend on meeting the demands of white segregationists? She decried the need to defer to "the mean-hearted nuts among us."⁷¹

A forum that the Greater Atlanta Council on Human Relations sponsored at the Interdenominational Theological Center in late September addressed two big issues at Grady: the admission of blacks to internships and training programs, and the naming of the nursing residence halls. Appearing with Dean Richardson of Emory and Grace Towns Hamilton were Dr. Heyward Hill, the former president of the medical staff at Hughes Spalding Pavilion, and Dr. Clinton Warner.⁷² One of the main issues was the tone-deaf suggestion from the FDHA to name the new dormitories for African-American nurses after the states of Mississippi and Alabama—two states that hosted notoriously vicious responses to the civil rights movement. (The authority would soon back off from what seemed like an intentionally provocative suggestion.)

Early in October 1961, Dr. Bell and representatives of the NAACP, Atlanta Council on Human Relations, and the Atlanta Medical Association raised the question of desegregating Grady with the Fulton-DeKalb Hospital Authority.⁷³ The FDHA quickly referred the potentially explosive topic to a special committee.

Appearing to still have faith in the Atlanta way, most members of Atlanta's civil rights leadership seemed willing to wait for the committee to make its recommendations. Other supplicants found the situation more urgent. James O. Gibson, the executive secretary of the Atlanta NAACP, said that unless the authority acted, litigation would follow.⁷⁴ Dr. Bell also was in a hurry. His continued outspoken advocacy for Grady's immediate desegregation seemed to chill Dr. Bell's relationship with other black leaders. While he pressed forward, they stayed behind, waiting for the FDHA and its special committee.

By the fall of 1961, desegregation of public space was still beginning in Atlanta. It had been only a few months since student sit-ins at lunch counters forced the Atlanta Chamber of Commerce to the negotiation table. Sitting-in at lunch counters and boycotting grocery stores and department stores were plausible tactics. Boycotting the only hospital available to indigent and working class blacks seemed impossible. The hospital was a necessity; there really were not any alternative sources for hospitalization. Nevertheless, informational pickets and protests began. Certainly few people would have bothered trying to desegregate Grady if the hospital was irrelevant. Indeed, desegregating Grady mattered precisely because the hospital was important—as much as the place of birth and healing as a symbol of public life whose significance nearly rivaled that of public schools.

In November, more than 75 students joined Dr. Bell in picketing outside of Grady. Marching peacefully, they carried signs that read "Disease and Death Know no Race" and "Give the Other 1/3 Of Atlanta An Equal Chance to Live." Where the picketing of restaurants and stores came in conjunction with boycotts, the protest outside of Grady was different. The chairman of the Committee On Appeal for Human Rights (COAHR), Charles A. Black, told a reporter, "We certainly don't want to keep anyone from receiving medical care." The point of the protest, he said, was "seeing that Atlanta's Negroes get an even share of existing medical facilities.'"[75] Coming on the heels of statements from local civil rights organizations condemning Grady's exclusion of black physicians, the direct action was a counter to stagnant behind-the-scenes negotiation. (Fred Turner, the chair of the hospital authority, said that the matter of desegregation at Grady "was in the hands of the U.S. Civil Rights Commission," and he had nothing else to add.)[76]

A week later, *The Atlanta Inquirer* sent a telegram to President Kennedy and members of Congress asking them to help wipe out the segregation clause in the Hill-Burton Act. Essentially, it was supporting Senator Jacob Javits of New York who was preparing a bill to rid the act of a loophole that allowed for segregated medical facilities.[77]

A short time later Grady announced that it had approved an African American candidate for a residency at Grady. The step did not satisfy Dr. Bell or other activists, and flare-up protests took place at Grady early in 1962. On February 6, demonstrators led by the COAHR accused the hospital authority of offering token integration, claiming it was not really allowing black interns to be accepted at Grady. Picketing outside of the hospital continued into the next week. On February 13, twenty-three protestors (including Dr. Bell) were arrested at Grady.[78] The editorial page of the *Constitution* admonished the demonstrators, saying that "the time for general protest ends when specific remedies begin." Dr. Bell and his friends, however, would not be dissuaded.[79]

Students and other activists kept pressing for change. For example, in February 1962, four men from Morehouse College attempted to desegregate Grady's white emergency room and its waiting room. Two "ill" students, Allen R. Coleman and Tom Southern, entered the white clinic without any problem. They made it up to the receptionist without being stopped. She politely asked them to fill out a blue patient information form and they complied. Things were going surprisingly well until Mr. Horace Bearden, the night administrator, intercepted the young men. He asked them to follow him, but before he could take them to the "colored" entrance they asked to be treated in the white emergency room, which was closer and, they pointed out, less crowded. Revere Rogers and George Poole, two students accompanying the ill men from Morehouse, stood quietly in the hallway until they were told to wait elsewhere. Their asking where that should be prompted Bearden to consult with a police lieutenant. Eventually, Bearden directed the four students to use any waiting room that they wished. They entered a white waiting room holding about a dozen people, all of whom left under the calming influence of policemen. After sitting in the room by themselves for about a half-hour, the four men from Morehouse left the hospital.[80]

The next month, on March 5, 1962, the Fulton-DeKalb Hospital Authority announced that Dr. Asa Yancey, who earned his M.D. degree at The University of Michigan School of Medicine in 1941 (and served as Chief of Surgery at Hughes Spalding Pavilion), had become the first African American elected to Grady's staff by the FDHA. By playing down Dr. Yancey's election as "part of the reorganization of Grady and the Spalding Pavilion," the authority hoped to avoid making any waves in White Atlanta.[81] The black press praised the move, repeating the message anti-segregation pickets outside Grady carried on their placards: "disease knows no color lines."[82]

The day after Dr. Yancey was elected to Grady's visiting staff, Sam Phillips McKenzie, a superior court judge for Fulton County, praised the hospital authority for its action as he instructed the new seating of the county's grand jury. After congratulating the people of Atlanta, Fulton County, and the State of Georgia for dealing with desegregating public schools, he noted that the issue also needed to be resolved at Grady hospital. He expressed hope that it would be undertaken there "as intelligently and as gracefully" as the desegregation of the city's public schools, which had recently started with the integration of students in four high schools.[83] (His idea that the school problem had been handled gracefully might have surprised the parents of black children.)

Judge McKenzie told the jurors about to investigate Fulton County's public institutions that the rulings of the United States Supreme Court were the law of the land, and that "ultimately discrimination must, and should be, removed from all areas of public life."[84] Given that the two prior grand juries avoided looking into racial matters at Grady, calling the hospital "well-run," Black Atlanta doubted that the new panel would follow the judge's promptings. In his charge to the grand jury, Judge McKenzie was preparing them for the likelihood that African American citizens would ask to appear and make suggestions about improving public services.[85] Dr. Bell and friends, however, were unlikely to seek the quiet of the grand jury room. Their's was a visibly public protest.

While applauding the FDHA for naming Dr. Yancey to Grady's staff, Dr. Bell reminded everyone he could that it was not enough. He and his fellow activists were still expecting desegregation of the nursing school, improved facilities at Hughes Spalding, and would find "nothing short of total desegregation of all [Grady's] facilities" as the "just and honorable solution." The civil rights community would not be satisfied until there was "complete desegregation for doctors, patients, and staff."[86]

At its meeting exactly 52 weeks earlier, in 1961, the FDHA revealed a remarkably generous act that may have dissipated any concerns the authority's members might have had about black interest in the institution. In the same week that the controversy over desegregating lunch counters in Atlanta's downtown seemed to be resolved, the FDHA announced that Ada Gholston, a 76-year-old black woman who had worked as a cook, had bequeathed her life savings of $3,627.22 to the institution because she had received wonderful treatment there.[87] While Grady had received all manner of gifts before—from land to a billy goat—this appears to have been the first major financial gift from a black patient. The rarity of the act stands out in light of patient attitudes toward the hospital. Whatever loyalty such deeds may have implied, Black Atlanta's recognition of Grady's vital role could be seen in the move to desegregate the hospital in the year following Ms. Gholston's passing.

In the same week that the FDHA removed the color barrier that had blocked black physicians from practicing at Grady, several major civil rights organizations rejoined Dr. Bell's effort to end all segregation at the hospital. Leaders in the NAACP, the SCLC, and the Student Nonviolent Coordinating Committee (SNCC) together with officials from the Atlanta Medical Association and the North Georgia Dental Society joined Dr. Bell in asking for Grady's complete desegregation.[88]

Leading a delegation of speakers before a special session of the Fulton County Commission, Dr. Bell warned that a lawsuit was coming unless the county created a systematic plan for fully desegregating Grady. (The three-member commission had called the special meeting to hear complaints about racial discrimination at Grady. All but two members of the board of the Fulton-DeKalb Hospital Authority also attended the meeting.) Dr. Bell claimed the FDHA had failed to act in good faith with Black Atlanta. Indeed, the special session of the county commission only took place after the FDHA had refused to hear Dr. Bell and others several times. At the commission meeting, a remarkable coalition of old and new leaders from Black Atlanta joined to press their case.

Dr. Hezekiah Lewis, president of the Atlanta Medical Association, told the commissioners that his group strongly supported the complete desegregation of Grady. Dr. Martin Luther King, Jr., announced that the SCLC was fully behind Dr. Bell, and he urged the commissioners to rely on "moral stamina and moral courage" to press the authority and hospital officials to desegregate Grady. The Reverend Ralph David Abernathy, pastor of West Hunter Street Baptist Church and treasurer of the SCLC, and the Reverend Martin Luther King, Senior, also addressed the commission. The Reverend King, Sr., bluntly told the commissioners that Black Atlanta was

Dr. Gwendolyn Cooper Manning

Seemingly stepping up the pace of its efforts, a month after Dr. Yancey's inclusion at Grady the hospital announced Dr. Gwendolyn Cooper Manning had joined its visiting staff. The daughter of a distinguished dentist in Atlanta, Dr. A. B. Cooper, Sr., she became the second African American and the first black woman named to that position. A graduate of Spelman College and Meharry Medical College, Dr. Manning had served as an intern at Chicago's Provident Hospital and as a resident at the Veterans Administration Hospital in Tuskegee, where she eventually became Assistant Chief of Medical Services. Having worked with Dr. Yancey at Tuskegee, she was drawn to Atlanta late in 1961 to enter private practice in internal medicine.[101] Other African American physicians appointed to Grady's staff following Dr. Manning included Dr. William W. Stewart and Dr. James D. Palmer. They were named to Grady's visiting staff in August 1962.[102]

"only asking for first class citizenship like anyone else."[89] This would include, according to a petition delivered by Charles Black, a student leader with the COAHR, accepting black physicians to full staff membership, admitting "all qualified persons" to the schools of medicine and x-ray technology, desegregating the nursing school, admitting black nurses to the post-graduate program, appointing an African American to the hospital authority, and fully desegregating all of Grady's facilities.[90] While the meeting seemed to have little immediate impact on the county commission or the FDHA, it looked like Dr. Bell and Black Atlanta's old guard stood unified.

Within two months, however, the relationship between Dr. Bell and established leaders in Black Atlanta fractured again. In an article in *The Atlanta Inquirer,* Dr. Bell "denounced a sniping campaign against him" by "Negro leaders."[91] He thought they were afraid that he would challenge their leadership in the community. Whatever worries they might have had about Dr. Bell, it would have been hard for them to match the headaches he was causing the Fulton-DeKalb Hospital Authority.

The public, insistent, and often abrasive nature of Dr. Bell's protest violated local customs. He was breaking unspoken and unwritten rules that had governed official race relations in Atlanta since the race riot of 1906. For the members of the FDHA, who saw themselves as following the Atlanta way of taking gradual, safe steps toward desegregation, Dr. Bell was radically impatient. The FDHA didn't want to move too fast.

The hospital authority was worried about the consequences of desegregating Grady. While wealthy whites had their own hospitals to turn to—like Piedmont Hospital—where else could people who relied on the public hospital turn to for medical treatment? The circumstance for many in the middle class was mitigated to some degree by the increasing use of hospital insurance as a benefit of employment. While more people were enjoying that benefit, and fewer paid the whole cost of hospitalization out of their own pocket, it was far from universal. Given the shortage of available options for lower income whites, the hospital authority continued to believe that desegregating patient care at Grady could unleash severe social conflict.

Much of the FDHA appeared anxious about the potential response of white patients to desegregation. Would patients from White Grady accept integrated hospital rooms? Would they even agree to, much less be comfortable, sharing a hospital room with someone with whom they would not share a public restroom or water fountain? Especially given the potential personal intimacies involved in hospital treatment, the board's white members—the only sort it had—doubted that White Grady's patients would embrace the hospital's integration. All this seemed vexing to the board before anyone could even stop to ask if white patients would accept care from black physicians. While concerned about the response of white patients, the FDHA had a greater fear of the wrath of white friends and relatives in the hospital's waiting rooms. Given the city's racial history, the hospital authority seemed to have plenty to worry about—at least from white residents. To the FDHA, the prospects for whites peacefully acquiescing to the consolidation of White Grady and Black Grady seemed dim. While the board worried about the concerns of whites, its members assumed black residents would embrace desegregation.

The effort to desegregate the publicly owned hospital took place at the same time Black Atlanta was pushing the city's board of education to enforce the U.S. Supreme Court's ruling in *Brown v. the Board of Education of Topeka, Kansas*. The speed in desegregating Atlanta's schools was proving far too deliberate for the parents of black children. Similarly, after several months of lobbying for change at Grady, Dr. Bell and his colleagues found the FDHA far too languid in addressing the fiercely urgent issue.

On June 19, 1962, Drs. Roy C. Bell and Clinton Warner, Miss Ruby Doris Smith and her mother, Alice Banks Smith, the Reverend John Middleton, Ms. Edwina M. Smith, Mrs. Dorothy Cotton, and Mrs. Septima Clark, all "Atlanta residents and taxpayers," filed a lawsuit in federal court to desegregate patient care, the medical staff, and medical training at Grady. In addition, the suit sought to desegregate state and local medical societies in Georgia.

Although he had gained backing from civil rights organizations, publicly Dr. Bell had been "a virtual one-man gang" since the meeting with the county commissioners three months earlier.[92] By the time he filed the suit, Dr. Bell had become a familiar face in Atlanta. Unpredictable and sometimes outrageous, Dr. Bell seemed out of control not only to whites, but also to other activists. Civil rights veterans, like the distinguished A. T. Walden, held Dr. Bell at arms length, as did younger activists, because they worried his often harsh and provocative comments would undercut the movement.[93] As a result, Dr. Bell waged a fairly lonely battle for many

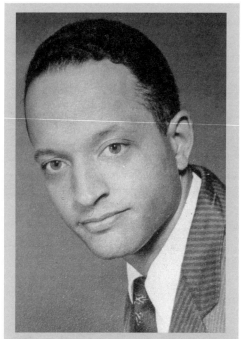

Dr. Lee Shelton, a graduate of Howard University College of Medicine and a well-respected general surgeon in Atlanta, was one of the first two physicians to integrate the Fulton County Medical Society.

months, only joined occasionally by students from the COAHR. The most important support he received came from members of the SCLC.

Dr. Bell was active in the Southern Christian Leadership Conference, as were Mrs. Cotton, Mrs. Clark, and the Reverend Middleton. Mrs. Cotton was a member of the SCLC's staff who would direct its citizenship education program. Mrs. Clark was the daughter of a slave and a legendary civil rights figure known for her literacy programs and citizenship schools. Reverend Middleton was president of the Atlanta chapter of the SCLC and wrote a weekly column on the Bible for *The Atlanta Inquirer*. While the SCLC could not contain Dr. Bell's tendency to be outspoken and, sometimes, somewhat outrageous, Dr. Warner, the surgeon and fellow plaintiff, had a moderating influence on Dr. Bell and served as an important bridge between him and black business leaders. Another plaintiff in the case, Ruby Doris Smith, a Grady Baby and graduate of Atlanta's public schools, was a student at Spelman College. Her relative youth should not obscure her significance. A rising leader in the civil rights movement, and a veteran of picket lines and jail cells when the suit was filed, Smith brought energy and important student support to Dr. Bell's cause. (A courageous and effective leader, she became the most powerful woman in the Student Nonviolent Coordinating Committee until she was felled by cancer in 1967 at the age of 25.)[94] As vital as the plaintiffs were to the lawsuit against Grady, the case obviously depended on their lawyers.

The National Association for the Advancement of Colored People (NAACP) became involved in Dr. Bell's case, just as it had engaged in civil rights activity since its founding more than a half-century before (three years after the Atlanta Race Riot of 1906). The NAACP had led the successful fight against Georgia's whites-only primary two decades before the NAACP Legal Defense and Educational Fund (LDF) took the lead in legal efforts to desegregate Grady. Attorneys Jack Greenberg, James M. Nabrit III, and Michael Meltsner of the LDF in New York joined local attorneys Donald Lee Hollowell and Horace T. Ward to serve as the plaintiff's legal talent. The lawsuit named the Medical Association of Georgia, the Northern District Dental Society, the Fulton County Medical Society, the Georgia Dental Society, the Fulton-DeKalb Hospital Authority, and Grady's Administrator, Frank Wilson, as defendants.

The lawsuit was ambitious. According to the Chicago *Defender*, the LDF considered the suit to be "the broadest legal attack on medical segregation to date."[95] The plaintiffs claimed that Grady violated the Fifth and Fourteenth Amendments to the United States Constitution by remaining segregated while getting more than 85% of its operating budget from public funds. The hospital, they noted, had received $6 million in public money towards its $7 million operating budget in 1960.

Only two months before the case's first scheduled hearing in federal court, the Fulton County Medical Society met (on July 5, 1962) to review a proposal from Dr. Ebert Van Buren, a distinguished physician who created Grady's first diabetes clinic in the 1930s. He suggested that the society remove all racial restrictions on its membership. Acting with relative quickness, the society passed Dr. Van Buren's proposal the next month. Within weeks, and in the same month of its first scheduled appearance in court as a defendant in the lawsuit, the Fulton County Medical Society quietly admitted two black physicians. Dr. Lee Shelton, a general surgeon who graduated from the Howard University College of Medicine in 1951, was one of the black doctors brought into the society's fold. Dr. Asa Yancey was the other black physician honored with admission to the society. Since the society had removed its racial barriers to membership, the court dismissed the Fulton County Medical Society as a defendant in the lawsuit.

Momentous legal and political developments helped further undercut Jim Crow between the time Dr. Bell and his fellow plaintiffs filed their lawsuit in the summer of 1962 and when the U.S. District Court issued its final order in the case more than two years later.

The federal courts continued to follow the precedent established by the Supreme Court's unanimous decision in *Brown*. Even in southern areas where federal district court judges upheld forms of institutional segregation, the U.S. Court of Appeals for the Fifth Circuit—led by the outstanding jurist Elbert P. Tuttle—reversed lower courts, regularly affirming racial equality.

Politically, the U.S. Congress began considering legislation that would lay out extensive federal protection to civil rights. Among other provisions, the projected bill would prohibit discrimination in public accommodations on account of race. Significantly, it also blocked racial discrimination by entities that received federal funds. While the bill's details hardly were set in stone, its intentions were plain when, in 1963, support for federal civil rights legislation emerged among white businessmen in Atlanta. Indeed, Atlanta's political leadership stood out as Congress debated the law.

On July 26, 1963, thirteen months after Dr. Bell filed his federal lawsuit against Grady, Mayor Ivan Allen, Jr., testified before Congress in favor of the proposed civil rights legislation. To help get his civil rights law through the Senate, President Kennedy wanted a respected southern politician to testify in favor of the pending legislation, and Atlanta's mayor fit the bill. Because he had come to reject segregation, Mayor Allen stood at odds with most southern white politicians. He had defeated the strident segregationist Lester Maddox in the mayoral election only two years earlier, shortly after having a change of heart concerning Jim Crow. To overcome Maddox's overwhelming support among Atlanta's white middle class, Allen had relied on the long-standing coalition of blacks and upper class whites. Mayor Allen's support for what became the Civil Rights Act of 1964 was as pragmatic as his political coalition.

Mr. Allen was born into Atlanta's closely connected white elite—a community of leaders who lived in a geographically small area that largely governed the city. Allen's family business, the Ivan Allen Company, prospered by selling office supplies. Eventually assuming control of the company from his father, Ivan Allen, Jr., did business with his neighbors and childhood friends—who just happened to run the city's leading commercial and civic enterprises. Before becoming mayor, Ivan Allen, Jr. served as president of the Atlanta Chamber of Commerce; he practically embodied White Atlanta's power structure.

Like most Atlantans whose family earned its fortune through hard-nosed pragmatism, Ivan Allen was a realist. He said as much when he testified in front of the United States Senate Commerce Committee. In the summer of 1963, Mayor Allen could do no less than admit that Atlanta's comparative "measure of success" in desegregation came "only because we have looked facts in the face and accepted the Supreme Court's decisions as inevitable and as the law of the land." Mayor Allen warned senators that "cities like Atlanta might slip backward" unless Congress laid out the civil rights law.[96] It is hard to overestimate the significance of Mayor Allen's testimony in helping get the Civil Rights Act of 1964 through the United States Senate despite strong opposition from staunchly segregationist senators.

In 1963 the FDHA fully understood what was happening in the city and across the South. Its members recognized that change was on the way. Like other white leaders in Atlanta they faced the facts, but their highest priority was to prevent racial violence. For that reason the FDHA worked toward a relatively modest, step-by-step desegregation of Grady. While the authority seemed somewhat willing to move on the issue, it also had to deal with Grady's superintendent, Frank Wilson, an otherwise highly effective administrator who resisted desegregation. After a heart attack felled Wilson in 1964, the hospital authority promoted assistant superintendent Bill Pinkston to run Grady.

Bill Pinkston was a smart, optimistic man who was well liked and highly respected by the people he dealt with and led. Raised as a Methodist in Valdosta, Georgia, Pinkston imbibed his denomination's ethos of social justice and adopted his parents' capacity for empathy. He also endured the economic reality of the Great Depression as he watched his father lose nearly everything during those years. At the time Bill Pinkston became Grady's acting superintendent, he already had worked at the hospital for seventeen years, developing an untarnished reputation for fairness and integrity. During those years Pinkston learned the hospital's finances inside and out. By 1964, Bill Pinkston had almost become a native of Grady hospital. An affable man, he put the interests of the hospital first. Bill Pinkston would be as effective as his predecessor, but differ from him in two vital way. First, Bill Pinkston would get along well with the people from Emory University like Dean Richardson and, second, Pinkston was anything but a segregationist. Pinkston was, however, a realist: he knew that middle class whites were angry about desegregation, and that they believed judges and the federal government were taking "their" public spaces away from them. To take away their hospital could provoke them into the riots that city leaders had avoided during the desegregation of golf courses, parks, and swimming pools.

The legal and political landscape changed greatly in the first two years after Dr. Bell filed his suit. Thus, by the start of 1964, a reasonable person could assume that the federal court might find in favor of Dr. Bell and the other plaintiffs. In February 1964, Judge Frank Hooper ruled that the Georgia Dental Association and the Northern District Dental Society had to admit black dentists.[97] One year later, in February 1965, Judge Hooper ordered Grady to desegregate its facilities and services.

The hospital quietly implemented the court's decision. Without any extra fuss, the landmark action in Grady's history officially happened on June 1, 1965. To mark the event, Superintendent Pinkston simply announced, "all phases of the hospital are on a non-racial basis effective today. We are grouping patients strictly on their medical needs. All outpatients, all inpatients, and all heart patients, etc."[98]

The resolution to Dr. Bell's lawsuit lacked drama in its denouement. There were no outbreaks of violence among the patients or their friends and relatives. The hospital authority's anxieties proved unfounded. In retrospect, the board and hospital leaders realized they could have moved ahead safely much earlier. Nearly twenty years after his retirement, Bill Pinkston wistfully admitted that given the chance to change anything in his tenure at Grady, he would have fully desegregated the hospital earlier.[99]

While the court order, effectively negotiated by the parties, prompted the desegregation of Grady in 1965, recent federal legislation was offering hospitals a significant financial incentive to change their ways. The Civil Rights Act of 1964, which prohibited discrimination by entities that received federal funds, had little immediate effect on Grady's financing. After President Johnson signed the Social Security Amendments of 1965 into law, however, Grady's finances would be transformed.

The creation of Medicare and Medicaid provided a financial boon to hospitals that cared for people who were formerly unable to fully pay for their medical treatment. Under these programs, services long discounted or rendered for free began generating revenue. These programs also created incentives and opportunities for Grady and other hospitals to offer new services. The law providing for Medicare and Medicaid would also indirectly force the desegregation of American hospitals.[100]

As the previously all-white hospitals in Atlanta began taking non-white patients at the end of the 1960s, and started accepting federal money for treating the once medically indigent, they would find ways to prosper from the new federal regulations. Those same laws, over the course of a generation, would lead a host of rivals to compete for some of Grady's patients and further complicate the hospital's finances.

Pioneers in Children's and Maternal Health

In 1972 Dr. John Daniel (Dan) Thompson of Grady and Emory's GYN-OB* department convinced Governor Jimmy Carter to appoint a Maternal and Infant Care Council. From its founding, the state council became instrumental in establishing a regional prenatal care system, first locally and then throughout Georgia.

This was hardly the first time Dr. Thompson persuaded people of the virtue of a powerful idea. Since becoming chairman of the Department of Gynecology and Obstetrics in 1961, Thompson led Grady's GYN-OB department in generating a host of strong, innovative programs. Many of these were designed to combat the high rate of reproductive mortality in the community. Others were designed for "improved gynecologic and obstetric care for the indigent." All of them improved the training of residents and medical students.[1]

Expanding the idea of what gynecology and obstetrics are was central to Dr. Thompson's vision. Gynecology, in his view, covered "the whole concept of femaleness." Obstetrics went far beyond the biology of reproduction; it involved caring for the woman in full. In practical terms, this meant that patients with primary gynecological disease and obstetrics patients would no longer be transferred to the care of another department at Grady if they contracted an illness or developed complications. Also, the idea of total reproductive health care included assessing behavioral and social factors that affected the outcome of a pregnancy. Dr. Thompson envisioned an ideal world in which a patient's obstetric care began before conception. His vision insisted on physicians understanding and being involved in the broader community. If they didn't, how would they really know their patients? He also challenged the notion that the high rate of death and disease among the South's poor was inevitable. Most importantly, with the support of private foundations, federal funding, and the administrations of Emory University and Grady hospital, he embarked on a mission to do something about the problem.

Under the leadership of Dr. Newton Long, the GYN-OB department inaugurated the Maternal and Infant Care Project at Grady in July 1965.[2] A five-year, seven million dollar grant from the Children's Bureau of the federal Department of Health, Education, and Welfare allowed Grady to develop a program to care for "high risk" mothers and their infants. Grady added 25 obstetric beds in the program's first year and twenty-five more in 1966. In an effort to improve outcomes for indigent women—the women with the highest risk for complications—the program addressed a broad range of issues, including malnutrition, high blood pressure, diabetes, heart disease, and kidney disease. The program assisting indigent women was seen as improving "the total health level of the community."[3]

---

* Dr. Thompson insisted on the designation GYN-OB over the more commonly used OB-GYN.

In its portrayal of the Maternal and Infant Care Project, Grady put the program in the context of the common good. Dr. Malcom Freeman, an obstetrician and perinatal pathologist, noted in the hospital's employee newsletter that the program was "not designed to make it easier for poor folks to have babies…but to break the ring of poverty by helping high risk mothers have healthier, more normal babies who can grow to be productive citizens."[4]

The project rapidly gained recognition as the finest reproductive care program for indigent patients in the United States. It also won acclaim from its patients, over 2,000 of whom were cared for in the program's first 14 months. (They were treated during pregnancy, delivery, and the postpartum period.) The program also became a hub for research that would change lives. For example, in 1967 the project "reported that 12.3% (722) of all deliveries at Grady hospital were of patients from 11 to 16 years of age, and 122 of these patients were having their 2nd, 3rd, and 4th child."[5] This information led to the creation of Atlanta's Adolescent Pregnancy Program in conjunction with Atlanta Public Schools.

The GYN-OB department had also created a Division of Perinatal Pathology in 1963. This crucial program—and its subsidiary Social Research Section and Abortion Surveillance Section—collected crucial data about premature births and perinatal deaths. While it predated the Maternal and Infant Care Project, it became a crucial part of the larger effort. By 1976 the results of the Maternal and Infant Care Project were staggering. Grady Hospital recorded its lowest perinatal mortality rate, the lowest fetal death rate, the lowest neonatal death rate, and the lowest premature birth rate in its history.

The GYN-OB department also organized an important gynecologic cancer program. By 1966, out of all of Grady's cancer patients, one out of every five suffered from uterine cancer. While the most frequently seen malignant disease in the hospital, only a dozen patients were diagnosed in the disease's early stages. Half of Grady's patients with cervical cancer were at Stage III or Stage IV. Because many of Grady's patients with uterine cancer were first seen and treated only after it was in an advanced stage, screening more adult women for the disease would be vitally important to improving outcomes for Grady's patients. By 1970, half of the cervical cancer patients at Grady were in the initial stage of the disease—a remarkable shift from a decade earlier.

The department also created a renowned Family Planning Program whose roots were in a conference on "Community Organization for Family Planning" held in May 1962. Grady also established a family planning clinic that attracted a large number of patients. (Grady's family planning clinics saw 21,125 patients in 1970.) Designed simply to improve health, the voluntary program influenced the development of similar services throughout Georgia.

Yet, with all those achievements, the creation of the regional prenatal care system ranks among the most significant acccomplishments of Grady's GYN-OB department under Dr. Thompson's leadership.

Not to be forgotten, Grady's GYN-OB department continued to deliver babies into the world—at a rate of about one per hour during the late 1960s and early 1970s. In addition, between 1960 and 1970, 63 physicians completed training in its residency program—and more than half remained in Georgia. In 1971, more than one-third of the GYN-OB physicians in the Atlanta area had taken their residency at Grady (47 out of 132).[6]

In the context of the extraordinary initiatives Grady's GYN-OB department undertook, three physicians on the Emory-Grady faculty would make outstanding contributions toward alleviating the significant problem of low birth weight newborns and their subsequent high mobidity and mortality rates.

Dr. Luella Klein

Born in rural Walker, Iowa, Dr. Luella Klein was one of two women in her class at the University of Iowa College of Medicine. After graduating with her M.D. degree in

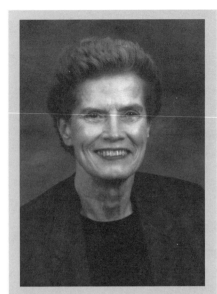

Dr. Luella Klein
An outstanding educator, gynecologist and obstetrician, and advocate for women's reproductive health

1949, Dr. Klein served a residency in gynecology and obstetrics at the Case Western Reserve University in Cleveland. From there Dr. Klein moved to Atlanta where she became a national leader in maternal and fetal medicine. Eventually she would head the Interpregnancy Care Project at Grady and, together with Dr. Al Brann, was an original co-director of the Emory Regional Perinatal Center. She later became director of maternal and infant care at Grady hospital. Known for expressing her views plainly, publicly, and vigorously, Dr. Klein has been a strong advocate of helping mothers of low-birth weight babies. Throughout her career she pushed colleagues to provide better prenatal care and sought increased state and federal funding to help make it a reality for as many patients as possible.

Through her efforts, and those of colleagues like Dr. Malcolm Freeman and Dr. Jacob Adams, physicians at Grady learned much about the problems that unplanned and unwanted pregnancies caused young teens. By the early 1970s Grady hospital annually saw nearly 900 deliveries to girls 16 and under.[7] Once they became pregnant, these girls were excluded from public schools—not only in Atlanta, but also across Georgia. Working with the Atlanta Board of Education, Dr. Klein promoted new policies designed to keep pregnant girls and those with young children in the public schools. Together with Dr. Benjamin Mays, then the president of Atlanta's school board, Congressman Andrew Young, Dr. Asa Yancey, and others, Dr. Klein promoted better nutrition and health care in addition to educational opportunities for teenage mothers. As a member of an *ad hoc* committee chaired by Dr. Robert A. Hatcher, Dr. Klein worked with a number of physicians and community groups trying to improve health services for teenagers in Atlanta.

Dr. Klein led a national campaign in the mid-1980s to reduce unwanted pregnancy in the United States. She urged American physicians to better explain the risks and benefits of various methods of contraception to their patients. She also spoke out against efforts to block teenagers from receiving birth-control assistance. One of the central elements in her campaign encouraged teenagers to learn more about sexual responsibility.[8] Based on her experience as the head of the teen clinic at Grady, Dr. Klein fully supported increasing federal funding for family planning clinics that served the poor and she consistently opposed efforts to reduce funding for family-planning services. Given that poor teenagers are among the most likely candidates for having high-risk pregnancies and low-birth weight babies, it made sense to help them avoid becoming pregnant. At the time, almost half of teen pregnancies in Georgia ended in abortion. Thus, she worked feverishly to prevent unwanted teen pregnancy through sex education and public health programs.

Her efforts were especially significant in Georgia because of the state's high rate of infant mortality during the mid-1980s. With an average of thirteen deaths for every 1,000 live births, Georgia had the fifth-highest rate of infant mortality in the United States. Sadly, by the mid-1990s, Georgia still ranked 48th in the nation in reproductive health.[9]

In the course of her career, Dr. Klein gained exceptional professional success and won numerous awards. Among other achievements, she was the first woman elected president of the American College of Obstetricians and Gynecologists. More significantly, she trained a large number of residents in gynecology and obstetrics at Grady Hospital. Most importantly, she successfully delivered many babies during her career.

Dr. Alfred Brann, Jr.

Dr. Alfred Brann, Jr., grew up in northern Alabama. Given that his mother died giving birth to him, it is fitting that Dr. Brann has devoted his life to improving the health of women and newborns. After extensive training in pediatrics and pediatric neurology, Dr. Brann was appointed Director of the Division of Newborn Medicine at the University of Mississippi in 1969, a position he held until 1975 when he became the director of the Division of Neonatal-Perinatal Medicine in the Emory University School of Medicine and Grady Memorial Hospital. He continued as its director until 1990 when he relocated to the College of Medicine at the University of Oklahoma to become the chairman of the Department of Pediatrics. Three years later he returned to the Emory-Grady system. In 2002, Dr. Brann was presented with the Lifetime Achievement Award from the Georgia chapter of the American Academy of Pediatrics.

While Director of Neonatal and Perinatal Medicine at Grady, Dr. Brann was involved in a highly successful regional perinatal program that was responsible for a 50% decline in the hospital's infant death rate between 1975 and 1996. Dr. Brann also helped create the Interpregnancy Care Program, a project focused on reducing the number of very low birth weight newborns by improving the health of reproductive age women. Through his efforts, together with those of Dr. Luella Klein and other colleagues, Atlanta achieved the lowest rate of infant deaths in the six perinatal regions of Georgia. (Albany, Savannah, Augusta, Columbus, and Macon were the other five regions.)

During the 1990s, Dr. Brann focused his efforts on lowering the staggeringly high

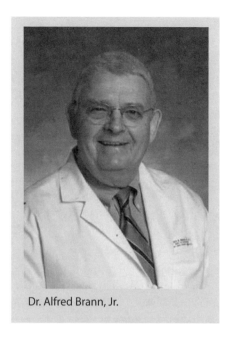

Dr. Alfred Brann, Jr.

infant mortality figures in countries around the world, including China, India, Pakistan, and the Republic of Georgia. As director of the World Health Organization/Collaborating Center in Perinatal Care and Health Services Research in Maternal and Child Health, Dr. Brann was able to help universities, government agencies, and health professionals worldwide measure perinatal success and improve outcomes for patients.

Dr. Andre Nahmias

Dr. Andre Nahmias arrived on Grady's campus in 1964 and was appointed Chief of Pediatric Infectious Diseases at Grady and Egleston Children's Hospital, positions he would hold until 1998. He earned his M.D. degree from George Washington University School of Medicine in 1957. He served the following two years with the U.S. Public Health Service, and then continued his training in Boston in the field of neurology and infectious diseases. In addition to his role in the infectious disease department, in 1970 Dr. Nahmias was appointed Professor of Pediatrics in the Emory University School of Medicine. He taught there until his retirement in 2003.

Dr. Nahmias authored or co-authored 281 highly respected peer-reviewed medical journal articles concerning subjects such as staphylococcus infections, meningitis, HIV, and herpes simplex diseases. His efforts with the herpes simplex virus received worldwide recognition and included research on the rapid diagnosis and treatment of this potentially deadly disease in newborns. His work with Dr. C. Alford of the University of Alabama Medical School in Birmingham and several other collaborators showed that early treatment of neonatal Herpes Simplex infections with the drug Vidarabine (adenine arabinoside) was beneficial but it clearly was not going to be the answer to this disease.[10] In a follow-up study reported in 1986, Drs. Nahmias, Alford, Richard J. Whitley, F. Y. Aoki, and several other participants proved that acyclovir, a selective inhibitor of herpes simplex virus replication, was the treatment of choice for herpes simplex encephalitis and a major improvement over Vidarabine.[11] These studies were major breakthroughs in therapy and gave Grady Memorial Hospital national and international recognition. During the years between 1965 and 1978, Dr. Nahmias was one of the thirty most cited virologists in the world.[12]

The last years of Dr. Nahmias's active career were devoted to the growing problem of HIV in newborns. He helped create the first pediatric AIDS clinic in Georgia (at Grady) in 1986. Along with other pioneering pediatric AIDS clinics, Grady's developed ahead of federal funding for pediatric AIDS clinics and before the first major national foundations to fund the fight against pediatric AIDS were organized. By the end of 1987, the Centers for Disease Control reported 737 pediatric AIDS cases across the nation, a figure generally considered to be low because of underreporting and late-reporting of the illness. That year Congress included $5 million for Pediatric AIDS Demonstration Projects for the 1988 fiscal year (October 1, 1987—September 30, 1988).

The next year, 1988, Elizabeth Glaser, a woman from California who unknowingly contracted HIV/AIDS from a blood transfusion and unwittingly transmitted the illness to her daughter (through breast milk) and her son (in utero), together with friends

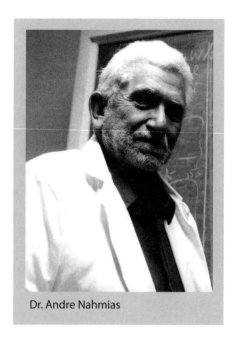

Dr. Andre Nahmias

Susie Zeegen and Susan DeLaurentis formed a foundation to fund and support Pediatric AIDS research. The Elizabeth Glaser Pediatric AIDS Foundation quickly began to play a major role in bringing hope to children with the disease and in helping prevent the spread of AIDS around the world.

Since its founding by Congress in 1990, the Ryan White HIV/AIDS Program has provided the bulk of federal funding for Pediatric AIDS care and research and has provided important financial support to Grady's clinic.

Private foundations and federal funding have provided crucial financial support for pioneering immunologists like Dr. Nahmias and his colleagues at Grady. Their research laid crucial scientific groundwork by investigating the disease and its implications for women and infants when the virus was first being uncovered. Dr. Nahmias also helped make Grady one of the first institutions in the nation to regularly test pregnant women for HIV/AIDS. This screening was vitally important in helping to prevent the transmission of the disease from infected women to their newborns.

Expanding Grady as Georgia Grows
1965 - 1989

"You know, when you take everything into consideration, you'd have to be crazy to run a general hospital."
—Grady Patient and Member, Health Subcommittee, Citizens Central Advisory Council, Economic Opportunity Atlanta, quoted in the *Atlanta Journal*, October 21, 1970.

If a historian had to select a single hinge year in Grady's history, there would be a strong argument for choosing 1965. Not only was it the year in which the long fight over Grady's desegregation finally ended, it also was a critical year in reorienting Grady's future. While white flight and desegregation reshaped Grady's social world, the passage that year of new federal programs (Medicare and Medicaid) to pay for the medical care of the elderly and the poor put the hospital's finances and ambitions on a new path.

The rise of Medicare and Medicaid altered Grady's economic reality and affected its relationship with other hospitals in the city. For generations Grady had been the safety valve for Atlanta's private hospitals by relieving them of much of the expense associated with charity care. In essence, Atlanta's private hospitals couldn't have lived without Grady. The enactment of Medicare and Medicaid, however, would turn the safety valve into something completely different: a competitor for serving the newly insured patients. Once the federal programs took hold, the formerly uninsured elderly and the poor would have an easier time being admitted to private hospitals. In 1967, hospital administrators widely assumed that the new federal programs would mean the end of public hospitals. Although at first fewer patients used public hospitals, the numbers quickly rebounded.[1]

As the new federal programs started offering hospitals reimbursement, older distinctions between private and public hospitals blurred. Gradually, private hospitals began accepting public dollars from Medicare and Medicaid to treat "private" patients. In addition, tax-exempt bond financing for private hospitals made the distinction between private and public hospitals even fuzzier. This shift in the character of private hospitals would have a large impact on Grady. At first, however, Grady had the advantage of suddenly receiving funds for treating people who had been charity cases. (The city's private hospitals were far from ready to absorb very many of the newly insured patients.) This meant a great deal of money for Grady and, together with federal grants for education and research, helped the hospital improve and expand its services.

Treating those with nowhere else to go—along with relieving private hospitals from much of the burden of charity care—had been a central part of Grady's mission. Those goals remained, but increasingly the working poor (rather than the indigent) had nowhere else to turn. The cost of treating the uninsured—people with too much income to qualify for Medicaid but who were denied or could not afford private insurance—would be a central concern for Grady in the coming decades, as would rising costs.

In the 1960s, ongoing demands for novel and increasingly expensive medical technologies required Grady to continue to adapt and spend. In addition, Grady would have to make substantial investments in its physical plant in the coming decades. Although in 1965 its facility was less than a decade old, new technologies, changing medical practices, and the increasing demands spurred by metro Atlanta's growing population would drive Grady to reorganize and improve its facilities.

Centralized air conditioning had become increasingly plausible for commercial space by the mid-1960s, in large part because the cost had fallen dramatically in the years since the new Grady hospital was built. By 1968, as air conditioning became an imperative for American hospitals, Grady began installing a cooling system. Estimated to cost $3.5 million, the project involved installing ductwork and chilled water lines throughout the building. On December 2 and 3, 1968, three giant chillers (each costing $70,000 and weighing 50,000 pounds) were placed on the roof of Grady's clinic wing. By the summer of 1970 the entire outpatient clinic and the rest of the hospital were finally connected to a central air-conditioning system.[2] At the same time that Grady was installing its mechanical cooling system—an important and still relatively expensive investment—it also was adopting another type of new and costly equipment, the mainframe computer.

The introduction of Medicare and Medicaid, together with the expanded use of commercially available insurance, led to a massive increase in the processing of claims by the hospital. The Fulton-DeKalb Hospital Authority noted that the new federal programs "led to a transition from the hospital's traditional charity service to a situation in which statements of charges must be prepared and presented to third-party payers in the cases of higher and higher [sic] percentages of patients."[3] Simply handling those demands meant the hospital would need to address its organization, systems, and management.

Following a study of the hospital's business office in 1967 by Arthur Andersen and Company, a national accounting firm, Grady purchased a mainframe computer system. The large RCA Spectra 70/35 computer would help with a broad range of administrative needs, including patient census, inpatient accounts receivables, outpatient accounts receivables, payroll, asset depreciation, accounts payable, storeroom and pharmacy inventory, general ledger, budget, and workload statistics.

Two year later, Grady bought a newer model of the RCA Spectra with twice as much available processing memory and double the processing speed. During that year, 1970, Grady's data processing department would generate the billing for 1,000,000 patients.[4] (Grady's computer was also used to manage nearly all of Spalding Pavilion's administrative needs except for receivables and inventory.) This technological advance, however, did not mean the end of paper files. In 1970, Grady added 58,706 paper file folders to the shelves of the Medical Records department—one for each new patient who came to the hospital that year.

The computer system required a huge room for the computer itself, numerous desks for clerical staff that used a keypunch system to enter data, space for a tape library, and an area for programmers. Over time, however, the space required for Grady's computers would diminish. While computers had become central to the administration of Grady's business affairs by 1970, it would be several more years before Grady began to computerize medical information.

The pioneering efforts of Dr. David H. Vroon, the chief of Grady's clinical laboratories, led to the computerization of the clinical laboratory in 1978. This made test results immediately available at computer terminals elsewhere in the hospital, saving time for physicians and nurses, and improving patient care.⁵

Long Range Planning

In 1968, the Fulton-DeKalb Hospital Authority hired Cresap, McCormick and Paget Management, a firm specializing in hospital management, to develop a long-term plan for Grady. Funded by the FDHA, Emory University, and an anonymous private source, the study provided Grady with a ten-year development plan. (The authority had hired the same firm for a similar project in 1960.) The study, coming in eighteen months later at over 100 pages, offered a roadmap for developing programs and services on the Grady campus. It also examined the relationship between Emory and Grady and the future of Hughes Spalding Pavilion. According to Grady's Medical Director, Dr. Douglas Kendrick, it was "imperative that a medical center such as the Emory-Grady complex take stock and determine the direction we should take in the future."⁶ According to the report, the Emory-Grady complex had much to consider.⁷

Among their many recommendations, the consultants suggested merging Hughes Spalding Pavilion's staff with Grady's. In the longer term, they proposed transforming the Pavilion into an extended care facility. In the short term, however, the consultants urged the hospital authority to meet the Pavilion's immediate needs for an intensive care unit, a coronary care unit, a new surgery recovery room, and a pharmacy.

The consultants also suggested erecting an Education and Research annex for Emory-at-Grady personnel. Estimating the cost at $12.35 million, the consultants thought the building should be built, financed, and maintained by Emory. Because the building would benefit Grady and its patients, however, they recommended Grady help Emory find funding for the project. The building would be built over a new 2,200 car parking deck. The proposal for Grady also included enlarging outpatient facilities, adding 132 hospital beds, and expanding services in ophthalmology, radiology, clinical laboratories, and anesthesiology. At the same time, the consultants suggested decentralizing Grady's clinics. Working together with the county health department, the new clinics would "get services closer to the people who use them."⁸

Shortly after the eighteen-month study was completed, the authority approved the firm's plan "in principle." Grady's superintendent, Bill Pinkston, noted that "while the Authority has adopted the report in principle, which establishes a sense of direction, none of the report can actually be implemented without the Authority and Emory University working very closely with many organizations, such as medical societies, health departments, local planning organizations, and our patients."⁹ Bill Pinkston would take an inclusive approach to planning for Grady's future.

Creating Clinics

In the late 1960s, Grady began planning a remarkable expansion of services. This was made possible in part by the influx of new money from the insurance for the poor and the elderly through Medicaid and Medicare. It was made necessary, in part, as a response to scientific advances, rising standards of care, the desire to provide the best possible medical education, and Atlanta's changing demographics. The key to Grady's strategy was to open new facilities within the hospital. By the end of the decade, these included the Muscular Dystrophy Clinic as part of the Physical Medicine Clinic, an Observation Ward for patients held in the Medical Emergency Clinic, a tuberculosis screening program, a Psychiatric Day Center, and a Hemophilia Clinic. In 1970, Grady opened five more new clinics and departments while expanding other services.

Nephrology Center

Grady brought together all of its kidney treatment clinics into a single area when it opened the nation's first regional kidney center in June 1970. Located on the hospital's seventh floor, the Atlanta Regional

Nephrology Center offered comprehensive service to patients. These included dialysis units, an area for critically ill renal patients, and a postoperative section for people who received a kidney transplant.

The Atlanta Artificial Kidney Center, one of the nation's leading home dialysis training centers, which began four years earlier, became part of the larger project. With expanded facilities, the center planned to train fifty patients each year on how to use artificial kidney machines at home. Other patients, however, needed to regularly visit the center for dialysis. (It had twelve beds.)

The regional center also included a kidney transplant program. (The first kidney transplants at Grady took place a month after the Atlanta Regional Nephrology Center opened.) The center's medical director, Dr. John H. Sadler, expected Grady to become a hub for kidney transplants in the South in part because it developed a regional (and computerized) system for acquiring kidneys. (Grady expected to obtain up to 150 donor kidneys each year, mainly from accident victims.) A novel computer program would allow Grady to match donated organs with recipients across the Southeast. After finding a match, Grady would fly the organ to the patient.[10]

The Night Clinic

A week after opening its center for kidney care, Grady unveiled a Night General Admission Clinic. This revolutionary clinic changed how patients used the hospital. The clinic allowed Grady's staff to direct patients who came at night with non-emergency complaints to a place of their own. Doing so helped reduce demands on Grady's hectic emergency room. Staffed with three internists, a pediatrician, a radiologist, two nurses, and support staff, the night General Admission Clinic brought relief to anxious patients who otherwise would be left to a long wait before being treated.

The idea for the night clinic sprang from a series of meetings between a panel of patients and Grady's administrators. Starting in 1969, Bill Pinkston and other top hospital officials regularly met with patients to plan improvements. Residents of low-income neighborhoods elected the members of the panel through Economic Opportunity Atlanta (EOA), a poverty-fighting program that evolved from Lyndon Johnson's Great Society. Instead of being a bureaucratic planning organization giving directions to others, EOA actively sought input from local residents on issues that mattered to them.[11]

The ten members of the Citizens Central Advisory Council of EOA's Health Subcommittee acted as a focus group for evaluating proposals for new services. The group also suggested ways to improve Grady. For example, the residents pleaded with Grady to expand its dental service. At the time Grady only extracted teeth and repaired jaw injuries. The patients wanted Grady to offer teeth cleaning, dental fillings, and tooth straightening. While that thoughtful suggestion proved impractical because of spatial and budgetary limitations, other ideas from the grass roots took hold. The Night Clinic was the first of these, and its impact was quickly felt by Grady and appreciated by outpatients. The EOA's advisory council's Health Subcommittee also helped improve communication between Grady and residents in local neighborhoods.

Psychiatric Emergency Clinic

The hospital had been involved in psychiatry for many years. In 1948 detention cells in the hospital were available for the violently mentally ill who were awaiting commitment hearings or transportation to the State Hospital in Milledgeville, located 100 miles southeast of Atlanta. When the new Grady hospital building opened in 1958, an 18-bed psychiatric unit was established on the eighth floor. The unit was a collaboration of the Emory School of Medicine, the FDHA, and the Georgia Department of Public Health.

Grady hospital also opened a psychiatric emergency clinic in 1970 that included six beds designated for patients referred from the Atlanta South Central Community Mental

Health Center. The psychiatric emergency clinic ran with little direct financial cost to Grady because the community mental health center reimbursed the hospital for the salaries of the thirteen people staffing the clinic.

Pediatric Intensive Care

In 1970 Grady also opened a pediatric Intensive Care Unit on the hospital's ninth floor. The pediatric ICU offered the community an important resource for improving the care and outcomes of seriously ill or injured children.

Poison Control Center

The care of children and some adults further improved when Grady opened the Poison Control Center under the direction of Dr. Albert Rauber in 1970. The system of Poison Control Centers started in Chicago in 1953 and over the following decades spread slowly across the nation. The Grady Poison Control Center quickly became an important health resource for Atlanta and, eventually, for all of Georgia. Patients, parents, and physicians increasingly turned to the center for its expertise and information. Grady initially funded the center's operations, but the state of Georgia assumed that role after it became obvious that the center served people statewide.

The Diabetes Treatment Center

On January 11, 1971, (the 49th anniversary of the first use of insulin in a diabetic patient) Grady opened its Diabetes Day Clinic. Under the direction of Dr. John Davidson, the center used a team approach to treating outpatients with diabetes. Patients would be diagnosed, educated, treated, and carefully followed by several experts in the Diabetes Mellitus field.

The dazzling success of Grady's pioneering Diabetes Treatment Center, the first hospital clinic in the United States to offer comprehensive care to diabetic patients, quickly became evident. Over 1,000 patients visited the center each year. In addition, Diabetic Nurse clinicians followed another 5,000 patients. The number of people treated tells only a small part of the story.

The rapid decline in hospital admissions for patients who lost control over their diabetes is a telling and remarkable indicator of the treatment center's success. Within three years of the center's founding, yearly admissions to Grady for patients whose illness had caused a diabetic coma plummeted from 500 to 100 patients. Many of the remaining diabetic coma cases occurred among people with previously undiagnosed diabetes. In addition to saving lives, the diabetes clinic helped Grady save money. In the early 1970s, Grady officials estimated that the decrease in coma cases saved the hospital $200,000 per year. Grady saved another $70,000 per year because it stopped using oral hypoglycemic medicines.[12]

The day clinic admitted six patients daily starting at 7:30 a.m. A physician, nurse, dietician, podiatrist, and laboratory technicians saw each patient. The experience proved intense for patients. The center designed individualized meal programs for each patient. The center also taught patients proper techniques for injecting insulin. When patients made a return visit to the center they underwent check-ups to make sure they

The Morrison Gift

Mrs. Ursel Warren Morrison volunteered for many years in Grady's Pediatric Outpatient Clinic. Devoted to the clinic and its clients, each year Mrs. Morrison sponsored a Christmas party for 500 needy children. Half of the children came in the morning, the other half showed up for the afternoon party. In addition to food and gifts, Mrs. Morrison arranged for local celebrities like Officer Don, the star of a local children's television program, to delight the children. Increasingly frail, Mrs. Morrison hosted her last Christmas party for the children in 1968. After her death in 1971 Mrs. Morrison's brother, Roy D. Warren, would sponsor Morrison Christmas parties.[139]

> ## Insulin
>
> Insulin, the principal hormone of the pancreas, is produced in the beta cells located in the pancreatic islands of Langerhans. These areas in the pancreas were first discovered in 1869. Diabetes mellitus had been known for centuries as a wasting disease characterized by a sweet urine. In 1889, J. Von Mering and Oskar Minkowski showed that removal of the pancreas produced the disease. This proved that the source of diabetes was a malfunction of the pancreas.
>
> Sir Frederick Grant Banting, a Canadian physician, working at the University of Toronto and aided by Charles Best, John Macleod, and James Colby, isolated the insulin hormone in 1921 from a dog's pancreas. Within eight months, Banting and Best produced insulin and treated their first diabetic patient. Banting and Macleod received the Nobel Prize in Physiology or Medicine in 1923 for the discovery that revolutionized the treatment of this deadly illness. Dr. John Davidson was born in 1922, the first year insulin was used to treat this disease.

were following their meal directions and that they were properly injecting insulin.

The new center did more than help patients manage their diabetic condition more effectively. The center became a source of education and training to health care providers. Under Dr. Davidson's direction, the Diabetes Treatment Center created education programs for physicians in the Atlanta area, conveying to them the latest scientific and medical information about diabetes. (Physicians gathered for the well-structured courses one day per week for a ten-week period.) The center trained 60 physicians and 350 nurses and dieticians from across the state of Georgia each year. As a result of this program, doctors returned to their private practices with the ability to provide patients with the latest and best methods for managing diabetes.[13]

Grady's care for diabetic patients had come a long way since Dr. Ebert Van Buren opened the hospital's first diabetes clinic in the 1930s. At that time fifty to sixty outpatients came in each week, monitored by nurses and physicians, and advised by a dietician.[14] Forty years later, the center gave hundreds of patients far more comprehensive care, monitored the progress of thousands of other patients, and trained physicians and nurses in the latest methods. Indeed, nursing moved closer than ever to the heart of the care that the center offered.[15]

Dr. John K. Davidson III

The care of Grady's diabetes patients changed dramatically after Dr. John Davidson III arrived on the hospital campus. A native of Lithonia, Georgia, Dr. Davidson graduated from the Emory University School of Medicine in 1945 under a special wartime program. He then served in the military for several years before entering private practice in Columbus, Georgia. In 1959 Dr. Davidson went to Canada in order to study physiology at the University of Toronto under Dr. Charles H. Best, the co-discoverer of insulin. After earning a Ph.D. in Physiology from the University of Toronto in 1965, Dr. Davidson was appointed to the faculty of the university's departments of physiology and medicine.

At the request of Dr. J. Willis Hurst, Dr. Davidson returned to Atlanta in 1968 to join the faculty of Emory's medical school. He immediately became the founding director of the diabetes unit at Grady Memorial Hospital. Although probably underreported, it was estimated that Grady's patient population at the time included at least 8,000 people suffering from diabetes. Annually the hospital was admitting hundreds of people who were in a diabetic coma; in addition, each year approximately 250 of Grady's diabetes patients required some type of amputation. It was a tragic and costly situation that Dr. Davidson would turn around.

Dr. Davidson, who himself developed diabetes in his youth, stressed dietary weight control and an exercise program more than medicine in the treatment of the disease. This approach was especially important

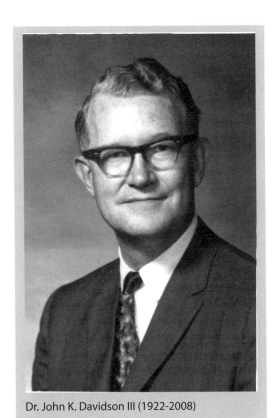

Dr. John K. Davidson III (1922-2008)

since approximately 90% of Grady's diabetic patients were obese. In his program, insulin was used as a last resort.[16] Recognizing that many of Grady's patients were illiterate, Dr. Davidson authored a picture book to guide them through the disease and its treatment. In addition to educating patients, Dr. Davidson was renowned for educating thousands of professionals. His textbook *Clinical Diabetes Mellitus: A Problem-Oriented Approach* went through three editions and became an invaluable reference tool for physicians around the world.[17] Patients also benefited from the substantive research conducted at Grady's diabetes unit. Dr. Davidson's contribution to patient care for this debilitating and deadly illness may be unsurpassed in Georgia.

Dr. Davidson received numerous honors for his work, including the Upjohn Medal from the American Diabetes Association. Dr. Davidson, who retired in 1991, died in 2008 at the age of 86 and is buried at Decatur Cemetery.[18]

Against the City

Letters of appreciation sometimes found their way into the hospital's employee newsletter. The published letters tended to be from those who had been seen as inpatients (or their loved ones) rather than as outpatients. While letters of complaint did not receive similar publicity, there was ample dissatisfaction during the late 1960s, especially among outpatients, emergency room patients, and people using the pharmacy. Long waits, rudeness by some staff, and crowded conditions turned people off. Yet, few patients had anywhere else to turn. Some patient voices were muted by fear. Worried that complaining would lead to being denied treatment in the future, many black patients held their tongue—a longstanding habit that was becoming less pervasive in the civil rights era. Those who relied on "Mother Grady" were not necessarily satisfied with how they were being treated.

Grady's administrators and staff knew about the dissatisfaction in the community. They even seemed to realize one of its main causes. As one physician told a reporter, "Grady is a good hospital—but it has bad manners."[19] Those bad manners, however, reinforced deep-seated anger toward the institution. The Gradys had always been two hospitals, separate and unequal. Until the new "H" Grady was completed in the late 1950s, Black Grady had far worse facilities. Even in the new building, Black Grady appeared to get less than its equal share of resources. Until Grady desegregated, the black wards continued to be overcrowded and understaffed at the same time that the white wards had empty beds and full supply closets.[20] In theory the Gradys finally became singular when patient care was officially integrated in 1965. In reality, something else made Grady whole.

It wasn't so much that Black Grady and White Grady were united through desegregation as that White Grady all but disappeared. In the white flight that started in the 1950s, much of White Atlanta effectively seceded from the city.[21] By 1960, the patient mix at

Grady—which had long been almost evenly divided between black and white—had become mostly black. Only 30% of the patients at Grady were white in 1960; the proportion steadily declined for a decade, falling to about 10% by 1970.

Ensconced in the safety of the suburbs, White Atlanta wanted little to do with the city it had left behind. It didn't want the schools, it didn't want the crime it feared, and it didn't want the city to annex the suburbs—a move that whites within the city limits promoted. After the city acquired three major professional sports franchises between 1966 and 1968, whites would drive downtown for entertainment, if not for shopping. By 1970, whites had been moving out for over a decade at the same time the black population grew. In 1970, Atlanta was residentially more than twice as segregated as it had been in 1940. While white enclaves remained in the north of the city, much of the white middle class had migrated to Cobb and Gwinnett counties and to northern Fulton County. Those areas boomed during the 1960s and 1970s as the area attracted tens of thousands of people from far beyond Atlanta. Few suburbanites were interested in paying taxes for the benefit of people living in the city.[22]

Harry West, the manager of Fulton County, bluntly told the Buckhead Kiwanis Club in July 1970 that most citizens in the county didn't know "what services their tax dollars [were] buying." White suburbanites might think Atlanta would be forced to solve "its ghetto problems" with its own money, but West intended to correct that misunderstanding. "In reality," he said, "it is Fulton County tax money that pays for welfare, public health, Grady Hospital, the courts and probation services while the federal government pays for most of the Model Cities, public housing and Economic Opportunity Atlanta programs."[23] With 25 cents of every county tax dollar going to Grady, West wanted his audience to know that they were paying for a service they weren't using. His appeal was reminiscent of the arguments made a decade earlier when the city's parks and swimming pools were being desegregated. Once again, many whites believed they were paying taxes for the benefit of black communities rather than their own.

West didn't want the county to pay for Grady; he wanted the State of Georgia to be responsible for the hospital. If it did, he would have another $12 million in Fulton County's budget. More than that, he believed state funding would be more fair to Fulton taxpayers since, he claimed, people from throughout the state came to Grady for treatment.[24]

At the time West prepared his remarks, white fears about black ghettoes remained high. Terrible riots devastated black communities in cities like Detroit, Cleveland, and Newark in 1967. More riots in American cities following the assassination of the Reverend Martin Luther King, Jr., in April 1968 further stoked white fears. Although Atlanta was largely calm after the assassination, whites remained anxious about black communities at the time Harry West made his case to the Kiwanis two years later. It was not that whites were callous about the causes of black unrest. While they cared about the problems, few whites would accept that they had anything to do with the problems of ghettoes they didn't inhabit.

The Kerner Commission, appointed by President Johnson and headed by Otto Kerner, the governor of Illinois (1961-1968), investigated causes of the riots among urban blacks in 1967. The conclusions it presented only weeks before Dr. King's murder fit Atlanta as easily as they did the rest of the nation. The two Atlantas had become increasingly separated from each other for more than a decade. The Kerner report warned that the entire nation was "moving toward two societies, one black, one white—separate and unequal." Ultimately, the Kerner Commission reported, White America didn't understand that "white society is deeply implicated in the ghetto."[25] It was already evident, and the pattern would be reinforced as Atlanta's suburban secession continued in the coming decades: Suburbanites didn't want to pay for the services they didn't use.

Three years after West's speech in Buckhead, the Fulton County Commission tried to get the state legislature to follow through on West's proposal. With the county spending $15 million per year on Grady, the commissioners passed a resolution asking the state to relieve it of Grady's costs. Their argument had little to do with sharing burdens; the commissioners said little about Grady's role in training one-fourth of the physicians in Georgia, or its services being used by residents beyond Fulton and DeKalb counties. The rhetoric centered not on what Grady did for Georgia, but on what Grady did to property taxes in Fulton County. Commissioner Milton Farris believed that if the state took over responsibility for Grady, property taxes in Fulton County could be lowered by 20 percent.[26] (He was also following through on a proposal from Governor Jimmy Carter that the legislature appropriate money for health programs so that counties could cut property taxes.) Since the legislature, which was dominated by rural interests, failed to see the benefit in assuming full responsibility for Grady, Fulton County remained financially obligated for the hospital.

Appointing Mrs. Hamilton and Mr. Russell to the Hospital Authority

In January 1971 the Fulton County Commission appointed John F. Ingram, Jr., Grace Towns Hamilton, and Herman J. Russell to the Fulton-DeKalb Hospital Authority.

John Ingram, Jr., was a vice-president with The Citizens and Southern National Bank. He had worked there for twenty-seven years and was an established figure in the city's civic leadership. Like the long line of distinguished white businessmen who came before him, Ingram voluntarily served on the board in the hope of doing something wonderful for his community. Adding him to the board wouldn't raise any eyebrows. Neither would the appointment of two African American board members. Seven years after Clayton Yates became the first black member of the FDHA, the naming of people like Mrs. Hamilton and Mr. Russell wouldn't surprise. To the leaders of White Atlanta, it seemed prudent. The Fulton County commissioners were counting on their new appointees as crucial allies in solving serious problems confronting Grady and Hughes Spalding Pavilion.

Mrs. Hamilton had remained extremely active in the community long after her instrumental role in creating Hughes Spalding Pavilion. At the time of her appointment, Mrs. Hamilton was serving as a representative to Georgia's General Assembly. The Fulton County Commission, however, wanted the hospital authority to have more than a friend in the state legislature.

Because of her essential role in creating Hughes Spalding Pavilion, Mrs. Hamilton carried remarkable moral authority concerning its fate. The Cresap, McCormick and Paget management report, completed a year and a half earlier, recommended closing the Spalding Pavilion by 1980. While it might meet a need in the community by reopening as a long-term care facility, the Pavilion seemed to have outlived its usefulness as a public hospital for Atlanta's black middle class. Passage of civil rights laws (plus civil rights provisions in the Medicare law) had forced white hospitals like Crawford Long, Georgia Baptist, Piedmont, and Emory into accepting black patients. These hospitals began planning for expansion in the late 1960s, and it appeared the need for a "small short-term general hospital" had waned.[27] A few years after desegregation, budget-conscious officials from Fulton County saw little reason for Spalding's continued existence. But Spalding was causing bigger headaches for the Fulton-DeKalb Hospital Authority than the logic of its creation.

The Joint Commission on Accreditation of Hospitals accredited Grady for only one year in 1969. While citing a few administrative problems at Grady, the commission focused on numerous problems with Spalding Pavilion. In order to fix the problems, the FDHA would have to spend money it didn't have. While most of the hospital's original raison d'etre faded with the integration of Atlanta's private hospitals, any steps that might be taken to close Hughes Spalding Pavilion were fraught with political danger.

Although Spalding Pavilion had yet to live up to its original promise of becoming a center for training black physicians, the potential remained. If the hospital were closed, where in Georgia would African Americans gain medical training? In a state still suffering a severe shortage of black physicians—and Emory University School of Medicine having at best an extremely weak track record—closing one of the few hospitals welcoming to black physicians would be difficult. Accomplished physicians on the Pavilion's staff, like Dr. William Holmes Borders, Jr., were vocal about the hospital's continuing relevance. Spalding Pavilion kept attracting patients and, its supporters argued, its occupancy rate would improve dramatically if the FDHA properly outfitted and supplied the hospital. Spalding's supporters remained angry that the FDHA continued treating the Pavilion as an afterthought.[28]

The commissioners of Fulton County could have no evidence that Mrs. Hamilton would support closing the Pavilion, but they seemed to hope she would be helpful in dealing with what looked like an unnecessary expense. In addition, they were confident that her appointment would help Grady resolve other problems with Atlanta's African American communities.

The Fulton County Commissioners also turned to Herman J. Russell, a lifelong resident of Atlanta (and Grady Baby), to serve on the hospital authority. He undoubtedly had a better chance to help solve Grady's problems with Atlanta's black communities than did Philip H. Alston, Jr., an influential lawyer whose resignation opened the seat Herman J. Russell filled. The son of a plasterer and a maid, H. J. Russell attended public schools in Atlanta. After graduating from Tuskegee Institute in 1953, he joined his father's plastering business (and took it over when his father retired two years later). In the next few years the firm prospered by building duplexes and apartments in Atlanta's African American communities.[29] But it also grew by being an effective subcontractor for white-owned general contractors on projects like the construction of Atlanta-Fulton County Stadium.

At the time he was appointed to the hospital authority, H. J. Russell had proven adept at negotiating and balancing the two Atlantas. Mr. Russell served on the boards of institutions that were prominent in Black Atlanta, including Citizens Trust Company, Morris Brown College, and the Atlanta Committee for Cooperative Action. He also served on the boards of institutions that cut across racial boundaries like the YMCA, the YWCA, the Atlanta Community Chest, and the Atlanta Chamber of Commerce Rapid Transit committee. H. J. Russell had broken a crucial color barrier in November 1962 when he became the first black member of the Atlanta Chamber of Commerce.[30] While he could navigate both Atlantas, the commissioners hoped his appointment, together with Mrs. Hamilton's, could help Grady run more smoothly and mend its strained relations with African Americans.

Black Atlanta's hostility toward Grady at the start of 1971 was rooted in perceptions of discriminatory care and the indisputable fact that the hospital had fought desegregation. At that point Bill Pinkston had been working for some time to solve the gargantuan problem Grady's past posed for the hospital's relationship with Atlanta's black communities. He did this in part through regular meetings with the EOA's health subcommittee starting in 1969. One outcome of those conversations was the "privately funded" hiring of Wright, Jackson, Brown, Williams & Stephens, Inc., a public relations firm owned by African Americans, in the summer of 1970.

After investigating the hospital's relations with its patients and its employees, Wright, Jackson declared that "there is very little fundamentally wrong with the Grady Hospital complex."[31] Nevertheless, the firm suggested nineteen ways for Grady to improve. These included installing directional signs and floor plan outlines for visitors, streamlining the check-in process at Hughes Spalding, and making certain that the patients' meals were actually warm when served.³² The study focused on Grady's relations with people who went there for work or medical care.

Naming Mrs. Hamilton and Mr. Russell stood as part of Grady's larger effort to improve relations with Black Atlanta. Even with their addition to its roster, the overall makeup of the authority had changed little from earlier years. To someone who played pool with the Reverend Martin Luther King, Jr., at the Butler Street YMCA, serving on the authority may have been less fulfilling than hoped. Mr. Russell left the board after two years. Two years later Mrs. Hamilton also left the board when the Fulton County Board of Commissioners removed her from the Fulton-DeKalb Hospital Authority.

Mrs. Hamilton was off of the FDHA as of February 19, 1975, only two weeks after the Fulton County Commission had reappointed her to the authority. The commissioners reversed course because they were miffed that she had introduced a bill in the state legislature to shorten their term in office. She had done so in order to resolve an electoral muddle. The commission had recently been expanded to include commissioners elected at-large from throughout the county. Unfortunately, the rules for electing at-large members had come in dispute before a recent election because of ambiguity about whether at-large members could be elected by a plurality rather than a majority of voters. An ad hoc ruling by a judge had left the matter unsettled when at large-members were elected with only a plurality of the vote. To solve the problem, Mrs. Hamilton proposed that the legislature expedite the end of the new commissioners' term of office.

In addition, Mrs. Hamilton long had a dispute with commissioners Charlie Brown, Goodwyn (Shag) Cates, and Henry Dodson, an African American who abstained in voting both for her reappointment and for removing her from the hospital authority. Richard H. Johnston, the commissioner who made the motion to rescind her recent reappointment, said Mrs. Hamilton "does not properly

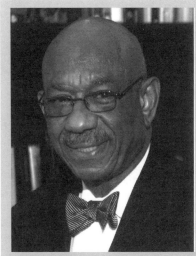

Herman J. Russell developed the largest African-American owned real estate and construction firm in the United States. As a business and civic leader, he provided crucial bridges between Black and White Atlanta.

represent our thinking." The commission claimed that it removed Mrs. Hamilton because she had not been supportive of Grady during her time in the legislature. This rationale was suspect since Mrs. Hamilton had vigorously and steadfastly pushed for more state funding for Grady. The underlying reason for the commission's action seemed obvious to anyone paying attention.³³ Political tit-for-tat had trumped the needs of Grady and its patients.

The state general assembly was not amused by the commission's retaliation against Representative Hamilton. State Representative Mike Egan from Fulton County, the minority leader in the state house, said in response, "I think they ruined any chances of getting anything from this legislature. We have been working to get money in the 1976 budget for Grady, but it appears the county commissioners want to block that."³⁴

State Representative Sidney Marcus, the chairman of the Fulton County legislature and a great friend of Grady who worked hard behind the scenes to get the state legislature to appropriate money for the hospital, sponsored a resolution honoring Mrs. Hamilton for her decades of public service. It referred to her time on the hospital authority as "one of the highlights of her career as a public servant."35

The significance of Grace Towns Hamilton and H. J. Russell being on the FDHA board is two-fold. It represented an overdue recognition by White Atlanta that Black Atlanta deserved more representation at the FDHA board table. It also suggests that in 1971, as the Fulton County Commission faced reorganization and an expansion from three to seven members, the commissioners wanted to mend fences with Black Atlanta. Both Mrs. Hamilton and Mr. Russell cared deeply about Grady; indeed, their passion may only have been exceeded by a man whose tenure on the FDHA board started in the year that Mrs. Hamilton was removed from her post.

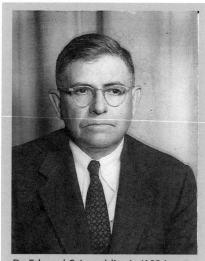

Dr. Edward C. Loughlin, Jr. (1934-2011): His love for Grady was known by all who knew him.

Dr. Edward C. Loughlin, Jr.

The Fulton County Commission appointed Dr. Edward C. Loughlin, Jr., a distinguished orthopedist, to the FDHA in 1975.

Born in North Carolina in 1934, Dr. Loughlin enjoyed a photographic memory and had a deep commitment to his family, his patients, and Grady hospital. He graduated Phi Beta Kappa from the University of North Carolina in three years. Following a clinicial clerkship at the historic Saint Bartholomew Hospital in London in 1958, he graduated with an M.D. from the University of Pennsylvania Medical School in 1959. Dr. Loughlin enjoyed a surgical internship at Emory and then completed his residency in orthopedics at Grady hospital.

Dr. Loughlin entered private practice in 1964, joining the highly respected group of Funk, Wells, and Dimon—the forerunner of Peachtree Orthopedic Clinic, one of the most prominent orthopedic practices in Georgia. At the same time, he also served on Grady's medical staff. Widely respected as a surgeon, Dr. Loughlin's passion for Grady hospital and his interpersonal skills helped him gain the appointment to the FDHA board.

Quick-witted and sociable, Dr. Loughlin used his substantial charm to full advantage as he led the FDHA's budget committee and became involved in the complex negotiation of a new thirty-year contract between Emory and Grady.

Dr. Loughlin became chairman of the hospital authority in 1983. The first physician to serve in this capacity, Dr. Loughlin held the position for eight years, until his term expired in 1991. His tenure as chairman coincided with a growing effort by some members of the Fulton County Commission to exert greater influence on the hospital's operations. Indeed, one of his greatest challenges as chairman was to fight off meddling politicians who saw in Grady an opportunity to advance their own interests.

Dr. Loughlin was a forceful advocate of the passage of a crucial bond issued in the 1980s to finance a badly needed renovation and expansion of the hospital. During a bitter conflict between the hospital authority and the Fulton County Commission over Grady's renovation, Dr. Loughlin played a major role in keeping the needs of Grady's patients in the foreground of the debate. In a controversial move, the Fulton County Commission, with whom he had sparred during his chairmanship, refused to reappoint him to the authority's board at the end of 1991. Despite having the support of

Tom Lowe, a prominent commissioner, Dr. Loughlin could not win the endorsement of the commission's chairman, Michael Lomax, who effectively prevented Dr. Loughlin from continuing his service to the board. Two months later, with Lomax casting the only dissenting vote, the commission returned Dr. Loughlin to the FDHA for one more term.

After he retired from the Peachtree Orthopedic Clinic in 2007, Dr. Loughlin continued to volunteer at Grady two days per week, helping patients and training medical students and residents.

Dr. Loughlin became a Fellow of the American Academy of Orthopaedic Surgeons and was awarded the Emory University School of Medicine's Medical Alumni Association's Distinguished Professional Achievement Award. The Medical Association of Atlanta awarded him its highest honor, the Aven Cup, in 1988. Three years later it presented Dr. Loughlin with its Distinguished Service Award.

Grady hospital's Loughlin Radiation and Oncology Center, with 15,000 square feet of clinical space and 10,000 square feet of laboratory space, was dedicated in his honor in 1992.

Dr. Loughlin died following a stroke in March 2011.[36]

The Trouble With Spalding Pavilion

Hughes Spalding Pavilion faced vital challenges in the late 1970s, many of them a result of its past. Throughout its history, the hospital had been shadowed by questions about its future. While every institution moves into the unknown, unexpectedly low physician and patient usage rates raised questions about the hospital's future in its first years. Not until about 1960, when the training program for physicians was getting off the ground and the hospital had started running near full capacity, did its future seem secure. Yet, even then a fundamental question remained: What would happen to Black Atlanta's hospitals when White Atlanta's hospitals desegregated?

Created as a civil rights weapon for integrating medical education, the pavilion was presented to White Atlanta in part as meeting Black Atlanta's severe need for more hospital beds. Although the pavilion's beds could satisfy only part of the deep want imposed by segregationist restrictions, would they still be needed once racial limitations at other hospitals were lifted? Would there be a use for Spalding Pavilion's teaching program after Emory's medical school became integrated? It is unclear if Spalding Pavilion's planners ever stopped to consider what would happen to their institution when Jim Crow died. What could you do with a separate hospital in a desegregated world?

The irony in Spalding Pavilion's founding ideal—that separate hospitals would by definition become relics of the past in a desegregated world—went unaddressed. As White Atlanta's hospitals finally desegregated in the late 1960s, however, it became clear that Spalding Pavilion would have to compete for the loyalty of white physicians and attract young black physicians. Suddenly, nearby institutions from which its clients had long been excluded, in particular Crawford Long and Georgia Baptist hospitals, were becoming Spalding Pavilion's rivals. The changing demographics of Black Atlanta also posed a challenge to the pavilion.

In the late 1950s and early 1960s, much of the Pavilion's patient base and staff began moving from the center of the city toward the west and southwest sides. Those who did, like Dr. Yancey, faced a long commute to Hughes Spalding.[37] As these areas grew, new medical facilities emerged. The expanding African American middle class in southwest Atlanta gained a new option for hospitalization after Archbishop Paul Hallinan dedicated Holy Family Hospital on September 13, 1964. Open to people of all races (and funded in part with federal money) Holy Family grew out of the Catholic Colored Clinic that Catholic laywomen organized in 1941. (They turned the clinic over to the Society of Catholic Medical Mission Sisters in 1944.)[38]

Established a half-mile west of its parish church, St. Paul of the Cross, Holy Family Hospital was developed with strong support from people intimately connected to Hughes Spalding Pavilion. Clayton Yates, a member of the Advisory Board for Hughes Spalding Pavilion, served on Holy Family Hospital's fundraising Campaign Steering Committee as did Hughes Spalding, Sr., who joined the committee in March 1959, shortly after he resigned from the Fulton-DeKalb Hospital Authority.[39] As it was being planned and built in the late 1950s and early 1960s, Holy Family seemed like a complement to Hughes Spalding Pavilion; by the late 1960s it was starting to look like a competitor. The growth of Holy Family together with the desegregation of White Atlanta's hospitals and the Emory University School of Medicine raised the long-ignored question: Should Hughes Spalding Pavilion close once the goal of desegregated medical care and education was achieved?

The Cresap, McCormick and Paget consulting report completed in 1969 said yes. While the pavilion might draw both white and black patients if it updated and expanded its services, it would still suffer severe financial trouble. The best course of action, the consultants said, was to close the hospital by 1980. Ideally, they suggested, the building would be expanded and renovated for use as a rehabilitation and extended care facility—the same suggestion that Cresap had offered in 1960. The recommendation to close the pavilion in 1980 depended on there being enough hospital beds in the city. Even as the study was being conducted, Grady added window air conditioners to Spalding's patient rooms. What it did not do, however, was satisfy the demands of either the Pavilion's physicians or of the Joint Commission on Accreditation of Hospitals.[40]

The Joint Commission cited numerous problems at Hughes Spalding as one reason it granted Grady only one year of accreditation in 1969 rather than the usual three years. The trouble went beyond inadequate patient charts and discharge summaries. According to the Joint Commission, Spalding Pavilion and Grady needed to operate under the same rules and regulations. FDHA chairman Robert Regenstein thought the the solution would be for Emory to provide medical supervision at Spalding Pavilion—an option resisted by both the medical school and physicians at Spalding. While Dr. Douglas Kendrick, Grady's Medical Director, was unconvinced that Emory offered the answer, he did foresee a movement "toward an amalgamation of Hughes Spalding and Grady."[41] While this had long been the dream of Black Atlanta, the idea didn't necessarily sit well with physicians at Spalding Pavilion. Dr. James Palmer, former president of the Atlanta Medical Association, argued that physicians at the pavilion preferred to make their own rules and run their own hospital.[42] At the same time other people in Atlanta were considering an option that the consultants had not addressed. Ironically, given the formal desegregation of the Emory University School of Medicine several years earlier (it had only one African American graduate by 1970), the proposal seemed separatist: develop a medical school for African American students.

Morehouse School of Medicine

Early in 1968, the Georgia Comprehensive Health Planning Council, part of a state agency responsible for identifying health needs and priorities for Georgia, organized a task force to study "physician manpower" in the state. Examining demographic and statistical data for more than a year, the eight-member committee issued a critical report in the summer of 1969. It recognized a host of problems, many rooted in a dramatic increase in the "demand for medical services."[43] Recognizing that Georgia continued to suffer from a shortage of physicians, the committee recommended ways to increase the number of doctors in the state and make a more efficient use of them. Concerned by the possibility of "a continued snowballing demand for health care" in Georgia, the report also contained recommendations for patient education.

Chaired by Dr. William W. Moore, Jr., a well-respected neurosurgeon and President of the Fulton County Medical Society (1967), and including among its members Bill Pinkston, Dean Arthur Richardson from Emory, and Dr. Louis C. Brown, representing the Georgia State Medical Association, the committee recommended increasing medical school enrollments in Georgia. It suggested further study of three options: expanding existing medical schools, starting a two-year medical school, and creating a four-year medical school. In addition, it recommended that "specific opportunities should be developed to provide for the education of more black medical students."[44] Among the other problems it addressed was the crying need for more physicians to serve rural communities and the poor.[45] One member of the task force, Dr. Louis C. Brown, came away from the experience as a man with a mission.

His work with the committee reinforced Dr. Brown's belief that Atlanta could support a second medical school; in particular, one located at the Atlanta University Center, a consortium of six historically black institutions of higher learning. Dr. Brown spread the gospel of the need for a new medical school designed to train physicians who would serve minorities and the poor. He seemed to bend the ear of everyone he could find. While some saw him as a "voice crying in executive suite wilderness," his persistence and persuasiveness brought others to the cause.[46] Working with Dr. Calvin A. Brown, Jr., an alumnus of Morehouse who in the 1960s became one of the first African American faculty members at Emory's medical school, and with other physicians in the community, Dr. Louis Brown steadily gained support for the project.

The future medical school would be designed to address problems caused by the history of racial discrimination in medicine and medical education. There continued to be a serious shortage of black physicians in Atlanta. The ratio of black doctors to Atlanta's African American population had barely improved since the Atlanta Urban League conducted its study shortly after World War II. More broadly, too few physicians served the poor and minorities in the United States. The new school would attempt to address both concerns. While it expected the student body to be predominantly African American, it would admit a mix of students interested in serving the rural and urban poor.[47]

In 1970, shortly after desegregation had finally become the standard for all of Atlanta's hospitals, Dr. Bernard Hallman, Associate Dean for Community Affairs and Professor of Medicine at Emory, and a crucial figure in the development of medical education in Atlanta during the 1970s, repeated the task force's finding that while 26 percent of Georgia's population was black, only 2.4 percent of Georgia physicians were of the same race. He would work hard to get the problem solved. The crying need for black primary-care physicians in Georgia continued.

Dr. Hugh Gloster, who succeeded Dr. Mays as President of Morehouse in 1967, wanted the challenge of changing the way things were to the way they ought to be. In 1971, President Gloster gained permission from the Morehouse College Board of Trustees to explore establishing a medical-dental education program at the school. (Two trustees, Thomas Kilgore and Calvin Brown, were especially interested in the program.)[48] As the school looked into options, it held conversations with the National Institutes of Health, black physicians in the community, Emory's Associate Dean Hallman, and others. Morehouse faculty members Dr. Joseph N. Gayles and Dr. Thomas E. Norris, together with Mrs. Alice G. Green, analyzed options and helped the college win a grant of $100,000 from the National Institutes of Health in February 1973 for a feasibility study.[49]

In 1974, Morehouse won a two-year planning grant worth $806,964 from the federal Department of Health, Education, and Welfare to develop an educational program that would lead to the opening of a new medical school. Announced by President Gloster of Morehouse College and Congressman Andrew Young in ceremonies at Morehouse, the grant offered substantive hope that a full-fledged medical school would be opened within a decade. The new medical school would not be exclusively for blacks or males, but it was expected to be a predominantly black school.[50]

In 1975, Dr. Louis Sullivan was appointed the school's first Dean and Director of the Medical Education Program at Morehouse College. More than any other individual, Dr. Sullivan would shape its development. He set its policies and high standards, he recruited faculty and students, and he brought effective trustees to its board. Of course, he did not work alone. He had broad support from the Atlanta Medical Association, the National Medical Association, Mayor Maynard Jackson, the trustees of the schools associated with the Atlanta University Center, and many large national foundations.

The black caucus in the Georgia Legislature played a helpful role in getting funding for the medical school at a crucial point in its development. In 1976, while the school was still being planned, Governor George Busbee designated $100,000 for the school from his emergency fund. Two years later, months before the Morehouse School of Medicine was about to open, black caucus members struck a deal with legislators from middle Georgia who were eager to create a new medical school at Mercer University in Macon. Following the agreement, Governor Busbee included $2 million dollars (divided evenly between Morehouse and Mercer) in the state budgets for each of the years 1978, 1979, and 1980. The amount for each school rose to slightly more than $1.5 million for the 1981 fiscal year. State funding for Morehouse increased again after Joe Frank Harris became Governor of Georgia in 1983.[51]

In April 1978, the Liaison Committee on Medical Education, which accredited medical schools in the United States, voted to give Morehouse School of Medicine provisional accreditation for a two-year program in the basic medical sciences.[52] The class of 25 students that started in September 1978 would be the first for the only predominantly black medical school created in the United States during the twentieth century. The next year Morehouse's medical school would open its first new building. Two years later, in 1980, Emory University School of Medicine accepted half of the new Morehouse School of Medicine's charter class. The other students from Morehouse School of Medicine transferred to medical schools at Howard University, Meharry Medical College, the University of Alabama at Birmingham, and the Medical College of Georgia. Morehouse School of

---

Volunteers Still Vital

In late 1968, Dr. Harlan Stone, the Director of the Burn Service, asked Mrs. Virginia Herring, Director of Volunteer Service, for a favor. He needed volunteers to assemble a type of dressing that was commercially unavailable. Until then Dr. Stone had been preparing the dressing for burn patients while they were under anesthesia. Unfortunately, he couldn't use cotton cushioning when making dressings in the operating room because the cotton lint tended to fly everywhere. As result, the dressings he assembled were only made from cotton cellulose and gauze—an uncomfortable dressing for a severe burn.

In December 1968, the Woman's Society of Greater Travelers Rest Baptist Church signed up for the job. Grady prepared a room for them with a large table and racks for huge bolts of cotton batting, gauze, and cellulose so that the women could make the dressings.

Working there, the women put together a dressing with a layer of gauze at the bottom, several layers of absorbent cellulose, a layer of cotton several inches thick, and then topped with a final layer of gauze. Made in sizes from 36 x 50 inches to 10 x 20 inches, the dressings were wrapped and taped in brown paper for placement in a gas sterilizer before being stocked in the operating room and in central supply.

Before long, a team of women from All Saints Episcopal Church also began to make dressings for burn victims.[118]

Medicine's first four-year class entered in 1981. A major milestone occurred in 1985 when the Morehouse School of Medicine graduated its first class of four-year students, most of which would devote their careers to primary care. Morehouse had planned to open a surgery residency program on July 1, 1991, but because of factors involving residency accreditation the program was delayed for another year. The Morehouse Medicine Department began residency training for thirteen physicians in Internal Medicine on July 1, 1992, the same day that Morehouse opened its Obstetrical-Gynecological service.

Dr. Louis Sullivan

Dr. Sullivan was born at Grady in 1933. He grew up, however, in Blakely, a small town in southwest Georgia. The son of a schoolteacher and an insurance salesman—both of whom attended college—Louis Sullivan excelled in his studies. Eager for him to be able to attend better schools, his parents sent Sullivan (along with his brother) to junior high and high school in Atlanta.

Louis Sullivan would be the class salutatorian when he graduated from Atlanta's Booker T. Washington High School. Continuing his studies a short distance away at Morehouse College, Sullivan again succeeded, graduating magna cum laude. The only black in his class in medical school, he graduated third in a class of 76 from the Boston University School of Medicine in 1958. Following graduation he had an internship and residency training at New York Hospital-Cornell Medical Center. During his career he served on the faculty of Harvard Medical School (1963-1964), Seton Hall College of Medicine (1964-66), and the Boston University School of Medicine (1966-1975) where he became full professor.

He also founded and directed the hematology section at Boston City Hospital. He co-authored numerous articles for medical journals and served on many professional committees and editorial boards. Dr. Sul-

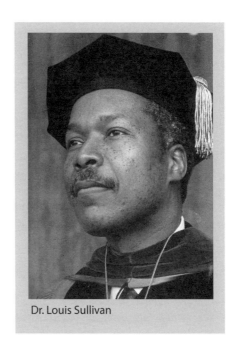

Dr. Louis Sullivan

livan would serve the Morehouse School of Medicine for fourteen years until, in 1989, he became Secretary of Health and Human Services under President George H. W. Bush. In 1993 he returned to Morehouse School of Medicine and continued as its president until he was appointed President Emeritus in July 2002.

Dr. Sullivan led Morehouse School of Medicine from being a two-year program of medical education to a fully accredited four-year medical school. An astute politician, Dr. Sullivan managed to recruit the wife of the Vice President of the United States to be a member of the Morehouse School of Medicine Board of Trustees. In her time serving there, Barbara Bush was known as an active, highly involved member of the board. Dr. Sullivan, known to be a workaholic himself, wouldn't have had it any other way. He has been awarded more than 50 honorary degrees and served on the corporate boards of several Fortune 500 companies.

The Burn Center

A new Burn Center facility opened at Grady in July 1974. Offering acute and specialized burn care (126 patients were treated during its first year) it led to a major reduction in the burn death rate. (The death rate fell from an average of 15% of patients prior to the opening to 6.4% after opening.) Perhaps less astonishing, but still notable, thanks to reduced infections and fewer complications, the burn unit's cost per patient also dropped.[53]

Eighteen of the Burn Unit's 28 beds were occupied when an urgent call came from the telephone company at 4:44 p.m. on April 4, 1977. Grady was requested to send "as many ambulances as possible out to the New Hope School on Highway 92." Southern Airways Flight 242, headed toward Atlanta from Huntsville, Alabama, had crashed in the small community of New Hope, about thirty miles northwest of Grady hospital. A few minutes later, the telephones rang again. This time the ambulance crews at Grady were told to relax. The request for help was being cancelled since rescue workers at the crash site "already had more ambulances than survivors."[54] Sixty-three people aboard the DC-9 died and 8 people on the ground suffered the same fate. (One other person on the ground would die from injuries several weeks later.) The 22 surviving victims were taken to local hospitals, including Kennestone Hospital in Marietta where approximately 25 physicians responded to the tragedy. Within hours, half of the plane crash survivors were transferred to Grady's burn unit. With the patient load increased by more than half, and patients being placed in an overflow ward, Grady's physician staff came to assist the burn unit director, Dr. Harlan Stone.[55]

W. Horace Bearden, Grady hospital's night administrator, was proud that Grady was there to help the crash victims. He told a reporter, "even though we might have a spillover, we still have better medical care because our people have specialized training in burn treatment. I'm not bragging but it's true and the other folks must think that, otherwise why would they send [the burn victims] here?"[56]

It was the worst aviation disaster in Georgia history and the first crash in Georgia involving a scheduled airline flight since 1941. After a severe hailstorm caused both engines to lose power, the crew tried to glide the jetliner in a forced landing on a rural highway. The pilot and the first officer died in the crash but the two flight attendants, Sandy Ward and Anne Lemoine, survived and were lauded for their heroism in helping other survivors get out of the burning wreckage.

Opening the Rape Crisis Center

The Rape Crisis Center at Grady Hospital opened in 1974 under the direction of Dr. Ann MacAllister. Dr. Peg Ziegler assumed the position of director in 1977 and would head the Rape Crisis Center until 1996. In its first year, the center saw, treated, and counseled 475 victims. Within two years, the number of victims treated would increase to 862, and by 1978 the center was helping over 1000 victims per year; about one-fifth of whom were under the age of 16. The Rape Crisis Center attracted many volunteers to its service. In 1984, when 83 individuals volunteered their time to the center, administrators estimated they needed twice as many volunteers to help with the approximately 1,200 victims receiving care annually. Volunteers stayed with the victim while in the hospital and also assisted victims as they prepared to testify in court against the rapist. The Center also provided a 24-hour telephone line to provide counseling and support.

Contraceptive Research

In 1983, the *Journal of the American Medical Association* published a study concerning 5,003 patients at Grady who had used an injected contraceptive, Depot Medroxyprogesterone [DMP A], between 1967 and 1976.[57] The research study examined whether the new contraceptive, whose dose was intended to be effective for three months after being injected in a woman, caused an increase in cancer. The study's results showed that patients using the contraceptive did not suffer from higher rates of cancer. On the contrary, patients using the drug proved less likely to develop cancer than would be expected for people of the same age in the general population.

The next year the *Journal of the American Medical Association* also published the results of a ten-year study conducted at Grady by the United States Centers for Disease Control and the Emory University School of Medicine. Examining the medical records of 30,580 women between the ages of 15 and 44 who were patients at Grady between 1967 and 1977, the study concluded that the current use of IUDs, oral contraceptives, Depo-Provera, or barrier methods of contraception revealed no evidence of harm to women. Not only did contraceptives not elevate the risk of death, they actually lowered the death rate by preventing pregnancy and its complications. The paper did recommend a longer study on possible adverse contraceptive effects such as cancer.[58]

Dr. Peter Symbas

Dr. Peter Symbas arrived at Grady in 1964 as the Director of the Thoracic and Cardiovascular Surgery Division. Born in Greece in 1925, Dr. Symbas earned his M.D. degree from the University of Salonika School of Medicine in Greece in 1954. From 1956 to 1961 he continued his training at Vanderbilt University. He followed his residency in surgery there with a one-year cardiovascular surgery fellowship at St. Louis University.

An outstanding research scientist and prolific author, he published 19 scientific papers in peer-reviewed journals before arriving in Atlanta. In the years since coming to Grady, from 1964 to 1992, Dr. Symbas authored or co-authored 140 more scientific papers. He also contributed chapters in 71 medical books. In addition,

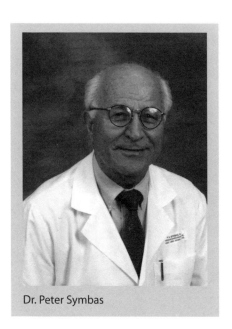

Dr. Peter Symbas

he wrote three highly acclaimed textbooks, including *Traumatic Injuries of the Heart and Great Vessels* (1972), which was translated into Japanese.[59]

Dr. Symbas was a leader in showing that autotransfusion is a safe way to save the lives of people arriving in the emergency room with massive chest bleeding. With time being of the essence for such patients, Dr. Symbas demonstrated the safety and effectiveness of collecting the patient's own blood and returning it to his veins. Previously physicians would only use the technique when matching blood wasn't available for patients who were bleeding rapidly. Dr. Symbas and his colleagues showed the procedure was safe—and perfected it—using dogs. Before Dr. Symbas published his results in 1972, autotransfusion was used more than 350 times at Grady without side effects.[60]

His outstanding contribution to surgery and its literature enhanced Grady's national (and international) reputation as an institution that provided high quality care to its patients, whose physicians made important contributions to the understanding of medicine, and that offered outstanding training to future surgeons.

Dr. Nanette Kass Wenger

A daughter of Russian immigrants, Nanette Kass Wenger graduated summa cum laude from Hunter College in 1951 and three years later earned an M.D. from Harvard Medical School. Following a stint at Mount Sinai Hospital in New York, Dr. Wenger joined the staff of Grady hospital as a resident in cardiology. In 1960 she was named the head of Grady's cardiac lab (started by Dr. Stead a generation before) and later became the head of Grady's cardiac clinics. In 1998 she became Chief of Cardiology at Grady hospital.[61]

Dr. Wenger served Grady hospital for more than a half century. During her remarkable and distinguished career as a physician, teacher, and researcher, the prolific Dr. Wenger published more than 1,100 journal articles, book chapters, and reviews in the medical literature. In addition, she authored or co-authored several books, including *Exercise and the Heart*, *Women & Heart Disease*, *Rehabilitation of the Coronary Patient*, *The Women's Heart Book*, and *Women, Stress, and Heart Disease*. She also chaired numerous panels during meetings of professional associations, advised and appeared on television programs, served on the editorial boards of national and international medical journals, became editor of *The American Journal of Geriatric Cardiology*, and made substantial contributions to the World Health Organization. She has been so remarkably productive during her career at Grady that some students and colleagues jokingly wondered if she had ever taken time to sleep.

Although not all of her time was devoted to professional activities—she has been involved in local associations, including Atlanta Hadassah and the Jewish Children's Service—her professional contributions have attracted interest in the popular media. At the end of 2009 *Woman's Day Magazine* named her—along with Oprah Winfrey, Michelle Obama, and many less-famous people—as one of fifty women who are changing the world. More than thirty years

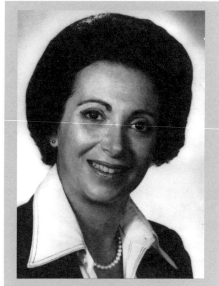

Dr. Nanette Wenger is an eminent cardiologist who served Grady for over fifty years.

earlier, in 1976, *Time Magazine* named her one of its "Women of the Year."

Dr. Wenger started out in cardiology at a time when few women were physicians (fewer than 10% of her class at Harvard Medical School were women) and even fewer served as faculty in medical schools. As Dr. Wenger's career evolved, she paid increasing attention to cardiovascular disease in women. In later years, she attended to cardiovascular disease in the elderly and to preventive medicine. She also became an expert in cardiac rehabilitation.

Being named Physician of the Year by the American Heart Association in 1998 was one of many honors awarded Dr. Wenger. In 2000, the American Medical Women's Association gave her its highest honor, the Elizabeth Blackwell Medal. In that same year, the American College of Physicians presented her with the James D. Bruce Memorial Award for her many contributions in the field of preventive medicine. In 2001, the American Heart Association presented her with the R. Bruce Logue Award for Excellence in Medicine. In 2004, the American Heart Association gave her its highest honor, the Gold Heart Award. She won the Georgia

Chapter American College of Cardiology Lifetime Achievement Award in 2009. Perhaps even more significant than her publications and awards, Dr. Wenger has been an inspiration for patients, students, and colleagues.

The Sickle Cell Center

In 1979, Grady introduced another major contribution to health care by establishing a sickle cell research and treatment program. Grady's pioneering effort would play a major role in furthering understanding of this devastating inherited illness. Grady's program soon became recognized as one of the premier sickle cell research centers in the United States.

While Grady already was researching the disease, it would take the determination of a mother, Berrutha Harper, for the hospital to realize a broader vision.[62] The organizer of the Sickle Cell Patient/Parent Group, Ms. Harper did everything she could think of in the early 1980s to pressure the Georgia legislature to fund a comprehensive sickle cell center. Neither a professional politician nor a physician, Ms. Harper showed the power of a mother. Her son, Kerry, suffered from the disease, and she wanted to create a place where he and thousands of other Georgians could get comprehensive treatment. Educating nearly everyone she met about the painful illness, Ms. Harper also pushed the state legislature to provide funding. At first it refused to fund such a center. In 1984, however, Georgia's General Assembly provided a $50,000 grant; within a year it provided another half-million dollars to establish a 24-hour acute care facility in a designated area of Grady hospital named the Sickle Cell Center. The Georgia Legislative Black Caucus played a crucial role in getting the sickle center at Grady to be funded by the state. In classic horse-trading, the caucus supported the bid of the Speaker of the House, Tom Murphy, to have the interest earned on the state's gasoline tax put into the general fund rather than dedicated to the state's Department of Transportation. In return, Speaker Murphy let the sickle cell funding move forward.[63]

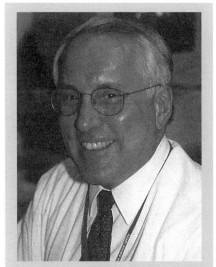

Dr. James Eckman is Professor of Medicine at Emory University School of Medicine and director of Grady's Sickle Cell Center.

At first the center was stuck in cramped quarters on the hospital's fifteenth floor. A little more than a decade later, the Georgia Comprehensive Sickle Cell Center enjoyed spacious quarters on the hospital's first floor. The around-the-clock center held a twelve-bed emergency room for Sickle Cell patients with an infection or other serious complications of the disease like anemia, retinal detachment, stroke, and the severe pain that comes when the sickle cell blocks oxygen getting to limbs or organs. The center also offered special programs targeted at the unique needs of sickle cell patients. These include genetic counseling and job training.[64] The center's creation represented a major political victory; more significantly, it became a major help to its patients.[65]

One of every six hundred African Americans in the United States is afflicted with sickle cell disease, making it one of the most common genetic problems in the country. On average, a patient with sickle cell anemia will suffer from intense pain, requiring hospital care, a couple of times per year. Those with more severe cases may need pain treatment once per month or more. The new center developed a dedicated staff, created new

The Great Condom Caper

Someone, or some group, stole sixteen thousand condoms from Grady's Family Planning Clinic at the end of 1989. While it probably is not a seminal incident in the history of Grady Memorial Hospital, the event did more than raise eyebrows at the time. Popularly dubbed "The Great Condom Caper," the incident prompted many humorous comments among Atlanta's citizens in the days that followed. Of course, writers and comedians in the Atlanta area used the episode to amuse their audiences. The manufacturer re-supplied the items at no cost to Grady. The crime has remained unsolved for more than two decades. If any researchers looked for a sudden decline in the local birthrate nine months after the crime, they have yet to disseminate the results of their research.

therapies, and provided education and support to patients throughout Georgia. Under the leadership of Dr. James Eckman, the center became an international leader in the care of sickle cell patients.

Through Dr. Eckman's efforts, Georgia began statewide sickle cell screening for newborns in 1999. Early detection means early treatment, often preventing death. This program saved the lives of many children who otherwise would have died from pneumococcal sepsis. The program has also saved money. Thanks to the center, the number of hospital admissions for sickle cell complications fell by two-thirds while the number of outpatient visits more than doubled. A decade after its opening, the cost of treating adult sickle cell patients at Grady had dropped from about $16,000 to $5,000, a decline of more than sixty-five percent. In 2000, Dr. Eckman was awarded the National Distinguished Clinician Award for his work with underserved populations. He shared the the same award with Allan Platt two years later when they were honored for inventing a new multidimensional pain assessment method that involved using a hand-held electronic device.[66]

Closing The Grady Hospital School Of Nursing

Following the recommendations of the long-term planning study from 1969, The Grady Hospital School of Nursing stopped admitting students in 1980 because of an impending merger with Georgia State University scheduled for 1982. The school provided Atlanta and the South with over 4,000 skilled professional nurses in the eight decades since its first class graduated in 1900.

The Trouble With Spalding Pavilion, Again

Political and medical clouds formed over the Fulton-DeKalb Hospital Authority in 1979 when a report surfaced that the Hughes Spalding Pavilion's occupancy had plunged during the 1970s. The daily patient census fell in half during that decade, plummeting to 34.4 in 1979 from nearly 70 in 1970.[67] Two major factors stood behind that dramatic decline: the desegregation of medical care in Atlanta and a large demographic shift in Black Atlanta. During the 1970s a large portion of Atlanta's black middle class moved from the city to the rapidly expanding suburbs. As a result, Spalding Pavilion became a relatively distant option for hospitalization. Besides losing much of its patient base, Hughes Spalding also faced new competition. Blacks with health insurance simply had more options than before. Thanks to the desegregation of medical care, the black middle class that remained in the city could choose Piedmont, Emory University, or one of the other hospitals that in the previous decade barred them from being patients on account of race. In addition, many medical groups integrated, with black physicians becoming part of larger white practices.

With its declining patient census, Hughes Spalding was a dramatic financial drain for the hospital authority during the 1970s; it lost at least one million dollars every year from 1974 through the end of the decade. In

1980 a formal study committee addressed the issue of what to do with Hughes Spalding Pavilion. Made up of distinguished physicians including Dr. Asa Yancey, Dr. Clinton Warner, and Dr. Samuel Atkins, the president of the Atlanta Medical Association, the committee also included representatives from the community, members of the Fulton-DeKalb Hospital Authority, Bill Pinkston, and state Representative Grace Towns Hamilton. The committee addressed basic questions: How many inpatients did the hospital need to be viable? How would it get to that level, and at what cost? If it couldn't reach an occupancy level that made the hospital financially viable, what would happen to the facility? The answers depended on the research.

After conducting "market analysis," consultants to the committee concluded that the pavilion's "primary service area" was stable and even beginning to grow. The hospital's base, it turned out, was not the black middle class but the black working poor. Notably, Hughes Spalding had a higher proportion of Medicaid and Medicare patients than any hospital in the Atlanta area except Grady, but as personal income levels rose, the reliance on Spalding Pavilion fell. Residents in wealthier areas of Black Atlanta were more likely to go to Southwest Hospital and Medical Center (formerly Holy Family Hospital) or Crawford Long Hospital than to Spalding Pavilion.[68]

The consultants also analyzed where the hospital was losing money and what it could do to generate revenue. Although it was the hospital's largest source of admissions, the obstetrics department regularly lost money for the pavilion. Even if it tripled its admissions and substantially raised room rates and the delivery charge, the obstetrics department would remain unprofitable. The consultants recommended closing the department and the study committee agreed.[69]

The easiest ways to enhance revenue were to reopen the third floor as a renovated ward for surgery and medical patients, establish an emergency room, and create a psychiatric ward. All of these would contribute to a major increase in hospital admissions. The consultants noted that, in general, emergency rooms provided 30% of the patients a hospital admitted. Spalding's lack of an emergency room put it at a serious competitive disadvantage. Modernizing the facility, adding more beds for general patients, and opening an in-patient psychiatric unit, the consultants projected, would increase the daily average number of inpatients from 35 to 76—an 82.2% occupancy rate if the hospital expanded to 92 beds. (It had cut back to 67 beds by closing the third floor in 1975—a move that increased its occupancy from 51% to 70%, even as the average daily number of inpatients dropped from 65.6 to 51.4.)[70]

The pace of integration in Atlanta remained slow and uneven. From 1975 to 1978, the number of African American physicians with privileges to admit patients at Piedmont Hospital stayed steady at 5, grew from 6 to 10 at Georgia Baptist, but jumped at Crawford Long from 25 to 37. In 1979, only twelve white physicians had staff privileges at Spalding Pavilion, and only one of them was considered active—defined by having admitted 40 or more patients that year. Even among African American physicians, participation at Spalding Pavilion had dropped significantly. Only two of sixteen members of the Atlanta Medical Association who were in general or family practice were active at Spalding. While fourteen of Atlanta's nineteen black physicians specializing in internal medicine were on Spalding's staff roster, only two of them were active. Although more than three times as many were on Spalding's staff, only thirteen surgeons had admitted at least forty patients to the Pavilion in 1979. None of the seven psychiatrists in the association actively used Hughes Spalding. While OB/GYN was the busiest area at Spalding, only five of 32 obstetricians belonging to the Atlanta Medical Association actively used the hospital.[71] The hospital built for African American patients was having trouble attracting black physicians.

Kurt Salmon Associates, the consultants to the formal study committee, explored a series of options for what to do with Spalding Pavilion. These included upgrading the pavilion to a full service general hospital, turning it into an extended care facility or skilled nursing unit, making the pavilion an outpatient clinic, or having it be a private primary care hospital with a stronger affiliation with Emory.[72] The FDHA's decision about what to do with Spalding would take several years.

The Press and Grady

National magazines honored Grady for its excellence during the early 1980s. In 1981, *Business Week* listed Grady as one of the 25 most outstanding hospitals in the country. The following year, *Family Circle* named Grady one of the top twenty health centers in the United States while the *Ladies Home Journal* called it "one of the South's great hospitals" as it included Grady in its list of 13 of the best hospitals in the region.[73] Accolades from the national press continued in July 1985 when *Reader's Digest* reported that a national group of medical experts voted Grady as being among one of the eighteen best trauma treatment facilities in the nation. The selection committee judged hospitals by the length of commitment to trauma care and a record of providing excellent care. It was an impressive honor but more so when it was noted that no trauma centers were listed for Boston, New York, or Los Angeles.[74] (Two years later Grady's Trauma Center earned a Level I Center designation, the highest achievement trauma centers can attain.)

Funding Trouble

Despite becoming relatively flush with cash immediately after Medicare and Medicaid were created, Grady's funding woes reappeared with vigor in the early 1970s. The root of its financial troubles was already apparent a decade earlier. Under state law, the two supporting counties were allowed to tax local property at a rate of up to 5 mills (0.5%) in order to fund the hospital. Grady first began to push up against that limit in the early 1960s when approximately one-fourth of Fulton County's budget was spent on Grady. The influx of federal funds that followed the creation of Medicare and Medicare allowed Grady to keep up with new technology and offer newly available diagnostic and treatment practices without asking the counties to come up with more money. Grady also turned to the State of Georgia for help, but it generally had a difficult time getting substantial support from the state legislature.

Part of the problem was that Grady, like public hospitals across the United States, seemed to have no identifiable constituency. The association of public hospitals (called the Council of Urban Health Providers), on whose board Bill Pinkston served, held a series of conferences in 1972 to examine the role public hospitals played in public health. Some of the main conclusions were predictable: public hospitals were vital for providing care to the poor and minority groups, served as major teaching institutions, were inadequately funded, overcrowded, and sometimes difficult for its patients to reach because of poor transportation. Another conclusion, however, stood out: "The public hospitals have no real constituency to which they can turn for active support." This surprises in part because a large number of patients depended on public hospitals for care and many medical schools relied on them for teaching. The problem, as one conference participant noted, was that the poor didn't like going to public hospitals, local officials didn't like to raise taxes to support them, and "taxpayers resent their taxes going into facilities for the poor."[75]

Like other public hospitals, Grady seemed to lack powerful support groups that would actively lobby the state legislature on its behalf. It seemed as if only the commissioners and legislators from Fulton and DeKalb counties had a vital interest in pressing for more state aid. With rural interests dominating the legislature, it remained challenging to get additional appropriations from the state.

By the late 1970s, the counties were again reaching the legal millage limits for supporting Grady. In a statement to a congressional committee, Bill Pinkston emphasized Grady's fundamental dilemma: "how to provide the improved level of care that was becoming available in the private sector to patients who could not afford to pay."[76] It touched on the heart of Grady's moral underpinning: all lives are equal, and those "who could not afford to pay" for their care ought to receive the same care as those who had access to insurance. (How they paid for that insurance—whether it was federally or privately funded—didn't seem to matter to Pinkston.)

Pinkston's testimony highlighted the cost of uncompensated care rather than the price of innovation. Although the rapid development of new ways to diagnose and treat illnesses led to rising expenses for Grady, making those available to its patients was at the heart of Grady's mission. In order to offer its patients the best possible care, Grady turned to new technologies or innovative procedures that could save lives. It also required the latest equipment for teaching. Residents and medical students needed to understand the latest procedures and techniques; they would be expected to know how to use them when they entered private practice. This meant Grady was practically forced to purchase newly available technologies. While keeping up with the modernization of medicine proved financially challenging, Pinkston's congressional testimony centered on the hospitals most crucial problem: paying for the care provided to people without private insurance, Medicaid, or Medicare. While the new federal programs contributed to an increased demand for medical services after 1966, state cutbacks in funding for Medicaid during the 1970s effectively increased the level of uncompensated care Grady provided.

Seeing little chance of getting more money through local taxes, Grady pinned its hopes on federal funding. The infusion of federal insurance for the poor and the elderly meant that Grady and other public hospitals in the United States were able to offer, in Pinkston's words, "as high quality health care as the state of the art would permit."[77] Even with that funding, Grady continued to rely on the two counties for much of its operating budget. Forty percent of Grady's revenue came from Fulton County through the 1970s. In 1978, Fulton's share of Grady's costs

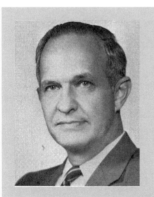

Robert Regenstein (1914-1998)

Julius Regenstein migrated from Germany at age 14 and settled in Alabama. Shortly after the Civil War he moved to Atlanta and in 1872 opened "the Surprise Store" on Whitehall Sheet in downtown Atlanta. The store quickly developed a reputation as a leading fashion center especially for young ladies. Robert Regenstein, a grandson of the founder, was appointed vice president in 1946 of the newly named Regenstein's. He later became chairman of the board and was in that role when the chain of stores was sold to outside investors in 1976. The chain closed its doors in 1994.

Robert Regenstein developed a reputation as an outstanding businessman; recognizing that, his peers elected him as President of the Atlanta Retail Merchants Association. He was also a member of the board of directors of Citizens and Southern Bank and president of the Kiwanis Club of Atlanta in 1976-77. (For 46 years he never missed a meeting.) He was also recognized for 38 years of active support for Pace Academy, a private school in Atlanta.

His greatest impact on his home city was his nineteen years of service on the Board of the Fulton-DeKalb Hospital Authority, including fifteen years as its chairman. During his tenure he led the incorporation of Medicare and Medicaid into the hospital's finances and was a major influence in the establishment of the Pediatric Emergency Clinic, the Burn Treatment Center, and the Drug Dependency Unit.

On Regenstein's death, Bill Pinkston stated, "Bob truly cared about all of the hospital's employees and patients and made sure that the medical students from Emory received the best education possible."[119]

amounted to $42 for every man, woman, and child living in the county.

Unfortunately for Grady and Fulton County, in the mid-1970s the growth in property tax revenues began to slow at the same time the hospital's expenses rapidly increased. The problem for Grady, according to Pinkston, was that the "cost of caring for patients not covered by Medicare and Medicaid—that is, those whose care has been financed from the local tax base—has simply outstripped the ability of the local tax base to support it." Putting it differently, Pinkston noted that "[t]he value of taxable property is not increasing rapidly enough to enable the tax system to cover our costs."[78] The counties understood that, too.

Arguing that Grady had become a regional hospital that served all of Georgia, in 1978 Fulton's commissioners asked the state to take over the county's payments for the care of the uninsured.[79] Uncompensated care had risen to such an extent that Fulton could not cover its share of the cost with its 5 mills of property tax. Just as in the early 1960s, Grady had come up against the limit of what Fulton County could fund. DeKalb County joined Fulton in asking the state to increase funding for Grady, noting that a growing number of patients from elsewhere in Georgia were using Grady's special facilities. Even if property values had been rising, or it had been technically possible to get more money from the counties in some other way, local taxpayers were in no mood to see their taxes for Grady increase.

A year before Pinkston presented his statement to a congressional committee, the Fulton County Commission had decided, for the first time, that a property tax bill would show the exact amount the property owner paid for Grady hospital. Two factors appear to have prompted the commission's decision: the failure to gain substantially more funding for Grady from the state legislature and the news that Grady's budget had risen an average of 16.6 percent per year over the preceding nine years.[80] Perhaps the county commissioners hoped the new line item would spark a taxpayers' revolt.

Suddenly informed property owners jammed the Fulton County government's telephone lines with angry telephone calls. The people who were persistent enough to get through the mass of busy signals protested that they could not afford to pay such a high amount of money for an institution they never used. In response to the outrage from constituents, Fulton board members once again pressed the state of Georgia to increase its funding for Grady. Indeed, the commission asked the state to assume all of the county's obligations for Grady. Getting a negative response, and seeing little hope of success with the state, the county commissioners hoped the Atlanta Chamber of Commerce would be able to put pressure on state officials to, if not completely assume the burden of funding Grady, at least provide more money.

In May 1979, the Fulton County Commission asked the Atlanta Chamber of Commerce to examine Grady's programs and funding sources.[81] Five months later the chamber declared that Grady was well managed. Good management, however, wouldn't solve Grady's fiscal problems. The chamber believed the hospital's shortfall in revenue would force Grady to cut services. If it didn't make cuts, the chamber's group predicted, Grady would face a $9 million annual deficit by 1984. Just as the county commissioners had hoped, the chamber focused on reasons for the state of Georgia to increase its funding for the hospital. These included Grady's role as a primary teaching hospital for physicians in Georgia and the services it provided across the state. Such reasoning resonated with Grady's advocates in the legislature. State representatives from Fulton and DeKalb counties, led by Sidney Marcus and including Paul Bolster, Robert Holmes, and John Hawkins, strongly supported giving Grady greater funding during the late 1970s. The Chamber of Commerce, however, wanted something more than an increase in direct funding: the chamber recommended the state broaden its Medicaid eligibility rules to cover all poor people in the state. If it did, Georgia would become eligible for more federal matching funds.[82]

In a controversial part of its report, the chamber claimed the relationship between Emory and Grady was tilted in favor of Emory. In short, the taxpayers were subsidizing Emory. In addition, the chamber charged that Emory physicians directed privately insured patients to Emory Hospital while sending the poor to Grady.[83]

Because of its funding crisis during the last half of the 1970s, Grady was unable to offer timely and adequate pay increases to its more than 4,000 employees. Although they received annual pay raises from 1974 to 1979, the salary increases were regularly delayed until the hospital became certain that it would get all of the money the counties were supposed to provide. Even worse for the workers, the raises Grady was able to offer were well below the rate of inflation. In the later 1970s, pay raises at Grady amounted to 5% or less at a time when inflation was in double digits. As Grady's compensation for its workers fell behind that of other hospitals in the area, employees started leaving for greener pastures. The financial turmoil subjected Grady to losing its best staff; it also complicated the hospital's effort to attract exceptional replacements.[84]

In 1980, Pinkston asked Congress to have "Medicare and Medicaid include, in the cost of doing business, a hospital's uncompensated services and bad debts."[85] In the prior year, 1979, those costs left Grady with a $29 million deficit. There was a precedent for federal programs taking care of bad debts, and Pinkston believed it was both reasonable and doable without adding bureaucracy. In 1979 that $29 million—funded by local taxpayers—was equal to the total amount Medicare and Medicaid paid to Grady. At the time, the state of Georgia's Medicaid program was limited to qualifying families with dependent children and to the disabled who qualified for Social Security's Supplemental Security Income program. The patients whose costs were covered by local taxes were just as poor as those who received federal assistance—they just didn't fit the categories established for those programs. Pinkston saw this as an inequity in Medicaid that could be resolved with "a more realistic income eligibility standard."[86]

As much as Pinkston might have liked more funding from the federal government, national political changes would dash his hopes. The election of President Reagan in 1980 suggested that an expansion of welfare payments of any type was unlikely. President Reagan had run on a campaign platform of reducing the nation's long-term debt by, in part, lower spending for the nation's system of public welfare. Once that policy was enacted, Grady could ill afford any loss of local tax funding.

In January 1982, a year after President Reagan took office, the Fulton County and DeKalb County governments announced a six million dollar decrease in their appropriations for Grady. The budget cuts led the hospital to lay off employees, close a 32-bed pediatric unit, lower the number of psychiatric beds from 36 to 24, eliminate 32 obstetric beds (which caused the early discharge of some patients), and discontinue convalescent ambulance services (which mainly involved shuttling the elderly and disabled to and from the hospital). Two-thirds of employees went without pay raises. Salaries only increased for positions where low pay hampered recruiting (including registered nurses, licensed practical nurses, and emergency medical technicians). Stagnant wages led Bill Pinkston to declare, "We simply cannot provide the same kind of care if we don't have the funds. … There is not a cut in this budget that we can do again next year."[87] As of February 15, the pharmacy would begin charging outpatient pharmacy patrons the full cost of their medicine instead of fees based on the ability to pay. The last maneuver alone was projected to save $1.2 million for the year. It also led to a public outcry when the hospital authority met in March. Once local governments restored twenty-seven percent of the cut funds ($1,600,000) in April, Grady restored the outpatient pharmacy's earlier fee structure. Because it had reduced its services, Grady managed to end the fiscal year with a surplus in its treasury.[88]

In 1982, 40 percent of Grady's funding came from Fulton and DeKalb counties, with Medicare picking up 21% and Medicaid 19%. Private insurance accounted for 9% of Grady's income while another 10% came directly from patients, state funding, and other third parties.[89] In the early 1980s, the increase in local tax digests continued to lag behind Grady's rising expenses; the digest rose 2% to 3% each year while Grady's costs continued to climb at an annual rate of ten to fifteen percent as they had since the late 1970s. High inflation together with the need to acquire new medical technologies meant that Grady needed more money.

When the Fulton County Commission proposed levying a one-cent sales tax, the hospital authority and Grady's administrators practically grew dollar signs in their eyes; they expected to receive about half of the anticipated $60 million revenue that the tax would generate. As a result, in Dr. Yancey's words, "Grady Memorial Hospital [expected] that yearly expenses will be met with greater grace for Fulton County income is likely to increase with general inflation more readily with the sales tax than with the property tax alone."[90] Although the tax would fall more heavily on the poor, the hospital authority and Grady's administration supported the tax increase because it would, according to Robert S. Regenstein, the authority's chairman, "help us avoid increasing patient charges to the poor in the future." In short, they hoped the sales tax would make the hospital financially more secure and help it better serve indigent residents.[91] Even with a new local sales tax, however, Grady would continue to pin its fiscal hopes on the state.

Grady seemed to have reason for optimism after the Georgia Statewide Health Coordinating Council met with several gubernatorial candidates during the summer of 1982. Both Republicans and Democrats supported having state revenues fund hospitals that cared for the indigent. State Representative Joe Frank Harris (later Governor of Georgia) also endorsed providing state money to teaching hospitals. A few months later, however, on October 28, 1982, Tom Murphy, the Speaker of the House in Georgia, dashed any hopes that may have been raised. Speaking to the Georgia Legislative Forum, he declared that the Georgia General Assembly would not increase aid to Grady. This did not mean, however, that other legislators were giving up the fight.

Renegotiating the Emory-Grady Relationship

Controversy developed in December 1983 when the contract between Emory and Grady expired without being renewed. Several issues capturing headlines revealed underlying conflicts that long existed between the two institutions. The contract's length was crucially important to the people running Grady. As the contract neared its end, Grady's negotiators pressed Emory to agree to a thirty-year contract as they had in 1953. A long-term contract would enhance the Fulton-DeKalb Hospital Authority's ability to sell long-term bonds at a favorable interest rate. In addition to longer-term notes offering lower interest rates, institutional investors would be more at ease knowing the relationship with Emory University helped secure Grady's future. Other complications, however, affected the negotiations between Emory and Grady.

On February 12, 1984, Drs. Louis Sullivan and Clinton Warner asked the Executive Committee of the Medical Association of Atlanta to support Morehouse School of Medicine gaining access to Grady's facilities. At a meeting with the Medical Association of Atlanta, Dr. Sullivan stated that Morehouse was not interested in interfering with the Grady-Emory relationship; it only wanted to be eligible for staff opportunities and for the school to have access to patient care. Dr. Edward Loughlin, the chair of the Fulton-DeKalb Hospital Authority, noted that third-year students at Morehouse already used Grady, and that Morehouse played a central role at Hughes Spalding Pavilion. The Fulton County Medical Society decided to stay out of the conflict; it wanted the interested parties to settle the matter. (The parties involved were the Fulton and DeKalb county commissions, the FDHA, the Morehouse School of Medicine, and the Emory School of Medicine.)

For its part, Emory suggested it might pull out of Grady if it was forced to share the hospital with another medical school. Emory was hesitant to sign a thirty-year contract with Grady that included Morehouse in the equation because it was uncertain about the new medical school's future. On March 2, 1984, the two schools, represented by Dr. Charles Hatcher (Emory) and Dr. Louis Sullivan (Morehouse), agreed that Morehouse would participate at Grady, with the details to be worked out in the coming months. The agreement that Emory and Morehouse reached weeks later allowed faculty members from both medical schools to be on Grady's active medical staff. While the contract would be reevaluated after five years, it gave Morehouse equal standing at Grady (although not equal responsibility for patient care). The FDHA accepted the new contract by a 10-1 vote; Drew Fuller cast the sole nay as a protest against county commissioners injecting politics into Grady's affairs.[92]

The Fulton County Commission needed its own fresh thirty-year contract with Grady. Minority contracting would be an important issue, and the county sought to ensure that 20% of the hospital's business would go to minority-owned firms. More than that, it wanted the counties to determine their support for Grady according to population instead of the current utilization of the hospital. If this had passed, DeKalb's contribution would have jumped by 50% while Fulton's would have fallen.[93] The measure failed.

The Impact of HIV/AIDS on Grady Hospital during the 1980s

In 1986, the Georgia Task Force on AIDS endorsed establishing an outpatient clinic at Grady to care for people suffering from the disease. Dr. Carl Perlino, a Grady epidemiologist and task force member, estimated the cost to create the clinic at almost one million dollars. At the time Grady was treating sixty of the 200 diagnosed AIDS cases in Georgia. In addition, Grady spent $200,000 in 1986 to test its patients for HIV/AIDS.

Dr. Harry Keyserling, acting head of Grady's pediatric unit, testified before the General Health Committee of Georgia's House of Representatives about the rise in positive test results for AIDS among high-risk pregnant women. Fourteen pregnant patients at Grady tested positive for AIDS in 1986. The signs of an epidemic among poor women stood clear by the start of the following summer. More pregnant patients at Grady tested positive for AIDS during the first five months of 1987 (16) than during the entire prior year. The dramatic spread of AIDS in Georgia was hardly limited to poor women. At the start of June 1987, state officials said that the number of reported AIDS cases in Georgia had quadrupled in the last year. Children accounted for twelve of the state's 800 AIDS cases. Infants who acquired HIV antibodies from their infected mothers accounted for the majority of the AIDS patients in the pediatric age group.

As medical professionals became more aware that the number of cases in Georgia was rising, Grady started testing for the AIDS virus in its pregnant patients. (The tests cost about ten dollars per patient.) Expectant women met in small groups with trained HIV counselors during their initial prenatal visit. The sessions proved effective, leading a majority of pregnant women to agree to take the AIDS screening test.[94]

The DeKalb Rape Crisis Center

In January 1988, DeKalb County announced plans to open its own Rape Crisis Center. Although one-fifth of the victims seen at Grady's Rape Crisis Center were from DeKalb County, the number might have been higher if more victims in DeKalb had been willing to travel to Grady. The distance and anticipation of a long wait upon arrival deterred many victims from being seen at Grady even though such a visit was necessary if the patient wanted to have the perpetrator prosecuted.

The idea of an independent center for DeKalb County originated in 1986 with Sue Ellen Mears, a community activist, and the Decatur Cooperative Ministry, a collaboration of more than a dozen churches. Under Mrs. Mears' leadership, they created a task force with representatives from several interested groups, including DeKalb Hospital and its administrator Charles Eberhart. In March 1989, Mrs. Mears and Bob Wilson, the county's District Attorney, convinced the Junior League to make a three-year commitment to establish a rape crisis center for DeKalb County. In October 1989, under the direction of Virginia Vaughan, DeKalb established a hot line for rape victims (but it operated outside the hospital). Rape victims from DeKalb County continued to be seen at Grady until 1991 when DeKalb Hospital began providing physical care to the victims. Like Grady, the DeKalb center examined the victims and treated any injuries, dispensed the "morning after" birth control pills, prescribed antibiotics to prevent venereal disease, gave immediate and follow-up counseling, and referred the victim to a support group. Aid was also given in dealing with the police; this included sending someone to go to court with the victim. The clinic's staff also offered public education in rape prevention.[95]

Renovating the Grady Hospital Building

By the early 1980s an idea that hospital insiders of all stripes—board members, administrators, physicians, and patients—had talked about for several years became a public issue. Put simply, Grady had to be renovated and expanded. The needs of the community had simply outgrown facilities that had opened a generation earlier. As the talks took shape in public meetings during 1983, the project's advocates estimated it would cost about $57,700,000 to refurbish the facility.

Such projects often grow quickly in people's minds as they imagine what could be accomplished with additional resources. Only four years later, by 1987, the estimated cost had risen by over 400 percent, to $250,000,000. That September, Fulton County Commission Chairman Michael Lomax suggested that the authority erect a new structure rather than renovate the building. He estimated the cost for a new hospital at 300 million to 500 million dollars. A month later, Mayor Andrew Young endorsed the Lomax proposal. Claiming that Chairman Lomax and Mayor Young had vastly underestimated the cost of a new facility, hospital officials rejected the idea within two months. The hospital administration and its consultants believed the institution (and taxpayers) would save at least 50 million dollars through renovation rather than total replacement.[96]

In March 1988, the hospital authority asked the Fulton County Commission to approve the renovation and expansion of Grady hospital at a cost of $295,000,000.[97] The proposal included adding 600,000 square feet, mostly for Grady's clinics. But more than that was at stake. Anticipating renovated quarters, the hospital had delayed acquiring new medical equipment in the last few years. Thus, over forty percent of the money in the renovation budget was earmarked for new equipment. The Fulton County Commission refused the hospital authority's request because at that time the question of what to do with the ailing Hughes Spalding Pavilion remained unsettled.

Public discussion about the long-anticipated and much-needed project took on a racial cast almost as soon as the Hughes Spalding Pavilion's future became intertwined with discussions about improving Grady. Black physicians, some of whom were faculty members in the Morehouse School of Medicine, protested the proposed closing. While they were upset about not being consulted about the closing, they were far angrier about what shutting the hospital doors would mean for their students and patients.

Had they been asked, they said, they would have told the FDHA that the recent decline in the use of Hughes Spalding resulted from the hospital authority's failure to buy state-of-the-art medical equipment for Spalding Pavilion during the last decade. The FDHA's neglect had left Hughes Spalding in a weak competitive position. Their argument suggested that if the authority had been looking forward, it would have supported the hospital more generously in recent years, buying the most modern equipment rather than starving it of the best tools available for diagnosing and treating patients. These physicians, together with county commission chairman Michael Lomax, also accused the white-dominated hospital authority of insensitivity to the needs of black patients.

Within weeks the racial dimension of the discussion grew more heated as black doctors, nurses, some black members of the county commission, and a few concerned preachers made allegations of racism. Some claimed that the hospital's administrator, Bill Pinkston, was a racist. (The accusation was laughable to Pinkston's acquaintances.) Others charged Emory University's faculty and medical residents with racism. Going further, some argued that because the majority of Grady's patients were black, African Americans should control the hospital—from the authority to the administration to the physicians. At a time when Grady was seeking more funding from the state legislature—a place where it had few friends among the representatives from the rural communities that dominated its halls of power—the charges of racism and the call for a race-based Grady seemed fruitless at best and self-defeating at worst. Cynthia Tucker, associate editor of the *Constitution's* editorial page, argued that the polarizing rhetoric was counterproductive. In her view, injecting the language of race threatened to undermine an ongoing push by Grady's supporters to squeeze money from an already reluctant state legislature. Ms. Tucker observed, "the recent rhetoric and actions of some of the black members of the county commission threaten the tiny bit of goodwill toward Grady that currently exists [at the state capitol]."[99]

The Fulton County Commission had threatened to block the hospital's renovation unless the FDHA responded to internal and community complaints. The grumbling over officials' failure to consult black physicians about closing the Hughes Spalding Pavilion was growing into a public chorus. In addition to the doctors, three hundred nurses also complained that they were not consulted about closing the Pavilion. For good measure, critics alleged the FDHA had mistreated Morehouse faculty and students.[100]

The hospital authority responded that on an average day only 35 of the Pavilion's 124 beds were occupied and the hospital was losing one million dollars each year. An audit conducted several weeks later showed the $1 million figure to be remarkably cautious; Hughes Spalding Pavilion had lost $850,000 in the first four months of 1988.[101]

In June, the chairman of the hospital authority, Dr. Edward C. Loughlin, claimed the authority was having trouble paying "the obligations incurred in operating Grady Hospital as they become due" because of the costs associated with Spalding.[102] The deficit from the hospital for black patients with insurance (or who could pay for themselves) was threatening the authority's ability to care for the indigent at Grady. Because the black middle class had options for hospital treatment that had been unavailable a generation earlier, many observers argued that the Hughes Spalding Pavilion was an outdated remnant of Atlanta's long and deep history of racial discrimination in medical care.

With the original reason for the Spalding Pavilion's existence largely withered away, the hospital's supporters sought a new rationale for keeping the facility open. The closest they could come was an argument put forward by Dr. Louis Sullivan—Spalding could serve Morehouse faculty members, giving them a place to treat private patients. The idea of using a publicly owned and funded hospital for the private benefit of a handful of physicians met quick and stout resistance. There was no need for them to use Hughes Spalding when Morehouse faculty could gain staff privileges and serve their patients at other hospitals in the city. Grady itself could be an option. With that last reason failing to gain support, Spalding became a piece of nostalgia.

The hospital seemed to have become nothing more than a giant "colored" sign in a society where the most obvious symbols of segregated public space had disappeared. Manuel Maloof, the celebrated tavern owner and DeKalb County commissioner put it succinctly: "It was built in the right time for the wrong reasons. It should go now."[103] But there was a different kind of urgency for another stakeholder at Spalding Pavilion.

The Morehouse School of Medicine saw that closing Hughes Spalding meant ending its fledgling program for training physicians. Because there would be no way for Morehouse to enlarge its training program without access to a large hospital, the school wanted to keep Spalding Pavilion alive. The FDHA, however, had other concerns: if Morehouse's need for Hughes Spalding dictated the hospital authority's actions, the result would be an unsustainable budget crisis. If, in order to meet Morehouse's needs, the FDHA gave Morehouse full access to Grady, there would be a duplication of services given Emory's role at the hospital. Two of everything medical at Grady would return the hospital to a form of racial division it ended twenty years earlier. More than that, duplicating services would intensify the hospital's budget woes. With costs rising, hospital administrators also worried that the added burden would cause Grady's quality of care to decline. While the FDHA believed that giving Morehouse full access to Grady would threaten the hospital's budget and quality of care, it recognized that closing Spalding Pavilion would leave the Morehouse School of Medicine desperate for additional access to Grady.

In the spring of 1988 the Fulton County Commission conceded that the Hughes Spalding Pavilion had become unafford-

able. By the end of April the Fulton County Commission held Grady's renovation hostage to only one demand: assuring the survival—and therefore fuller participation in Grady—of the Morehouse medical school. To meet Morehouse's need, the existing agreements between it, the FDHA, and Emory's medical school would need to be reworked.

The arrangement between Emory and Grady—sealed in a contract between them and the Fulton-DeKalb Hospital Authority only a few years earlier—gave Emory exclusive rights to faculty privileges at Grady. Under that contract Morehouse started sending about two-dozen third-year medical students to Grady for training, adding about ten percent to the teaching load of Emory's Grady faculty members. A new arrangement would substantially expand Morehouse's presence at Grady.

The Emory and Morehouse schools of medicine agreed to assign 25% of patients admitted to the five main departments of Grady to Morehouse faculty, residents, and students. They also agreed that the percentage eventually could rise to fifty percent. The Morehouse School of Medicine's size, however, was an important concern. Compared to Emory, the Morehouse School of Medicine provided only a small number of Grady's staff. Morehouse had twelve faculty members at Grady compared to about two hundred from Emory. Morehouse's hope to develop an accredited residency program would depend (among other things) on vastly increasing the size of its medical faculty.

Any hope for reviving the dying Spalding Pavilion vanished in June when the FDHA announced that it could not pay the financial obligations of the Pavilion as well as care for patients at Grady. It was revealed that from 1973 to May 1, 1988, the Pavilion had lost $7,305,998. Both county commissions reacted with shock at the losses. More than that, each rejected requests the FDHA made for reimbursement. (The authority had funded the pavilion's debt out of its operating funds.)

In September, the Fulton-DeKalb Hospital Authority voted to close Hughes Spald-

> ## The Wedding in the Emergency Room
>
> In 1988 a man arrived in Grady's Emergency Room suffering from severe gangrene. It had progressed so far that he was sent immediately into surgery. Before he could be whisked into the operating room, however, he begged, "I want to get married while I still have both my legs!" It turned out that he was serious. (His fiancé had accompanied him to the hospital.) A nurse in the emergency room contacted the hospital chaplain, found a surgical resident to be best man, and offered herself as the maid of honor. The chaplain promptly married the couple with the staff tossing confetti momentarily before taking the bridegroom into the operating room.[120]

ing Pavilion and instead use the facility for patient overflows during the renovation planned for Grady. Supported by the county commissions, the FDHA announced the closing of the Hughes Spalding Pavilion as of October 28, 1988.[104]

During the turmoil, some black officials intensely criticized the majority white hospital authority and Grady hospital's administration. Fulton County Commission Chairman Lomax asserted that having three out of the ten board members be black was insufficient. To outside observers, Lomax's conversion to using race as a qualifying condition for being a member of the hospital authority seemed awfully late in coming. This was because before the brouhaha over closing the Spalding Pavilion erupted, the last person Lomax had appointed to the board was a white banker.

Commissioner Lomax stated that the hospital authority was disinterested in the black community and that its members had little experience dealing with elected black politicians. He seemed to be pushing for the county commissioners to have greater influence in managing the hospital. Manuel Maloof, the outspoken Chairman of the DeKalb County Commission, responded, "If politicians run the hospital, the quality of care will go to hell."[105] You can almost see the ghosts of Samuel Candler Dobbs and Thomas K. Glenn nodding their approval and raising their glasses in a toast to the tavern owner.

The Fulton-DeKalb Hospital Authority knew that improvements were essential for Grady's future success. The building had significant problems, some of which might have been comical except for their seriousness. The elevators, which had been problematic from the start, were slowed because of crowding. This proved especially inconvenient for pregnant women who had to take the elevator up thirteen floors in order to reach the Labor and Delivery department. Pointing to the desperate need for renovation, Dr. Edward Loughlin joked that more babies were born in the Grady elevators than those in any other hospital in the United States.

As the hospital authority and Fulton County Commission battled over the proposed expansion, the county hired Arthur Young & Associates to conduct a management review of the hospital. Pushed by Chairman Lomax, the study (which cost $300,000) indicated that members of the hospital authority were not "as accountable or as well-informed" as they ought to be.[106] Apparently the hospital's trustees also needed to do a better job of keeping the Fulton and DeKalb county commissioners informed. The conclusions drew fire from the chairman of the hospital authority. Terming the report "worthless," Dr. Loughlin observed that much of what the Arthur Young study noticed had been identified earlier by other consultants.[107]

The report also recommended that the hospital start raising money from private sources. Over the years, Grady often had relied on private philanthropy and volunteers for many of its services. Yet, to systematically cultivate new, sustainable sources of outside funding would be a significant challenge. Professional fund-raisers and hospital leaders already knew that it would be nice to have a successful fund-raising campaign for the hospital. They also knew that it would be difficult to convince major philanthropies to give to Grady.

Cocaine Babies

Grady's newborn service started noticing a new problem in 1986. The intensive-care nursery, which usually admitted approximately 100 infants each month, began seeing a growing number of newborns with signs of cocaine addiction. The infants were small, had lower Apgar scores,* and required two to four weeks to withdraw from their addiction. Local media started paying more attention to the "cocaine epidemic" over the next few years. By 1990, nurses at Grady were reporting that at times almost half of the babies in the intensive-care nursery had cocaine in their urine.

While much of the public's attention was devoted to "cocaine babies," the infants represented a larger problem of cocaine use across the United States. An extremely addictive drug, cocaine was relatively expensive in powder form. As a result, the drug's use was mostly a middle-class phenomenon in the United States until the mid-1980s. At that point a new, cheaper form of the drug started becoming more widely available. Affordable and very addictive, crack cocaine became increasingly widespread in lower-income urban and rural areas with devastating effects for communities and users alike. An inexpensive "rock" smoked in a pipe, the intense "high" crack gave its users came with harsh physical consequences.

Desperate for a high, female crack addicts sometimes sold themselves in order to buy the drug. As a result, a dramatic increase in sexually transmitted diseases became associated with the spreading use of crack cocaine in the late 1980s. But crack inflicted other medical damage. By 1990, nearly half of the patients in Grady's burn unit were there because of accidental fires associated with making and using crack. That same year, nearly 40% of the male patients between the ages of 18 and 39 who came to Grady's triage desk for immediate care during weekdays tested positive for the presence of cocaine in their urine. (Their average age was 29.5 years.) A study of parturient women who delivered a baby at Grady in 1992 showed that 483 out of 3,641 who participated in routine voluntary drug screening tested positive for the drug. A retrospective study of these women showed that those who used crack cocaine were also much more likely than nonusers to deliver low birth weight infants.[108]

In 1990, nurses at Grady would create a newsletter filled with detailed stories about the horrible impact of cocaine and crack. They reported on children who became gunshot victims when crack dealers fired weapons at each other. They told of pregnant women who started to bleed in their brains after using the crack. They wrote about the "cocaine babies" at Grady. More than a compilation of disasters, the newsletter was an attempt to fight the problem. The nurses hoped that distributing their reports would lead local officials to do something about the spreading use of cocaine. In short, they were telling what they knew in order to improve public health. They were joined by physicians like Dr. William R. Sexson who published papers on the impact of cocaine use on newborns. Local newspapers picked up on the stories and reported about children like Pumpkin, a crack baby who weighed less than a pound when she was born in September 1991.[109]

Abortion At Grady

Abortion was illegal in Georgia during the late 1960s, except in cases of medical necessity. As a result, hospitals only performed therapeutic abortions. That legal nicety, however, did not stop women from having induced abortions elsewhere. Unfortunately, illegal abortions often caused medical problems. Many women who had complications

---

*The Apgar Score was developed by Virginia Apgar, M.D., in 1952. It is a quick appraisal of the initial health of a newborn. It is performed at one minute and again at five minutes after birth. Five criteria are observed: the newborn's Activity, Pulse, Grimace (reflex irritability), Appearance (skin coloration), Respiration. The maximum score is 10 with each category ranging from 0 (worst) to 2 (best).

following their abortion went to Grady for treatment.

In 1968 researchers decided to systematically survey all post-abortion patients at Grady. In a single year, sixty women came to Grady with complications after an illegal abortion. (Another thirty women were treated for complications from a therapeutic abortion.) Most of the post-abortion patients Grady treated, however, were unusual for Grady: they were white women from wealthier areas of the city and suburbs. Remarkably, not a single one of the white women had ever been to the hospital until they came to Grady to be treated for complications that followed an illegal abortion. Reporting the results of their survey at a scientific conference in December 1969, the researchers noted that women who chose illegal abortions did so earlier in pregnancy than did women who received therapeutic abortions. They also reported that white women tended to be less accepting of contraception.[110]

A little more than three years later, on January 22, 1973, the Supreme Court of the United States issued its historic decision in the case of *Roe v. Wade*. Ruling that citizens have a constitutional right to privacy, the court overturned state laws that prevented abortions during the first trimester of pregnancy. The controversial decision prompted a backlash among abortion opponents. Four years after the court's decision, Congress enacted a law blocking the use of federal tax money to pay for non-therapeutic abortions. Known as the Hyde Amendment, the law meant that women couldn't use Medicaid to pay for the procedure.

While Medicaid didn't pay for abortions, low-income women wanting to end a pregnancy still turned to Grady hospital. In 1978, Grady performed 1,527 abortions. The number continued to hold relatively steady for the next decade. Over the four-year period from 1985 to 1988, there were 6,045 first trimester abortions performed at Grady.[130] Since Medicaid did not reimburse Grady for the procedures, the cost usually fell into the category of uncompensated care. Because the local counties reimbursed Grady for unpaid treatment, many abortions performed at Grady were effectively paid for out of local taxes.

In a decision handed down in the summer of 1989, the United States Supreme Court ruled that states could restrict abortion in several ways. The court ruled states were free to end abortion in public hospitals. They also could block public health clinics from educating women about the procedure. Almost instantly county funding for abortions became a hot political issue in Georgia. Abortion opponents quickly pushed the legislature to limit abortion in the state. Others warned that doing so would lead more women to take matters into their own hands. As the only hospital in Georgia using tax money to provide abortions, Grady stood at the center of the controversy. At the end of September nearly two hundred anti-abortion protestors demonstrated outside the hospital; they didn't want local tax dollars to fund elective abortions. In response, Grady noted that many women coming to the hospital for an abortion suffered from AIDS; others were addicted to cocaine. Cautious since the court's ruling, legislative leaders seemed to retreat from the issue the closer they came to the opening of the General Assembly's new session in January 1990.[111]

Mr. Bill Pinkston

John William "Bill" Pinkston, Jr., was born in Valdosta, Georgia, on August 11, 1924, and grew up in that city just north of the Florida state line. He was enrolled at Emory University when he was called to active duty during World War II. After his discharge from the military he returned to Emory to complete a bachelor degree in business administration. Upon graduation in 1947 he went to work for the Western Electric Company. He left a year later to become the assistant controller for Grady. He held several other administrative positions before being named the hospital's Chief Executive Officer following Frank Wilson's death in 1964. He served effectively in that position for a quarter-century, retiring in 1989.

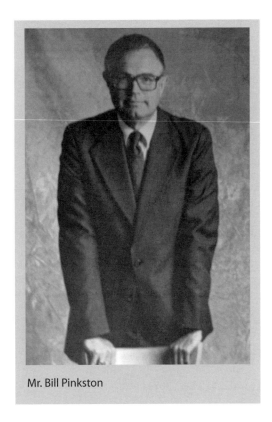

Mr. Bill Pinkston

Bill Pinkston steered Grady through very rough waters. Outside forces seemed to make the largest waves—ones that hit urban charity hospitals across the nation. The rise of Medicare and Medicaid had drastically altered the financing of the American hospital by suddenly providing specific monetary reimbursement for the care provided to indigent, low-income, and previously uninsured patients. The new programs also demanded fresh administrative systems for handling mountains of new paperwork. Because a host of new technologies for diagnosing and treating illness emerged during the Pinkston era, Grady regularly needed to purchase new equipment, reconfigure the hospital's spaces, and find money to pay for both.

Together with all this, the emergence and recognition of new diseases, most notably HIV/AIDS, created a series of significant challenges for the hospital. How to treat and manage HIV/AIDS seemed especially daunting after the virus first became identified. The public's understanding of transmission was clouded and it worried, needlessly but sometimes hysterically, about casual transmission. For large parts of American society, fears about AIDS (and ignorance about causes and prevention) spurred discrimination. The handling of HIV/AIDS also was a medical conundrum before the first effective pharmaceutical treatment strategies emerged. It could be a nightmare for hospitals as staff worried about blood contamination. The disease prompted new safeguard measures for hospital workers, including protective clothing and new waste disposal strategies. The new disease also prompted pharmaceutical research—although not quickly enough or effectively enough to suit activists. It took several years, but eventually medicines were developed to help patients manage the disease.

Hospital costs grew dramatically during Pinkston's tenure at Grady in part because of major advances in pharmacology that extended the life expectancy of patients with chronic illnesses. Gunshot wounds and traffic accident injuries continued to fill the trauma center. Starting in the 1980s, the cocaine epidemic provided additional challenges, especially with the "crack baby" phenomenon. New awareness of the impact of drugs and alcohol on infants together with new diagnostic capabilities and amazing advances in neonatal technologies also meant new administrative challenges. Together with all this, the population Grady served was increasing. The city was one of the fastest growing in the nation, and with that growth came a vast increase in the number of patients seen at Grady.

Rising public expectations about the facilities, services, and comforts a hospital would provide also affected Mr. Pinkston's work. As central air-conditioning systems spread rapidly in public spaces during the 1960s, it became apparent that the hospital's reliance on window units, or on a breeze blowing in from above the highway nearby, was insufficient. Installing central air-conditioning became a medical imperative and a public expectation, one that would improve medical outcomes and heighten patient comfort. Other public demands concerned specific services. In response to citizen suggestions, Grady would open its night clinic and establish the Rape Crisis Center. Changing medical standards also altered the physical configuration of the hospital, especially as the movement toward having more clinics inside of hospitals intensified. So too did patient and professional demands for nursing care. Throughout Pinkston's years at Grady, the hospital had nursing shortages that never seemed to subside.

In 1965, under Pinkston's leadership, the hospital finally became fully desegregated. Nearly two decades later, Pinkston would welcome students and faculty of the new, predominantly black, Morehouse College School of Medicine to the educational, patient care, and research mission of Grady. By the time he announced his retirement in the autumn of 1988, controversies swirling around Grady demonstrated yet again that there were, broadly speaking, two Atlantas—one black, the other white. The controversies surrounding Grady also showed how little each Atlanta knew about the other. Although Grady's patient services were racially integrated, the number of white patients had fallen dramatically since 1960. Non-Hispanic whites accounted for fewer than one in ten patients. In its role as a teaching hospital, Grady had students and faculty both from a predominantly white medical school and from a predominantly black one. For all of the efforts to overcome the hospital's division into two Gradys, by the end of the 1980s Grady continued to symbolize the city's racial contrasts.

Long after his retirement in the autumn of 1989, Bill Pinkston admitted that bitter public fights about closing Hughes Spalding and over the tripartite relations between Grady, Emory, and the Morehouse School of Medicine prompted him to leave the job he loved earlier than he might otherwise have preferred.[112] While he claimed to not be very good at the politics of hospital administration, Bill Pinkston was a master of the art he didn't much care for. He managed to keep the money coming from county commissioners who would have preferred to cull popularity by cutting taxes rather than spending the public's money. Keeping local tax revenue coming seemed increasingly important during the 1980s as federal spending for social programs declined. Bill Pinkston quietly navigated the public hospital past the shoals of inadequate funding, expensive medical innovations, escalating expectations, a sudden rise and then severe cutbacks in government programs paying for health care, competing political factions, battles over institutional prerogatives, and the ever-present issue of race. As a former member of the FDHA board observed, Pinkston was tough, and he cared about only one thing: Grady hospital and its people. When Bill Pinkston retired, the appreciative chairman of the hospital authority declared, "Bill Pinkston is Grady Hospital."[113]

Grady Medical Directors

Dr. Douglas Kendrick

Retired Major General Douglas Kendrick, a native of Atlanta, graduate of Emory University and its medical school, and a former commanding general of Walter Reed Army Medical Center, became Grady's Medical Director on May 1, 1967.

During his distinguished medical career, Dr. Kendrick practiced at the Mayo Clinic and then as the head of surgical research at Walter Reed. An active researcher, he helped develop the military's Blood, Plasma, and Albumin Program. Dr. Kendrick served in World War II and, after the war, became General Douglas MacArthur's personal physician during the time General MacArthur administered post-war Japan. After a time as executive officer to the Surgeon General of the United States, General Kendrick became commanding general of the 9th Hospital Center in Germany and then oversaw surgery in nineteen military hospitals in Germany, France, and Italy. A renowned surgeon, General Kendrick was involved in removing the gallbladder from former President Dwight D. Eisenhower in 1966. His massive history (922 pages) of military medicine during the

Second World War was published as *Blood Program in World War II*.[114]

Joining Grady hospital after retiring from the military, Dr. Kendrick also accepted an appointment as an associate dean of Emory's medical school. At Grady Memorial Hospital, Dr. Kendrick took responsibility for the areas of hospital administration concerning the organized medical staff and the hospital's affiliation with Emory. He quickly won praise for improving relationships between nurses and the medical staff. Following Dr. Kendrick's resignation, the hospital named Dr. Asa Yancey as its new medical director.

Dr. Asa Yancey

Asa Yancey was born in Atlanta on August 19, 1916. Educated in the local public schools through high school, he continued his education at Morehouse College from which he graduated in 1937. After earning his M.D. degree from the University of Michigan in 1941, Dr. Yancey took a surgical residency under the tutelage of the famed surgeon Charles Drew at Howard University. After military service in WWII, Dr. Yancey became an instructor of surgery at Meharry Medical College. He then served as chief of surgery at the Veterans Administration Hospital in Tuskegee, Alabama, from 1948 until he returned home to Atlanta in 1958 to become Medical Director of Hughes Spalding Pavilion. There he established the first accredited training program for black surgeons in Georgia. Seven young physicians completed surgical training at Hughes Spalding before the program was discontinued. In 1962, he became the first African American named to Grady's visiting staff. (He was not, however, the first African American to perform surgery at Grady. That honor belongs to Dr. W. Harry Barnes of Philadelphia who, during the annual meeting of the National Medical Association held in Atlanta in 1931, performed a bronchoscopy at Grady.)[115] In 1972, Dr. Yancey became Medical Director of Grady Memorial Hospital—a post he fulfilled with extraordinary skill and great distinction.

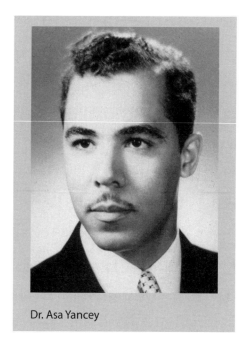

Dr. Asa Yancey

In January 1987, Dr. Yancey made an emotional speech to Fulton County's lawmakers. In hopes of easing the financial burden healthcare placed on county residents, he asked the state to extend Medicaid benefits to the working poor. He also asked the legislature to give Grady more money because the hospital cared for many people who lived outside Fulton and DeKalb counties. Dr. Yancey also argued in favor of tort reform. He claimed that excessive malpractice premiums absorbed funds that could be used to treat sick people. Grady was spending an amazing amount of money on its self-insurance program, and if it could reduce that spending—$13,000,000 in 1987—it might also be able to ease the taxpayers' burden.

Among his many achievements, Dr. Yancey was elected twice to the Atlanta Board of Education. He also served on the editorial board of *The Journal of the National Medical Association*. Dr. Yancey also was the first black physician allowed onto the staff of St. Joseph's Infirmary after Archbishop Halliman ordered the hospital's desegregation in 1963. The first patient Dr. Yancey admitted into St. Joseph's was the Reverend Martin Luther King, Jr. It was while a patient there that Dr. King first heard that he had won the Nobel Prize for Peace.

Dr. Yancey retired at the same time in 1989 that his friend Bill Pinkston left Grady. Dr. Yancey's remarkable legacy includes four children, three of whom–two sons and one daughter–became physicians.[116]

Dr. Hamilton E. Holmes

Dr. Hamilton E. Holmes, a 47-year-old orthopedist, was elected to replace Dr. Yancey as Grady's medical director. Dr. Holmes and the renowned journalist Mrs. Charlayne Hunter-Gault were the first African American students admitted to the University of Georgia. After graduating from the University of Georgia cum laude in 1963, Hamilton Holmes became the first of his race to enter the Emory University School of Medicine, receiving his medical degree in 1967. Dr. Holmes followed his graduation from medical school with a residency in surgery at Detroit General Hospital (later renamed Detroit Receiving Hospital). He then undertook a residency in orthopedics at Emory, which he completed in 1973.

He was an excellent choice for medical director, a position that he kept for six years. In January 1995, Dr. Holmes ran afoul of the hospital's new administration. Grady's new CEO, Edward Renford, initiated severe budget cuts soon after taking his position, and the response within the hospital was far from favorable. The controversial decision led three of the institution's vice-presidents to resign. Dr. Holmes was not likely to leave his position as medical director on his own. Although

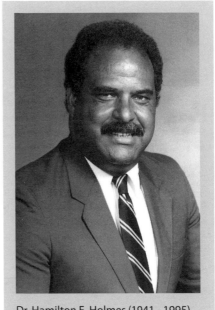

Dr. Hamilton E. Holmes (1941 - 1995)

he was an employee of the Emory University School of Medicine when he accepted the position, the hospital's new leadership suggested his affiliation posed a significant conflict of interest for Dr. Holmes at Grady. Apparently his working for Emory suddenly compromised his impartiality when mediating disputes between Emory and the Morehouse School of Medicine. Supportive of its new CEO, in January 1995 the Fulton-DeKalb Hospital Authority board refused to renew Dr. Holmes' contract as medical director. Sadly, Dr. Holmes died the following October, two weeks after undergoing quadruple bypass heart surgery.[120]

The Whirlwind
1990-2008

"Taking care of poor people who are sick, who don't have any other way to get care, is not pork."
—Manuel Maloof, DeKalb County CEO, September 11, 1994

Public hospitals across the United States faced a host of problems in the 1990s. Money was the root of most of their troubles: they just didn't have enough. The central struggle to have income keep pace with rising costs resulted from an underlying problem that affected for-profit hospitals and other non-profits as much as public hospitals: fewer people being treated in hospitals. In addition, those who came stayed for a shorter period than only a decade before. Changes to federal regulations also expanded the competition for patients insured through federal programs. More broadly, the traditional culture of medicine seemed to be under attack. What had once been defined in terms of a calling was becoming dominated by the culture of commerce and profitability.

Of course, American physicians had been businessmen throughout the twentieth century. Most physicians had private practices, and their leading professional organization, the American Medical Association, worked to protect the income of the physicians. Maintaining the physician's independence, however, had been an equally important goal for the association. This desire, more than economic concerns, drove opposition to the corporate practice of medicine during the first half of the century. In the last decades of the twentieth century, however, the pressure to engage in trade was challenging older ideals of following a calling. The high-minded ideals seemed to be giving way to the language and ideals of market culture.[1]

While this was beginning to affect the practice of some physicians, it was becoming endemic for hospitals. Non-profit hospitals faced increasing cost pressure and competition from publicly traded corporations during the 1990s. Because of the way the American health system had developed, calculating investors saw hospital corporations and other health care providers as offering large rewards relative to the risks. Indeed, publicly traded for-profit hospitals and health care companies had grown rapidly during the 1970s and 1980s and continued to expand in the 1990s. What critics derided as the "commercialization" of medicine—distinguishing it from the time when individual physicians acted as independent businessmen and many hospitals were run by religious institutions—appeared to be putting pressure on all hospitals to cut costs. The massive scale of hospital conglomerates gave them greater buying power with suppliers. Lowering the cost of materials, however, was only part of their strategy. The search for profitability also led to intense negotiations for better arrangements with insurance companies and a focus on reducing expenses that would challenge traditional ideas about the practice of medicine.

The drastic change in the environment was reflected in the language people used when talking about the delivery of health care. Patients were starting to be seen as customers, hospitals were beginning to serve markets rather than communities. What were once charity cases had become uncompensated care. As Dr. Rashi Fein warned in an essay in *The New England Journal of Medicine* in 1982, "the language of the marketplace" was "infecting the culture of American medicine."[2] A noble and humane service to humanity was being transformed into a commodity.

Concurrently, the cost of care was rising dramatically. Part of this resulted from investment in expensive new medical equipment. Hospitals across the country invested large sums in rapidly changing information technologies in the hope of achieving greater efficiency in everything from billing to ordering supplies. At the same time that costs rose, revenue fell as hospital usage declined.

According to the National Academy of Sciences' Institute of Medicine, the nation lost 198,000 hospital beds between 1993 and 2003.[3] It was a time of consolidation in the "hospital industry." Independent community hospitals in American suburbs struggled as did Catholic, Lutheran, Baptist, Seventh Day Adventist, and other non-profit hospitals. Many would close or become part of larger hospital systems. The reduction in the number of beds during the 1990s and the closing of hospitals resulted from several long-term trends.

Starting in the 1970s, Americans began using hospitals less often for outpatient services. Increasingly they received diagnostic tests at outpatient centers. In addition, more surgery was being performed on an outpatient basis.

Changes in hospital and medical insurance contributed to the declining use of hospitals. By the 1990s the popularization of new insurance plans, especially Health Maintenance Organizations (HMOs) and Preferred Provider Organizations (PPOs) pressed hospitals to behave differently in order to contain costs. Insurance companies pressured hospitals to reduce the length of a patient's stay. Not only was the number of hospital admissions falling, the patient's length of stay was becoming shorter. Insurance companies also helped push people to obtain a medical diagnosis and treatment in an outpatient setting.

In this environment, public hospitals, which had long existed in part to help relieve private hospitals of some of the costs associated with charity care, were competing with the institutions for which they had been a safety net. At the same time, Grady's traditional source of revenue—local tax-support—was reaching political limits.

For supporters of public hospitals, the list of failing public hospitals would become depressing by the end of the twentieth century. Legendary public hospitals would begin to fail in the 1990s. Others, like public hospitals in New York City, were privatized—a fate that Grady Health Systems narrowly avoided in the mid-1990s. Pressed by the state legislature that year, Grady hired APM Management Consultants to make what amounted to an efficiency study for the hospital.[4] The consultants were directed to come up with a strategy that would let Grady provide "low cost, effective health care" and, at the same time, "substantially reduc[e] local tax support."[5] This came two years after a powerful congressman from Atlanta's northern suburbs, Newt Gingrich, suggested Grady should be studied as a candidate for privatization.[6] In a difficult economic environment of declining support from the local counties and rising costs, Grady would have to scramble for every dime.

Grady began planning its major renovation in 1984, when the pattern of changing hospital usage was murky. The trend of declining hospital use had become clearer by the time the first phases of Grady's renovation and expansion were finished. In 1992, three years after construction began, critics were wistful. They started to argue that the money spent on construction at the hospital would have been better spent on creating and expanding neighborhood clinics. Their hindsight, while not perfect, would have been more helpful as foresight.

Since planning for renovation first began, the needs of the hospital seemed to be growing in tandem with the area's rapidly increasing population. By the time the project was approved, the plan for revitalizing Grady hospital involved renovating 1.2 million square feet and expanding the hospital by another 600,000 square feet. The size alone made it a complicated project. What made it more difficult was that the hospital would have to continue running at full steam during construction. It would be hard to do it on the cheap. Renovating what had been Atlanta's largest building when it was built would become the most costly public works project in Georgia's history. By the spring of 1991, Grady's renovation became the center of a political firestorm.

The Taxpayer Revolt

On February 15, 1989, the city of Atlanta and Fulton County created a Joint City-County Board of Tax Assessors to oversee the reappraisal of every piece of personal and business property in Fulton County. (A new state law prompted the action.) Like many local governments, the city-county board turned to a private contractor to conduct its reappraisal. In hiring Cole-Layer-Trumble Company (CLT) of Dayton, Ohio, the joint committee turned to one of the oldest and largest appraisal firms in the nation. As CLT was finishing its work early in 1991, county officials realized that the reassessment would result in much higher valuations of property—and higher tax bills. Fulton's officials tried to prepare the public, but their efforts were in vain.[7]

Residents and business-owners were outraged after their new property assessments arrived in the mail. While the numbers generally reflected the fair market value of property, the appraisals caused severe sticker shock. Property owners understandably were concerned about the dramatic increase in the assessment and, as a result, in their tax bills.

Residents who tried to appeal the county's appraisals quickly became frustrated both by a confusing process and an inability to reach the people who were responsible. Overwhelmed by the massive number of telephone calls from angry residents, the assessor's office provided only busy signals. Cole-Layer-Trumble, less familiar to residents than the assessor's office, seemed utterly unaccountable to county residents. Frustration with the reassessments, the appeal process, and access to county officials soon triggered a broad tax revolt in Fulton County.[8]

The sticker shock heightened citizen concerns about local government spending. Well before the reassessment was finished, many residents already were up in arms about a large county office and court building recently built in downtown Atlanta. Critics focused their arguments less on the need for a new facility than on its apparent excesses.

Far from austere, the Fulton County Government Center became a potent symbol of wasteful government spending. Among other things, the county had decorated the building's atrium with palm trees costing $8,500 each. Chairman Lomax's opponents and others seeking political gain quickly seized on the cost of the palm trees and on the building's relative opulence. Defending the building, Lomax noted that the county government center was part of the revitalization of Atlanta's downtown business district. Defending the pricey palm trees, Chairman Lomax explained that a federal grant used to acquire the property required creating a park as part of the redevelopment. To comply with the terms of the federal funding, Fulton County officials interpreted the building's indoor atrium—which contained the controversial palm trees and a fountain—as a year-round park. At first, the atrium seemed like an ingenious solution to a problem posed by the federal grant. What had looked like genius soon symbolized bureaucratic bungling.[9]

Critics complained about more than symbols. They seemed especially upset that the county had increased spending and raised taxes during a recession.[10] Commissioner Lomax might have countered them by noting that even with the growth in spending, the tax rates for unincorporated Fulton County remained lower than those in the north suburban cities of Roswell and Alpharetta.[11] He also could have highlighted that the county was driven to raise taxes in part because of funding cuts from the federal and state governments. The critics, however, may not have cared.

The Fulton County tax revolt was in large measure a reaction to rising costs for services. The county's budget rose by 20 percent in a single year, from 1989 to 1990.

The county's desire to match its services to the rapidly growing population in northern Fulton County helped drive much of the spending increase. Hoping to accommodate its residents, the county added staff for the library system and jail. It also made overdue improvements to the jail (mandated by court order). Fulton County also increased funding for the arts to $3.4 million. Critics shouldn't have been surprised. The Chairman of the Fulton County Commission, Michael Lomax, had a long track record as a great supporter of the arts. Indeed, more funding for the arts had been a consistent theme in his successful campaigns for county commissioner.[12]

Of all of the county's expenditures, Grady was the most visible target for angry taxpayers. Since 1979, every property owner's tax bill showed the precise dollar amount levied on his or her property to pay for Grady. It was the only line item on Fulton's property tax bill except for schools.

Chairman Lomax, however, gave credence to the criticism when he identified Grady as the leading cause for the county's increased spending. It may have been naïve on his part, but Lomax hoped that focusing on Grady would lead the county taxpayers to pressure legislators to increase state funding for the hospital. At the time, the State of Georgia provided about 5% of Grady's budget. Lomax thought that because Grady's services benefited all of Georgia, the state should bear a greater share of the hospital's expenses. As he told the chamber of commerce and anyone else who would listen, it was unfair for Fulton and DeKalb counties to shoulder the burden for the rest of the state.[13]

Lomax's argument was hardly new. Grady's supporters had long argued that Grady benefited the entire state. Their pleas, however, had fallen on deaf ears at the state capitol. Perhaps Lomax's argument would hit a nerve with constituents in northern Fulton County. Maybe they would press their representatives for help in having the state legislature take on more of Grady's financial burden.

Mark Burkhalter, a realtor and former staff aide to congressman Newt Gingrich, was one of eight residents of North Fulton who organized an anti-tax group in the summer of 1991. In line with Lomax's hopes, the Lower Our Grady Tax Coalition (LOGTAX) planned to lobby the state legislature to increase Georgia's share of Grady's funding. They agreed with Chairman Lomax that the state ought to pay a larger share of Grady's budget. Cynics might suggest they were simply shifting their tax responsibility from local to state government. According to the group, however, patients from elsewhere in Georgia had cost Grady $8.3 million in 1990. They argued that it was unfair for residents in Fulton County to subsidize other counties for the cost of treating their patients.[14]

While it first pursued increased state funding for Grady, LOGTAX soon shifted its focus away from pushing the state to give give Grady more money. Instead, it began asking the state to force Fulton and DeKalb counties to cut their collections for Grady hospital. Burkhalter quickly became the group's spokesman. Boasting to a reporter that "this thing [Grady] has a lot of life to it, and it hasn't been touched," he saw a political opportunity and he took it.[15] Burkhalter rode Grady and local tax issues to a seat in Georgia's General Assembly.

Another group of Fulton County homeowners formed The Task Force for Good Government in response to the appraisal and appeals process. At first a vehicle for pushing procedural reforms, before long the group's mission broadened. By the summer of 1991, its mission mimicked LOGTAX, lobbying the legislature to increase state funding for Grady. Like Mark Burkhalter, its spokesman, Mitch Skandalakis, would ride popular anger over taxes and Grady to political success. His platform suggested that shifting Grady's tax burden from the county to the state would be a winning political strategy.[16]

Residents in Fulton County were angry that their tax dollars were subsidizing healthcare for people from outside of Fulton and DeKalb counties. Although the number of people who came from elsewhere was relatively small, county residents—facing a large increase in property taxes—simply wanted whatever relief they could get. If the state began to fully pay for the care of patients from outside of the counties, then property taxes in Fulton might fall.

Lomax's strategy of generating popular support for greater state funding for Grady seemed to be working. Soon, however, the residents' appeals for a legislative solution faded, their energy turning elsewhere. LOGTAX began emphasizing the need to cut spending at the hospital and started portraying the hospital as yet another symbol of government excess. Perhaps Chairman Lomax anticipated LOGTAX's shift to focusing on Grady's spending. The other group of tax protesters and erstwhile supporters of state funding for Grady, however, gave Lomax more than he expected. Late that summer, Mitch Skandalakis and members of the Task Force for Good Government organized a drive to recall Chairman Lomax from office. Although they failed to get enough signatures within the allotted 45-day time period, the group could claim a victory for spurring what Dick Williams, a local columnist, presciently characterized as the unofficial beginning of the "dissolution of Fulton County."[17]

Accounting for more than a quarter of the county's budget, Grady looked like an obvious target for residents angry about their property tax bill. Even if the county's services might seem inadequate, people who saw their taxes in terms of fees for services could at least recognize tangible benefits from taxes paid for police, firemen, jails, the justice system, parks, and recreation. Those were services they expected and received from the county. By contrast, relatively few residents in prosperous northern Fulton County were likely to use Grady, except in a severe emergency. Even then, given its distance, it would have to be a certain type of medical crisis.

While the hospital's trauma care and burn unit were first-rate, those services did not symbolize Grady to people in north suburban Fulton County. Grady, to them, was a hospital for poor people. It wouldn't take long for residents to argue that the other services in the county also were being unfairly distributed. The old Atlanta belief that white taxpayers subsidized services for black areas reappeared with all the vigor that it had during the era of desegregation. While the issue was often put in economic terms, that the wealthy subsidized services for the poor, it was rarely put in terms of seeking the common good. Once more, taxes were viewed as fees for services. The line item on the property tax bill for Grady hospital stuck out as a service that wasn't being used. While few whites put the issue in blatantly racial terms, many black residents in southern Fulton County perceived the attacks on Grady's spending as racially motivated.[18]

The association of Morton Rolleston, Jr., with a legal battle against the county's property reassessment looked to black leaders like evidence that the anti-tax movement was racially motivated. Their view was rooted in Rolleston's legal history more than a quarter-century earlier rather than anything he said in 1991. During the early 1960s Rolleston owned the Heart of Atlanta hotel, an establishment that refused to serve blacks. He responded to the Civil Rights Act that opened public accommodations to everyone by filing a suit against the United States only two hours and ten minutes after President Johnson signed the bill into law. *Heart of Atlanta Hotel v. United States* was the first legal challenge to the new law. Rolleston was explicit that the *Heart of Atlanta* case was not about segregation but about unchecked federal power. In December 1964, the United States Supreme Court used the case to affirm the constitutionality of the public accommodations section of the civil rights bill.[19] Some leaders in Black Atlanta saw Rolleston's past and his connection with the lawsuit against Fulton County's property reassessment as a way to peg the anti-tax movement as racist. Yet, significantly, Michael Lomax went out of his way to reject that view. While he indicated that some protestors were racially biased, he denied that the tax protest was on the whole racially motivated. Instead, Lomax generally viewed the movement in economic terms.[20]

Not everyone viewed Lomax's remarks so charitably. Dick Williams thought Lomax had come "perilously close to real race baiting" in assessing the motivations of tax protesters. Williams claimed that by making "explicit allegations of racism," Lomax had "infuriated many white voters." Pointing to the commission's record in the prior year, Williams suggested Lomax should have been emphasizing that Fulton County had "cut actual spending by 2 percent across the board" in the prior year.[21] The drop in spending, however, may not have gone far enough to satisfy voters who were angry about the property reassessment in Fulton County.

By the fall of 1991, LOGTAX, the Grady tax and spend watchdog group, had set its sights on the costs of renovating Grady. After a great deal of research, the group claimed to have found ways to save $6 million during construction. Grady officials contended the group miscalculated; the suggestions would provide only $2.6 million in savings, less than one percent of the project's cost. More importantly, Grady had logical reasons to ignore some suggestions from LOGTAX. Responding to the group's idea that the hospital use less expensive materials for floors and walls, Grady officials argued that longer-lasting materials would save money in the long run. Other claims, however, proved more contentious, their refutation more complicated. For example, LOGTAX charged that the building renovation was extravagant. In its view the hospital required neither an atrium nor skylights—these were luxuries rather than necessities. In response, Grady's defenders argued that the people using Grady should have pleasant surroundings. In some ways, LOGTAX was arguing that enhancing the built environment for the next generation mattered less than a few million dollars.[22]

In late November, the Fulton-DeKalb Hospital Authority approved an operating budget of $285 million for 1992, an increase of 9.6% from the previous year. Fulton County would pay $72.8 million, and DeKalb would contribute $23.7 million. Together, the counties total contribution of over $96 million would be a 5.4% increase over the previous year. The hospital budget did not include money for the four satellite clinics, ambulance service, or the Crestview Nursing Home. Adding those figures in, along with debt service on bonds for the hospital's renovation, meant that the budget rose by $25 million. The total requested from Fulton was $100.3 million, from DeKalb $29.9 million.[23]

Angered by the hospital's spending, and what he saw as a lack of competitive bidding, Lomax sent a strong signal that the hospital's proposed budget for the next year would have to be reduced. In December, Chairman Lomax led the Fulton county commissioners in holding back three appointments to the Fulton-DeKalb Hospital Authority, including the reappointment of Dr. Edward C. Loughlin, whose term was to expire at the end of the year.

The hospital authority responded to Lomax's concerns about its purchasing practices by approving new guidelines to expand competitive bidding and lower the cost of supplies. It did little to change race-neutral guidelines it adopted in 1990, but the authority did adopt an ethics policy to address potential conflicts of interest. Significantly, the revised guidelines reinforced the idea that minority-owned businesses would get at least 30% of the hospital's spending on supplies and construction. The guidelines avoided racial terms; instead, they referred to "socially" and "economically" disadvantaged business owners.[24]

At the start of 1992, Chairman Lomax and the county commissioners held public hearings on Grady's budget. The first meeting, held in northern Fulton County, gave residents a chance to vent frustration with Grady's spending.[25] It looked like a deft political maneuver on Lomax's part. Although he survived a recall movement the previous fall, Lomax knew he was still in trouble with north suburban voters. He had publicly called for Grady to cut spending—and threatened to slash its budget—and he hoped the public meetings would pressure Grady to reduce costs by about $8 million. Even if the tactic failed, Lomax appeared ready to cut the county's contribution.

Before the meeting even took place, however, the county commission removed Dr. Edward C. Loughlin as chairman of the hospital authority. Normally it would have mattered little that Dr. Loughlin's term had expired eight days earlier. In ordinary times Dr. Loughlin would have stayed on as chairman until either his term was formally extended or someone else was elected to the board. By a vote of four to two, however, the commission removed Dr. Loughlin from the authority chairmanship. Chairman Lomax seemed to have rid himself of the complication of having an independent voice as chairman of the hospital authority. The bickering between the hospital authority and the county had devolved into a power play by Chairman Lomax. One of the commissioners who opposed the move, Gordon Joyner, referred to the maneuver as a "public lynching."[26]

If Lomax expected that engineering Dr. Loughlin's removal would endear him to north Fulton residents, he would have been surprised. Dr. Loughlin was about to be re-nominated by commissioner Tom Lowe, a member who represented North Atlanta and part of suburban Fulton County.

Dr. Frank L. Wilson, Jr., a distinguished physician in Atlanta and the son of a past Grady's administrator, publicly defended Dr. Loughlin. Noting that Dr. Loughlin had trained at Grady and was committed to the institution, Dr. Wilson observed, "It appears that his primary sin was that he would not be a yes man to the Fulton County Commissioners." Placing the commissioners' decision to vacate the position in historical context, Dr. Wilson noted that the Fulton-DeKalb Hospital Authority was supposed to help isolate Grady from politics and to ensure its excellence. His point was clear—the county should stop politicizing the administration of Grady hospital. If it didn't, the quality of care would decline. Reminding readers of Grady's reputation as one of the best public hospitals in the United States—both in terms of how it was run and in the services it provided to patients and the larger community—Dr. Wilson warned that Grady would become a lesser institution if a "yes man" for Fulton County became the authority's chairman.[27]

With Dr. Loughlin removed as chairman, the town-hall meeting in North Fulton turned from a hearing on Grady's budget to an attack on the hospital. Residents who attended the meeting were clearly angry about their taxes and about Grady's request for additional funds from Fulton County. (It wanted a big increase from the $89 million dollars Fulton paid in 1991.) In response, Mitch Skandalakis urged the formation of a citizen's panel to oversee the hospital's spending. Given that the hospital authority consisted of county residents, Skandalakis's proposal may have seemed a little odd. His words, however, indicated how dissatisfied citizens in north Fulton were with, in their view, paying for a service that only benefited other people.[28]

Many of the residents who showed up at a second meeting, held the next week in South Fulton, were dissatisfied hospital workers. Complaining about poor working conditions and low wages, the Grady

Fast Food Comes to Grady

In the summer of 1991, Grady hospital leased a space in the corner of its parking garage near the hospital's main entrance to McDonald's. It seems odd that a hospital with an internationally renowned diabetes center that preaches the importance of diet for controlling the illness would lease space to a restaurant selling hamburgers, French Fries, and milk shakes. In the 1980s, however, McDonald's had introduced healthier choices, including salads and a chicken sandwich. McDonald's also pledged to work with Grady's dieticians to create even healthier alternatives for the restaurant's menu.

Grady's decision was driven in part by the chance to make money from the restaurant's sales. But Grady also was competing with other hospitals in the area. McDonald's had reached an agreement a little earlier to place a restaurant at Northside Hospital in Sandy Springs. Apparently Grady hoped to keep the friends and families of inpatients happy with their meals. In addition, Grady's cafeteria continued to offer nutritious alternatives.[101]

employees blasted a new plan by hospital management to tie pay raises to performance. They feared that lower-paid workers would receive little benefit from the program. Other South Fulton residents, however, focused on the tax issue and seconded the complaints of their neighbors to the north.[29]

Given that Grady had been well run during the Pinkston years, and continued to become financially more efficient after his departure, hospital officials seemed to have a hard time taking Chairman Lomax's posturing very seriously. His accusations of poor oversight by the hospital's trustees, evidenced, he claimed, by the salaries of administrators and the prevalence of no-bid purchasing of supplies, seemed like little more than political theater to hospital trustees. To other observers, the bickering between Fulton commissioners and Grady trustees and administrators threatened to undermine the hospital's remaining public support in north Fulton.

Manuel Maloof, still the Chief Executive Officer for DeKalb County, defended Grady and its new director, Robert B. Johnson. While Maloof was a great fan of Grady—telling a reporter, "Grady is the heart and soul of what Atlanta has always been. God help us if it weren't here"—he also noted that in the preceding two years Grady had dramatically increased its revenue (thanks to better than expected payments from private insurers and the federal government). More surprisingly, Grady was on the cusp of giving back several million dollars to the counties. At the same time, the percentage of Grady's operating budget funded by the counties was falling to its lowest level in seven years.[30]

Following the public meetings, the Board of Commissioners of Fulton County adopted an operating budget designed to keep property tax rates steady. They did it by keeping funding for Grady level at $89 million—$16 million below the hospital authority's cumulative request for the next fiscal year.[31]

In April 1992, Grady adopted a revised budget for the year, increasing its spending beyond what Fulton and DeKalb counties had approved at the start of the year.[31]

In response, Fulton and DeKalb counties both stopped their funding for the hospital. The dispute centered on the counties' role. Officials from Fulton and DeKalb argued that the contract with the hospital authority empowered the counties to set Grady's budget. Grady's representatives, however, claimed only the FDHA could set Grady's budget. In their view, the counties could establish nothing more than their annual contribution to Grady. Robert L. Brown, the authority's new chairman, claimed it was the only sensible way to proceed. How would it work if the counties set the hospital budget? Suppose, for example, that the two counties disagreed about purchases detailed in a budget? If the counties wanted to control health care spending, they ought to figure out what they wanted to pay for indigent care and leave the budgeting to Grady.[32]

Robert Johnson, Grady's administrator, also defended Grady's budgetary authority. Eager to gain more independence from the two counties, he flatly asserted that the counties could not dictate Grady's budget. The hospital's revised budget—admittedly with increased spending—simply reflected an unexpected infusion of federal money. While Grady believed the windfall belonged to the hospital, county officials argued that the sudden arrival of $35 million should turn into a rebate for the counties. Under remarkable pressure from constituents angry about property taxes, Fulton's commissioners pushed for a rebate from the hospital. After failing to get the money, the county threatened to stop writing checks to Grady.[33]

Michael Lomax charged the hospital with irresponsibly expanding programs without taking into account how to pay for them in the future. Perhaps cutting off $8 million in payments each month seemed like the height of responsible behavior to Lomax. In any case, he was making a point—one in which he was joined by DeKalb County's CEO, Manuel Maloof.[34]

With the money blocked, Grady threatened massive cuts to its staff and programs. The counties claimed Grady was bluffing, that it could adjust its finances until the impasse was resolved. As an editorialist noted, if that had been the case, the argument would have been over why the counties needed to give Grady any money in the first place. The counter-argument was that unelected hospital officials were unaccountable to voters. In that line of reasoning, only the elected county commissioners could set Grady's budget.[35]

The issue was resolved after hospital trustees agreed to allow the counties to review and revise Grady's budget. In the end, the counties approved a $9 million increase. In return for hospital trustees agreeing to the review, the heads of the two counties agreed to support building a new AIDS clinic for the hospital.[36]

Minority Contracting at Grady

Tensions between the hospital authority and the Fulton County Commission intensified in the late 1980s as plans for the hospital's renewal developed. Less than two years after construction began, delays and cost overruns intensified conflict between hospital administrators and local officials. Even more important, however, was the hiring of minority-owned firms. Although the FDHA had promised that 30% of the construction funds would go to minority contractors, Chairman Lomax didn't take the authority at its word.

Once again Michael Lomax stood at the center of the controversy over Grady's renovation. The hospital authority and the county commission butted heads over who should manage the project. The hospital authority set up a formal bid process, overseen by a selection committee, to choose which firm would be paid $11.4 million to manage the project. None of the top three candidates were minority-owned, so Michael Lomax and other Fulton commissioners pressured the hospital authority to appoint a firm with minority ownership. Mr. Lomax was in a position to force the authority's hand since Fulton County underwrote 78% of the bonds sold to finance the project. According to Dr. Loughlin, who headed the FDHA at the time, Chairman Lomax and other commissioners had insisted that the hospital authority hire DPM-Heery to manage the project.[37]

The firm was a joint venture between Diversified Project Management, established by Herman J. Russell, a former member of the FDHA, and Heery International, a large contractor. Although Russell had proven successful with many projects, including the expansion of Hartsfield Airport, his track record didn't blunt the sense of unfairness White Atlanta felt when DPM's joint venture with Heery International leap-frogged other firms bidding to manage Grady's renovation and expansion. In a city where race remained front and center, racial preferences in selecting government contractors was a hot-button political issue. In light of recent federal court decisions that restricted "minority set-aside" programs, the selection of DPM-Heery rubbed White Atlanta the wrong way. While successful joint ventures with white firms had helped turn H. J. Russell & Company into an extremely successful conglomerate, the work with Heery at Grady hospital seemed troubled early on. Those problems, which gained substantial press coverage, seemed to intensify White Atlanta's concerns about the Grady project.[38]

In April 1991, the DeKalb County Commission made clear that it was disappointed in DPM-Heery's work. According to newspaper reports, and the commission, the project had fallen at least two months behind schedule. This was due in part to a delay in the awarding of the hospital renovation's first construction contract—reportedly costing the project $30,000 per day. Given such figures, the project seemed ripe for criticism. DPM-Heery blamed the delay on state fire marshals. (The favor was returned.) The project managers, however, were not terribly worried about early delays or cost overruns. In the context of a five-year project, there was, from their perspective, plenty of room to finish the project on time and under budget. The hospital's chief administrator, Robert Johnson, seemed to side with DPM-Heery, calling all of the political infighting over minority contracting a tempest in a teapot.[41]

During the 1970s the hospital authority had created a Disadvantaged Business Enterprise (DBE) set-aside program to ensure that businesses owned by women and racial minorities would get a share of hospital contracts. The program remained in place until 1990, when the United States Supreme Court ruled that minority set-aside programs are unconstitutional except when patterns of racial discrimination are demonstrated. Ironically, the hospital authority turned to DPM-Heery to develop a new disadvantaged business program. Following direction from the hospital authority, DPM-Heery aimed for a race-neutral program that would direct contracts to economically disadvantaged firms.[39]

While the new program followed guidelines set out by the Supreme Court's decision, Chairman Lomax opposed the outcome. He became outraged when a white-owned firm, Coleman Industrial Contractors of Atlanta, won a contract under the new race-neutral program. In a letter to Dr. Loughlin, Chairman Lomax threatened to pull his support for the renovation project unless the percentage of minority contracts rose. (It stood at about 26 percent.) Chairman Lomax reportedly instructed Dr. Loughlin that the DBE firms' majority owners "are presumed to be women or minorities." Coleman Industrial, economically "disadvantaged" because it was unable to secure a line of credit from banks, was paid almost $47,000 to subcontract $940,000 worth of work to minority-owned businesses.[40]

Emergency Crisis and the New ER

When Grady's new emergency room opened in 1992 it covered more than an acre. The contrast with the old emergency room was stunning. The new quarters were four times larger and had 30% more staff than the old clinic. The improvement couldn't come fast enough. A state inspection of the old emergency room a few months earlier revealed a host of problems, including the case of a heart patient attached to an empty oxygen tank. This came on the heels of a tragedy the previous autumn. In the fall of 1991, two patients died from neglect in the Emergency Room of Grady hospital. A federal investigation concluded that the patients had waited in the emergency room for twenty hours without receiving basic medical care. They had received so little attention in the chaotically crowded facility that they had been given nothing to eat or drink. At the time, Grady's ER was seeing 150,000 patients per year (an average of 410 patients daily) and, like so many times in Grady's history, patients had nowhere to wait but in the hallways.[42]

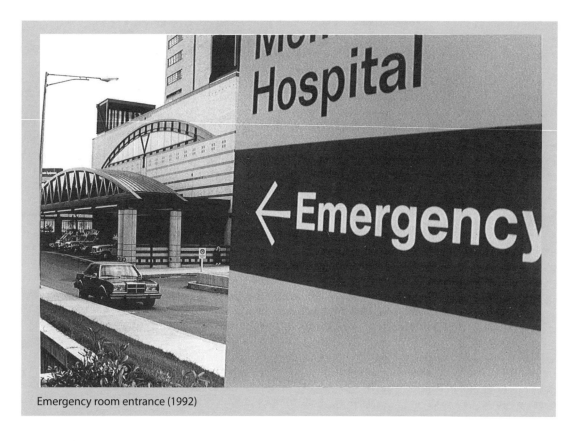
Emergency room entrance (1992)

The Infectious Disease Clinic

The Infectious Disease Clinic at Grady was, in 1991, the only place in northern Georgia where uninsured AIDS patients could receive treatment. At the time, the clinic could only accept 18 new patients per week, about half the number asking for treatment. This meant a long wait of up to four months before people with the illness could get their first appointment at the clinic. Cuts in state and federal budgets meant that Grady needed to look elsewhere to fund the clinic's expansion. Neither Fulton nor DeKalb counties were in any position to offer help. Funding from the federal Ryan White Comprehensive AIDS Resources Emergency Act, however, allowed Grady to renovate space in the hospital for an expanded clinic (which opened in September 1991) that could see up to 42 new patients each week. Despite this improvement, there was still too little room to serve patients in the way that Grady hoped or to handle the expected influx of new AIDS cases.

Shortly before being removed as chair of the hospital authority, Dr. Loughlin signed an option for the authority to purchase a seven-acre property on Ponce De Leon Avenue, less than two miles north of Grady. Local residents and business owners were outraged because they had not been consulted before Grady announced the agreement. Even Jim Martin, a state representative and an early and strong advocate of state funding for AIDS care in Georgia, decried the lack of neighborhood involvement in the planning.[43]

The selected site was in an area that had been struggling for years. While it was popular among the homeless and social service agencies, businesses in the neighborhood faced hard times. Believing that Grady's clinic would undercut their efforts to revitalize the area, business owners and nearby residents strongly preferred that the property have a different, commercial use.

If the neighbors were unhappy, local AIDS activists were delighted with the proposal. Atlanta's Aids Coalition to Unleash Power (ACT-UP) supported moving the clinic from the Grady campus to the new location. In response to neighborhood opposition, it organized marches outside of Grady and the Fulton County Government Center in support of the new Infectious Disease Clinic.[44]

The DeKalb County Commission, however, balked at supporting the new clinic, supposedly because it didn't like the location. The clinic also failed to obtain a majority when it came up for a vote in the Fulton County Commission in July 1992. Commissioners Emma Darnell and Milton Farris wanted to have other issues at Grady resolved first, including a contract dispute and a conflict over the hospital's budget.[45]

The deadline for the hospital to complete the purchase was July 27, 1992. The hospital authority could have gone ahead with the purchase on its own, but any bonds it issued would not have been guaranteed by the counties, and without taxing authority of its own, the authority would pay higher interest rates.

Less than two weeks before the deadline, on July 15, 1992, Fulton County commissioners signed off on the clinic, but only after directing Grady to keep neighborhood residents posted on what was happening. In addition, it limited the clinic's size to 30,000 square feet. Worried that the clinic would attract "outside" patients, it also demanded that Grady keep non-local patients "to a minimum."[46] The commissioners may have wished that, but the fact was that the Grady clinic would be the best place in Georgia for people suffering from HIV/AIDS to receive treatment. More than that, people coming from outside Fulton and DeKalb counties could establish residence easily enough. Without other treatment options, they would be left with little choice.

Five days after Fulton approved the clinic, the DeKalb County Commission again refused to give its blessing on the project. Instead, one week before the deadline DeKalb's commissioners urged Grady to find space on its existing campus or at an old Sears Roebuck building farther down Ponce de Leon (which the city of Atlanta had purchased a year earlier for a new police headquarters and other uses). Grady decided to go ahead with its existing plans. It would get DeKalb County's blessing later.

Grady dedicated the Ponce Center for Infectious Diseases on Thursday, October 14, 1993, with a gala event under a white tent in the clinic's parking lot. Headlined by

The Grady Rooters

People coming to the Emergency Room at Grady had a unique cheering section. Known collectively as the Grady Rooters, they got together on weekend nights at the ramp outside of Grady's Emergency Room to watch what more than one rooter considered "the best show in town."[33] Chatting amiably, and often drinking beer or liquor, they waited for ambulances to deliver patients. Typically a pleasant if generally disorderly bunch, they were there to watch accident victims and people with gunshot wounds arrive.

Much as people once went to the airport to watch airplanes take off and land, and audiences would gather to watch television programs about the dramas unfolding inside mythical emergency rooms, the Grady Rooters were fascinated by the drama surrounding Grady's Emergency Room. But they also participated in their own way, boisterously cheering as the ill and the injured arrived, and cheering again when patients left the ER.

The regulars also availed themselves of what came to be known as the Rooter Bar—a snack bar inside Grady where anyone could, and just about everyone did, wander in. The customers included patients, nurses, physicians, orderlies and other staff members and, of course, the Rooters. Over time the Rooters had become part of the life of Grady's ER, familiar to ambulance drivers and everyone who worked inside the emergency rooms.

The tradition of live entertainment that the Rooters at once enjoyed and provided ended in July 1992 when Grady's new emergency room opened at the opposite end of the building. There was no longer room for the Rooters.[102]

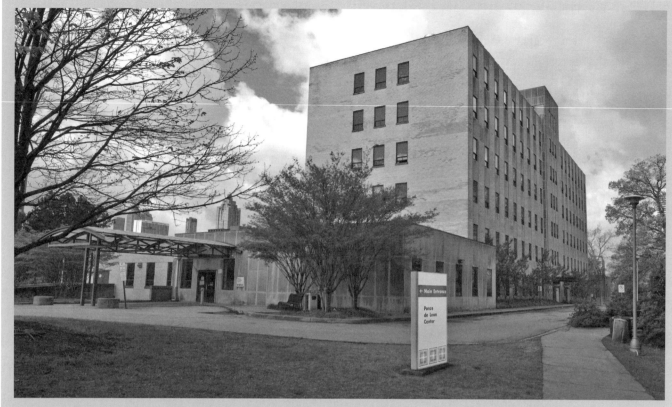

In 1993, Grady transformed the former Presbyterian Center into a comprehensive clinic for patients infected with HIV.

the prominent entertainer and AIDS activist Elton John, the event attracted more than 500 guests. A part-time resident of Atlanta, Elton John had established a foundation to fund AIDS research in 1992. A year earlier, Elton John performed for 22,000 participants in the first AIDS Walk Atlanta.[47]

The $7.5 million Infectious Disease Clinic was a comprehensive one-stop center. With its opening, Atlanta had gone in just a few years from having virtually no service for uninsured HIV/AIDS patients to having one of the finest comprehensive centers in the nation. It offered medical care, dentistry, psychological counseling, education, a pharmacy, and clinics for women, children, and teenagers. At the time the clinic opened the new facility, its medical director, Dr. Sumner Thompson III,* rightly referred to it as a "minor miracle."[48]

By 1993, eight years after the first AIDS cases were seen at Grady, nearly 9,000 residents in Georgia had contracted the illness. Officials estimated that another 50,000 citizens were HIV positive—a majority unaware of their plight. Where Grady's clinic had seen a few dozen patients in 1986, it cared for 4,000 patients in 1993. With 32.4 cases per 100,000 residents, Georgia ranked 11th in the nation in the number of reported HIV infections; Atlanta ranked seventh among American cities.[49]

Grady's clinic was at the center of a network of care that had slowly evolved in Atlanta. In the late 1980s, concerned individuals had created hospices for AIDS patients while others developed specialized housing like the Jerusalem House for low-income and homeless people affected by HIV. Still others organized early intervention

---

*Dr. Thompson was an internationally known and respected researcher on sexually-transmitted diseases. In 1987 Emory asked him to devote his efforts to lead the HIV/AIDS program at GMH. He cared for hundreds of patients. Sadly, Dr. Thompson died November 12, 1995, after a two-year battle with brain cancer.

clinics like one developed at Central Presbyterian Church.

Federal and state money paid for most of the operating expenses for the Infectious Disease Clinic. One reason that HIV/AIDS patients wound up at Grady and other federally funded institutions is that, at the time, most private insurance companies dropped patients who contracted the disease. That meant few HIV/AIDS patients were seen by private physicians, leaving them little alternative but public facilities.

At the end of 2003, the Centers for Disease Control reported on a study of 131 HIV-positive women who delivered babies at Grady Memorial Hospital in 1999 and 2000. According to the study, nine of the women delivered infants with the virus. Thanks to anti-retroviral drugs, the rate of transmission from mother to infant had been reduced dramatically since the mid-1980s. By 2000, the percentage of infants who were born infected with HIV from their mothers had dropped by 80 percent, falling from one in four to one in twenty infants of HIV-infected mothers. The most important reason that the generational transmission rate dropped was because HIV-infected women were properly taking the new anti-retroviral medicines. Testing for AIDS, together with counseling, also proved important in reducing the transmission rate. AIDS counseling made women feel more comfortable about taking the test for AIDS and the earlier they took the test, the sooner those with the virus would be able to start taking the medications. The sooner in their pregnancy that infected women took those drugs, the less likely they were to pass the virus on to their babies.

According to the CDC's study, none of Grady's infected pregnant patients transmitted the disease to their infants when they participated in all aspects of Grady's program. The Grady study showed the rate of generational transmission could drop further if the many low-income women who lacked prenatal care would receive medical attention throughout their pregnancy. The study also found that HIV-infected women addicted to illegal drugs needed earlier testing and prenatal care.[50]

Hughes Spalding Children's Hospital

Three years after it closed in 1989, Hughes Spalding Pavilion reopened as Hughes Spalding Children's Hospital following the major renovation and remodeling needed to make it suitable as a pediatric hospital. It opened with a capacity of 82 beds. As with the other parts of Grady, Emory University provided the medical staff for the hospital. In its first years the hospital was plagued with a low patient count. Often fewer than a quarter of its beds were being used.[51]

In August 2004, Children's Healthcare of Atlanta agreed to manage Hughes Spalding Children's Hospital. It made the announcement only a few days after Grady ended its opposition to the expansion of Children's Healthcare's two hospitals—Egleston Hospital and Scottish Rite Hospital. (In 1998, Egleston Children's Health Care System and Scottish Rite Medical Center formed Children's Healthcare of Atlanta—which instantly became one of the largest pediatric healthcare systems in the United States.) In 2004, Children's Healthcare also announced that it would spend at least $15 million to renovate Hughes Spalding. It would take a year to iron out the agreement.[52]

An affiliate of Children's eventually took over Hughes Spalding Children's Hospital in February 2006. Children's received $18 million from an anonymous donor in 2005 in the form of a challenge grant to help pay for its work at Hughes Spalding. Faced with an outdated structure, Children's Healthcare eventually opted to erect a replacement building for $43 million. The renamed Children's Healthcare of Atlanta at Hughes Spalding would have an 18-bed pediatric unit, a 24-hour emergency room, and a series of clinics—including facilities for children with asthma, Sickle Cell Disease, and those needing primary care. Staffed by physicians from Emory University School of Medicine and the Morehouse School of Medicine, Children's at Hughes Spalding remained an integral part of Atlanta's health ecosystem. By 2007, Emory residents in pediatrics would receive as much as 40% of their training at Hughes Spalding.

The Georgia-to-Georgia Initiative

Grady hospital was part of an initiative launched in 1992 to link physicians and scholars in the state of Georgia with the Republic of Georgia, formerly a part of the Soviet Union. During its first dozen years, the project—under the auspices of Grady, Emory, Morehouse School of Medicine, Georgia State University, and Georgia Tech—achieved remarkable success. The program brought forty medical school graduates from the republic to Atlanta for specialty training. It also addressed medical problems in the republic through the development of a women's wellness center in Kutaisi, Georgia, to educate women on breast health, perinatal care, and preventive medicine. Thanks to funding from the National Institutes of Health, the project helped set up a system for diagnosing and treating HIV/AIDS and tuberculosis in the Republic of Georgia. Remarkably, the program led to the discovery that nearly two-thirds of newborns in Tbilisi, Georgia, suffered from hypothyroidism because their mother's diets lacked iodine. The republic's government quickly acted on this finding by adding iodine to table salt. As a result, hypothyroidism among newborns became rare in the Republic of Georgia.[53]

Medicaid and Reform

Changes in Medicaid rules under President George H. W. Bush brought intense competition between public and private hospitals for Medicaid patients during the early 1990s. As a result, many of Grady's patients enjoyed fresh alternatives about where to be treated. Suddenly, Grady was competing with other hospitals in terms of quality, if not price. The profitable maternity business was especially appealing to private hospitals, and they aggressively sought obstetrics patients who were insured through Medicaid. By the mid 1990s, Grady's caseload began dropping dramatically as many patients who could go elsewhere took the opportunity.[54]

After President Clinton took office in 1993, many of the healthcare reform proposals he endorsed seemed to further threaten Grady with greater competition. In response, Grady planned to emphasize its lower cost of care on a per-admission basis. At the time, consumers didn't seem to care as much about cost when third parties paid for the health care. Grady anticipated that under universal insurance, it would have to compete with other hospitals on cost and quality.[55]

Grady officials believed that improving quality would draw new patients. In the early 1990s, some people were making political hay out of claims that the quality of care at Grady was in decline. While the assertion was generally debatable, the public perception had some basis in reality. In particular, the recent federal investigation into the death of patients in the emergency room continued to hang over the hospital.

While private hospitals were courting Medicaid patients, Grady became interested in attracting more patients with private insurance. At the time, only about seven percent of Grady's patients carried private insurance. This meant that fewer than one in ten patients paid for most of the cost of their care. Changing the mix of patients was important for Grady because privately insured patients tended to be far more lucrative for hospitals than those on Medicaid or Medicare.

In order to attract a larger number of paying patients, Grady would have to become more family and visitor-friendly. In addition to substantially improving amenities for the patient's visitors, this also meant efforts to keep its employees happy. Because it was under enormous cost pressure, however, Grady would be looking for ways to increase happiness without giving pay raises.

The biggest obstacle to attracting more privately insured patients, however, seemed to be the widespread perception that Grady was for the poor, that it was a place people went when they had nowhere else to turn.

Grady had been established to serve Atlanta's rich and poor alike. That noble dream, however, came under assault almost from the start. As a result, the vast majority of patients in Grady's history were people who had been unable to receive medical care anywhere else. Following the introduction of hospital insurance for many of the indigent through Medicaid, and universal hospital insurance coverage for the elderly through Medicare, more of Grady's insured patients were covered by federal and state programs.

It would be difficult for Grady to overcome its reputation as a hospital for the poor. To attract the middle class, Grady latched onto the idea of emphasizing that it offered a high quality of care. With its expanded and refurbished facilities, its excellence in acute care and other areas, Grady hoped to compete for what it had once called "private-pay patients." Repeatedly it looked for ways to increase the number of patients covered by private insurance. It would even create its own HMO programs. Although this was prompted by the state government's hope to push Medicaid recipients into managed care programs, Grady saw a commercial opportunity.[57] In the end, however, administrators seemed to believe that the best way to overcome the perception that Grady was for the poor was to compete for middle class patients on the basis of quality of care.

Crestview Nursing Home

Grady was asked to take on more responsibilities when the Crestview Nursing Home, an intermediate care facility owned by the county but operated by a private company, was accused of unsafe practices and unsanitary conditions. Founded in the early 1960s by Fulton County, Grady became the owner in August 1991, three years after Fulton County—with prompting from the state—fired the private management company whose health and safety violations had become notorious. Their management was so poor that the state forced nearly half of Crestview's patients into other nursing homes. After contracting out the running of Crestview to another private firm, the county turned the home over to Grady in 1991. Ninety-eight percent of its residents were paid for through the Medicare program. Recent state and federal efforts at budgetary reform had led government reimbursement for patient care to be reduced from $42 per day to $31.

In 1993, the state of Georgia took control of Crestview Nursing Home away from Grady because it deemed the home was a threat to its patients' well-being. In a nearly 100-page study, inspectors from Georgia's Department of Human Resources (DHR) reported that some patients were not getting food, water, or their medicines. Other patients were left lying in soiled sheets.

The largest nursing home in Georgia, Crestview was a no-frills place. There was little privacy for patients (some rooms slept four patients). While it was much improved in 1993 from what it had been before Grady assumed management—at least there were fewer rodents—many of the miserable conditions Grady inherited from the county proved hard to eliminate. According to the director of the DHR, David Dunbar, Crestview suffered from "widespread neglect for the basic health, safety and well-being of the residents."[103]

The biggest problem had to do with the nursing assistants—essentially the primary caregivers. It was the assistants who neglected some patients, tied others to their beds, and verbally abused still others. When it first took over the home Grady relied on a temporary staffing agency for nearly half of its nursing assistants. Following the DHR's inspection and sanctions, Grady made reforms and soon regained control of Crestview. Under the new regime, Crestview radically improved care and became an integral part of the Grady Health System. Financially, however, the nursing home would continue to be a financial drain in the years to come.[104]

Grady's Continuing Financial Crisis

In the summer of 1994, critics continued complaining that the money spent on the hospital's renovation—which they seemed to have forgotten was being paid for through long-term bonds—would have been better spent on adding community clinics. Not only Mitch Skandalakis, but also Robert Fulton, another county commissioner, rode anti-Grady sentiment to electoral victory. In his campaign literature, Fulton called for the privatization of Grady.[58] While not all residents in northern Fulton supported the proposal, most appeared to believe that they shouldered an unfair burden in funding the hospital.

Manuel Maloof, plain-spoken as usual, came to Grady's defense, saying that "taking care of poor people who are sick, who don't have any other way to get care, is not pork."[59]

In August 1994, reports surfaced that Edward Renford, Grady's new chief administrator, planned to cut 600 jobs in the following fiscal year. While he was expecting attrition to do most of the work for him, reducing the payroll from 6,600 to 6,000 would be a large cut for the hospital. He appeared willing to lay people off if needed. With the operating debt rising, Grady needed to cut where it could—and reducing labor costs looked like a relatively easy way to control the rapidly rising expenses. The problem was that labor costs had barely risen at Grady. In addition, nurses were already complaining about understaffing in parts of the hospital.[60]

By the fall of 1994, Grady was running an annual deficit of $20 million—although it was less than it would have been without an infusion of $45 million from the state of Georgia. The contract between the counties and the FDHA stipulated that the counties were to fund Grady—but only up to a maximum level set by the state legislature. Still, Grady was getting less than two-thirds of what was allowed by the state, and less than 10% of the tax money from Fulton and DeKalb went to funding one of the economic engines of the city.

The *Constitution* quoted Michael Lomax as saying that "the rhetoric of waste in government will provide a very large opening for a consensus to reduce funding for the hospital."[61] He thought it would be both biracial and bipartisan, expanding beyond county commissioners from the northern portion of Fulton County. Michael Hightower, the vice chairman of the Fulton County Commission, while remaining committed to Grady, pledged prudence. Yet, both Republicans and Democrats used fears about Grady to get out the vote. Heading into the elections in the fall of 1994, Democrats tried to get out the vote by raising fears about Republican efforts to cut Grady's funding. The issue continued to have a racial cast.[62]

Grady's HMO Experiment

In September 1999, Grady was forced to shut down the commercial and Medicaid HMO programs it had initiated only two years earlier. The HMO got its start in response to the state's effort to save money by driving Medicaid patients into HMOs. The end of Grady's experiment came when the state changed course.[63]

The Grady Coalition

At the start of 1999, Grady faced yet another shortfall in its annual budget. At the same time Grady faced rising costs, especially for medications, federal funding for Medicaid dropped thanks to the Balanced Budget Act of 1997. The state also cut its Medicaid reimbursement, and the amount of money taxpayers in Fulton and DeKalb counties contributed to Grady fell in real terms. Faced with stark reality, the board of Atlanta's charity hospital had a series of bad choices from which to choose in order to balance its budget. If it didn't raise prescription prices, the FDHA claimed it would need to close some clinics or even Grady's emergency room—which provided the highest level of trauma care in the city. The affable and highly capable board chairman, the architect Robert Brown, later explained in a public meeting, "This board is between a rock and a hard place.... the people who fund us have reduced funding."[64] In response to the cutbacks, the board offered several measures to raise enough revenue to meet the anticipated deficit.[65]

Grady's board proposed raising the price of medication for indigent patients from 50 cents to $10 per prescription. In addition, the once free clinics would charge $5 for each visit. On top of that, Atlanta's charity hospital was ending free shuttle transportation for patients. The poor would have to find and pay for their own way to the hospital or to one of Grady's neighborhood clinics. These dramatic price increases for the city's poorest, uninsured citizens was meant to help the hospital meet a $26.4 million shortfall.[66]

The city's leading advocates for the poor jumped into action and formed the Grady Coalition. Established activists in the city like the Reverend Ed Loring, a Presbyterian minister, and his wife, the Reverend Murphy Davis, also a Presbyterian preacher, who lived in the Open Door Community that ministered to the city's homeless, and Stewart Acuff of the Atlanta Labor Council, together with community activists and vocal black clergymen like the Reverend Timothy McDonald, pastor of a large congregation and a leader in The Concerned Black Clergy, organized, spoke-up, and held public demonstrations. This coalition quickly drew students, physicians, the homeless, business people, more community activists, and local politicians into its ranks. Organizing rallies in front of the hospital, the Grady Coalition attracted media attention to its cause.[67] The points it made were simple. If the proposed changes were put into place, the poor would stop visiting clinics and would be unable to afford their medications. One disabled grandmother with cancer and diabetes who lived in public, tax-assisted housing helped illustrate the issue for the Grady Coalition. According to critics of the proposed change, she would see the annual cost for her medications jump from $36 to $720.

To push their case, members of the Grady Coalition attended public meetings of the hospital authority and the DeKalb and Fulton county commissions. They waved placards, made noise, got arrested, and told the story of Grady patients whose ability to get medications would be affected by the changes. Coalition members created enough disorder at a meeting of the FDHA on March 22, 1999, that hospital security called the Atlanta police for help in restoring order. Before that boisterous meeting ended, the Grady Coalition met with its first success when Dr. Otis Smith* persuaded fellow members of the FDHA board to suspend the price hike for thirty days.[68] The state of Georgia and both local counties soon found additional money for the hospital. Grady's financial troubles were further eased later that year when Governor Roy Barnes facilitated a payment of $53.4 million in federal funds that Grady had not been paid in

> ## The Grady Health Foundation (1993)
>
> The Grady Health Foundation was formed in 1993 under the guidance of Robert L. Brown, the chairman of the Fulton-DeKalb Hospital Authority, Ann Cramer, an executive with IBM in Atlanta and a dynamo of civic leadership and community service, J. Veronica Biggins, Executive Vice President of Community Relations at NationsBank, and G. Lemuel Hewes, a partner with the law firm of King & Spalding. The foundation would provide important support for Grady hospital and its mission.

---

*Dr. Smith was one of the first African-American pediatricians in Atlanta. While attending Meharry Medical College, he ran out of funds. After a conversation with Dr. Benjamin Mays, Morehouse President, Margaret Mitchell provided an anonymous scholarship to Otis Smith. He was one of 40 to 50 African American medical students to benefit from the generosity of the author of *Gone with the Wind*. Dr. Mays revealed this information several decades after Mitchell's death.

previous years.[69] It would not be the last time that Grady found itself squeezed because of inadequate funding.

A Scandal: Charles Walker and Grady Memorial Hospital

Charles Walker was elected to the Georgia House of Representatives in 1982 from Augusta. He was re-elected three times to the same office and became the chairman of the Legislative Black Caucus. In 1990, Walker was elected to the state Senate and in 1991 was named chairman of the Senate Health and Human Services Committee. Two years later he served on the conference committee that wrote the state budget. An entrepreneur, Walker had established a firm that provided companies with temporary employees. Georgia Personnel was lucrative for Walker; he received $3.7 million in income from the personnel company from 1997 to 2001. Apparently Walker had begun placing substantial pressure on Grady Memorial Hospital to use his company's services as early as 1995. Walker's firms did more than $2.5 million in business with Grady and the Medical College of Georgia from 1996 to 2000. An investigation by the Georgia State Ethics Commission into Senator Walker's business dealings with Grady led to the imposition of a fine.[70]

In 2004, federal prosecutors indicted Charles Walker on 142 felony counts of corruption. Despite the allegations, Walker, who had lost his Senate seat in 2002, won back his old seat in 2004. At his trial, incriminating testimony came from Joyce Harris, a former human resources director at Grady who claimed to have been fired a few years earlier in retaliation for being a whistle-blower. She testified that Ed Renford, Grady's former CEO, told her that her department needed to hire temporary employees from Georgia Personnel because Senator Walker could help the hospital in the state legislature. Ms. Harris estimated that a recently passed bill was worth $40 million to Grady. She also testified that workers from Walker's company were relatively

Celebrating Volunteers

At the end of June 1994, Grady hospital celebrated a major milestone: over one million hours of volunteer help at the hospital. The volunteers came from all over the metro area. Some volunteers were students, others were retirees, and still others were homemakers. Some came through groups like the American Red Cross.

Some groups volunteered for areas of interest. Planned Parenthood directed volunteers to the Family Planning Clinic; the Arthritis Foundation provided volunteers for the Arthritis Clinic. Members of the Junior League had pioneered a Thyroid Clinic in the 1930s and later developed a crucial program in Labor and Delivery, giving patients in labor emotional support. The League's innovative program attracted attention from hospitals around the country.

Hundreds of members of the Junior League volunteered throughout Grady for a three-month period, later returning as regular volunteers. Many other volunteers were "free lancers" who came on their own.

Volunteers worked in nearly every area of the hospital. Those in the emergency room helped with intake of new patients. Others were in the ER to comfort patients, holding their hand and listening to their fears. Still others contributed time in the special care nursery. Among the most celebrated were the foster grandparents who came regularly to hold premature infants and rock them in a rocking chair.

When Grady celebrated its milestone of a million volunteer hours, almost 900 people were regularly helping out in 80 different areas of the hospital and clinics. There were never enough volunteers to fill all the needs—especially on weekdays. While hundreds of people came in at a regular time every week, others in the community volunteered their services for special occasions. Employees of SunTrust (formerly the Trust Company of Georgia) came regularly to help out at Christmas, decorating dozens of trees around the hospital. For decades employees of Rich's Department Store erected and decorated a large Christmas tree in the main lobby. In addition, each year the Council of Jewish Women provided a special Christmas party on the Pediatrics floor.

expensive. On June 3, 2005, Charles Walker was convicted on 127 counts, fined $150,000, ordered to pay $698,000 in restitution, and sentenced to 10 years and 1 month in prison. The extra month was added because under federal sentencing rules, a sentence longer than ten years must be served in full.[71]

In an associated case, Walker's daughter Monique Walker Hill pled guilty to a federal misdemeanor of tax evasion for failing to report $700 in income. She was sentenced to three years probation and fined $30,000. Separately, the Georgia Supreme Court suspended her license to practice law for 120 days and issued a public reprimand.[72]

The Steady Drop in Funding From Local Counties

During the 1990s and early 2000s, at a time when property values were rising, Grady's funding from local property taxes fell both in real terms and as a proportion of spending at the hospital.

In 1995, Fulton County contributed $76.82 million of Grady's $397 million in operating expenses. Almost a decade later, in 2004, Fulton had increased that annual figure by only $90,000. Grady's operating budget, meanwhile, had increased by $269 million. DeKalb County's story was similar. It had contributed $22.5 million to Grady's budget in 1995; in 2004, DeKalb's annual contribution was only $190,000 more than it had been a decade earlier.[73]

When adjusted for inflation, the funding from the counties dropped steadily during the late 1990s and early 2000s. When taking into account the rising property values and the substantial increase in total assessed valuation of property in the counties, the proportion of property tax that Fulton and DeKalb devoted to Grady declined even more drastically. At the same time, medical inflation was growing rapidly, its rate rising much faster than core inflation.[74] Although during that ten-year period, from 1995 to 2004, the counties cumulatively contributed about one billion dollars out of Grady's $5.2 billion in operating expenses, their proportion of Grady's operating budget dropped from 25% in 1995 to less than 16% in 2004.[75] Grady's skyrocketing costs, increasing by nearly 68% over ten years, were due to more than the inflation in the prices of medical goods and labor; metropolitan Atlanta's population continued to grow, as did the number of people in the area who were uninsured.

In addition to inflation, expanding population, and more uninsured residents in Fulton and DeKalb counties, Grady also had to deal with another reality. Since before the hospital was established, critics had warned that a charity hospital would attract the indigent to the city. In the early 2000s, few people moved to Atlanta in order to be treated at Grady. Instead, they could continue to live in their home county and commute to Grady for care.

According to a report from 2007, residents from every county in Georgia used Grady Hospital. During the prior year, Grady had spent $68.5 million to care for patients from outside of Fulton and DeKalb counties. Only $8 million of that was covered by payments from insurance and the state's other counties. Residents of Clayton County in south suburban Atlanta alone received over $11.8 million in care. Grady could only collect slightly more than half of that amount, even after making adjustments for funding from federal programs.[76]

Continuing Innovation and Research

Avon Cancer Center (2003)

The first Georgia Cancer Center for Excellence at Grady opened in 2003. Costing over $31 million dollars, the center occupied the hospital's ninth and tenth floors. It included exam rooms, scanning and therapy technologies, ten research laboratories, and room for forty inpatients. With comfortable waiting areas, a soothing garden, natural light, and a dedicated express elevator for patients, the facilities matched those of any private hospital in the country. Going far beyond a bare-bones, spartan look, the cancer center failed to spark an outcry among the budget-watching critics of spending at Grady. Somehow they overlooked the cherry wood magazine racks.

The Georgia Cancer Center for Excellence at Grady was the first regional center begun by the Georgia Cancer Coalition—a project started by Governor Roy Barnes to improve cancer detection and treatment among minorities, the poor, and the uninsured, and also to attract the best cancer researchers to Georgia. Funded by $28 million from the multi-state tobacco lawsuit settlement of 1998 and a $3.3 million grant from the Avon Foundation for Women, the center at Grady significantly contributed to the hospital's reputation for excellence in care and research.

In 2005, Dr. Otis Brawley, who founded the Avon Comprehensive Breast Center, recruited Dr. Sheryl Gabram-Mendola from Loyola University Medical Center in Illinois to direct the program. Prior to her staff position at Loyola, she was a faculty member of the University of Connecticut School of Medicine. Funded by the Avon Foundation for Women, the breast center provided low-income women with access to first-rate care. Thanks to the work of Dr. Gabram-Mendola and her team, and especially community outreach efforts guided by the Rollins School of Public Health at Emory University, the number of mammograms given at Grady increased dramatically. As a result, many women were diagnosed with the illness far earlier than they would have been otherwise. Instead of being diagnosed at Stage III or worse, the cancers were being found very early, dramatically improving the patient's chances of beating the disease. Dr. Gabram-Mendola and her colleagues started to treat hundreds of impoverished breast cancer patients each year. Thanks to the program, poor women were able to access the highest quality medical care at Grady's cancer center.[77]

Trauma Care

Dr. Arthur Kellerman emerged as one of the leading figures in efforts to turn Grady hospital around. The founding Chairman of the Department of Emergency Medicine at Emory, Dr. Kellerman developed a command of health care policy that extended beyond emergency medicine.

In an essay in the *New England Journal of Medicine* published in 2006, Dr. Kellerman claimed the quality of America's trauma care system had declined to an alarming degree during the previous decade.[78] Grady's emergency room reflected national problems. It overflowed and, in 2006, would be unable to handle the large number of severely injured patients from a terrorist attack as it did after the bombing at Centennial Olympic Park in 1996. Indeed, 90% of the nation's trauma centers were running at or above capacity. Like hospitals across the nation, Grady frequently was forced to board emergency patients in the hallways.[79]

Hospitals are interconnected organisms. If no beds are available in the Intensive Care Unit, emergency patients have to wait in the trauma center. When a trauma center becomes especially overwhelmed, the hospital alerts incoming ambulances to head elsewhere, a practice called diversion. As a result, it takes longer for patients to begin to get care—whether they are insured or not.

Hospitals, which faced a national shortage of nurses, often did not have enough physicians. Many specialists avoided taking emergency room calls out of concern about malpractice suits, little or no reimbursement for their efforts, and the loss of hours from their private office practices. The absence of specialists would lead hospitals to divert ambulances because they were unable to treat certain patients. In contrast, Grady, the only Level I trauma center for a hundred miles in any direction, always had neurosurgeons available. Because of this, people with severe traumatic brain injuries, which are extremely difficult and expensive to treat, were regularly sent to Grady, especially in the overnight hours.

Dr. Kellerman noted that many different analysts had documented that, ironically, the Emergency Medical Treatment and Labor Act passed by Congress in 1986 effectively worsened rather than improved emergency care. The law mandated that people have a legal right to emergency care. Congress, however, enacted the rule without new funding for emergency departments or trauma centers. In response, some hospitals shut their emergency rooms. Remarkably, over four hundred hospitals in the United States closed their emergency rooms between 1993 and 2003. (Many hospitals that kept them open found overcrowding and ambulance diversion more expedient than the costly expansion of facilities.) During the same decade, the number of visits to emergency rooms rose by nearly 25 percent.[80]

Being at Grady's Emergency Room has often been compared to being in a war zone. The analogy has been apt. Indeed, Grady hospital was so busy treating patients with gunshot wounds and other major trauma that, in 2004, army medics from Fort Stewart came to Grady's ER for training before shipping out to serve with the American military in the war in Iraq.[81]

International Medical Center

By 2000, more than one-half of the babies delivered at Grady were born to Hispanic mothers. In response to the changing cultural mix of Grady's patients, Dr. Inginia Genao, a young physician at Emory and Grady, spearheaded the creation of the International Medical Center at Grady hospital at the start of the new millennium.[82]

After Dr. Genao left to become a professor at Yale in 2005, Dr. Flavia Mercado became Medical Director of Grady's Department of Multicultural Affairs. Dr. Mercado had co-founded Grady's bilingual outpatient clinic in 2002, six years after she joined Grady Health Systems as a pediatrician at the Lindbergh Women and Children's Health Care Center, located in northeast Atlanta. The majority of its patients spoke Spanish with limited English. Many people from other immigrant communities, also with limited English language skills, also visited that clinic.

Dr. Mercado became responsible for the treatment of patients with language difficulties both at the hospital and its outlying clinics, especially the Lindbergh, North Fulton, and North DeKalb clinics. She also became responsible for training physicians to practice medicine with cultural competency.

Understanding patients and their circumstances had been a focus of Grady's social service department since the 1930s. In the 1990s, a physician's ability to work effectively with patients from other cultural backgrounds—and the ability to speak a second language—became increasingly important at Grady as immigration to Georgia expanded. Until the 1990s, cultural diversity in Atlanta was generally seen in terms of black and white. Unlike New York, Chicago, Los Angeles, and many other American cities, Atlanta historically had attracted relatively few immigrants. That began to change in the late 1980s as a large number of Asian, Mexican, and Central American immigrants began finding their way to the city. From 1990 to 2000, the Latino population in the Atlanta area tripled.

According to the National Council of La Raza, the number of Hispanic births in Georgia grew from 2,263 in 1990 to 16,819 in 2002.[83] Although Medicaid and Medicare were already limited to U.S. citizens and legal residents, federal welfare reform in 1996 further restricted the access of legal immigrants to programs like Medicaid. They would have to wait five years after becoming permanent residents (or getting a green card) before they could apply for federal benefits. As a result of the legislation President Bill Clinton signed into law in 1996, state and local governments took on more responsibility for the health care of poor uninsured immigrants.

As the demographics of the communities it served changed, the Grady Health System faced new challenges. Public hospitals in the northeast and midwest United States, like those in the far west and in Florida, had a long history of dealing with patients who spoke limited English. For Grady the issue was complicated by settlement patterns. Few of the immigrants lived near Grady hospital in downtown Atlanta; most of the newcomers took root miles away in northeast Atlanta or in nearby suburbs. As a result, the language and cultural competency of physicians, nurses, and everyone else who worked in the Grady Health System became increasingly important, especially for the GYN-OB department and the outpatient clinics.

Robert L. Brown

Robert L. Brown, a native of Dublin, Georgia, and a magna cum laude graduate of Tuskegee University, created R. L. Brown & Associates in 1984, providing architectural and construction management. His firm designed the Birmingham Civil Rights Institute, the Stone Mountain Tennis Center (the tennis venue for the Atlanta Olympic Games in 1996), academic buildings for local colleges, and the Drew Charter School and YMCA in Atlanta's East Lake community. A member of the Board of Trustees for Agnes Scott College and the The Georgia Historical Society, he sat on the boards of corporations including Georgia Power Company and the Citizens Trust Bank. Well-liked in the business community, Robert L. Brown also served on the boards of the Metro Atlanta Chamber of Commerce, The Georgia Chamber of Commerce, Wesley Woods Center, and the Georgia Shakespeare Festival. He became a member of the Fulton-DeKalb Hospital Authority in 1985 and served as its chairman from 1992 until 2006.

In 1991, Mr. Brown went undercover, dressed as though he were homeless, and accompanied an indigent patient to Grady. What he observed about the attitude of Grady's staff bothered him greatly. He would later report that the opinion of hospital personnel was, "you have no choice, so sit there and we'll get to you when we can."[84] Mr. Brown worked hard from that point to ensure that all of Grady's staff treated every patient with dignity and compassion. He also worked hard to keep the hospital thriving during a period of political conflict and declining financial support from the local counties.

W. Clyde Shepherd, Jr.

William Clyde Shepherd, Jr., was appointed to the Fulton-DeKalb Hospital Authority on January 25, 1972, to fill the unexpired term of Scott Candler. He was the secretary and treasurer of the Shepherd Construction Co., Inc., and served both as Chairman of the National Board of Governors of the National Asphalt Pavement Association and as President of the Georgia Asphalt Pavement Association. He also developed and owned the Toco Hills Shopping Center and several other local shopping centers.

Clyde Shepherd faithfully and actively served Grady's board for twenty-two years. He tirelessly worked to improve Grady and make it as effective as possible for its patients. He also used his considerable business acumen and experience to save the

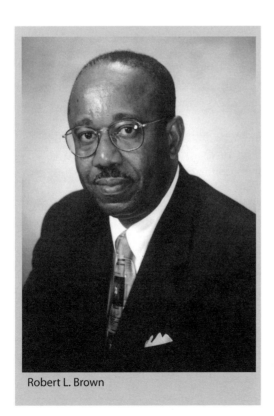

Robert L. Brown

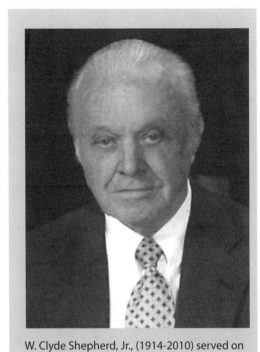

W. Clyde Shepherd, Jr., (1914-2010) served on the board of Grady hospital for 22 years.

hospital money. When he retired from the board, at the age of eighty-six, Robert Brown called him "the conscience of Grady."[85]

Robert Johnson

Appointed to succeed Bill Pinkston as Grady's chief administrator, Robert Johnson arrived as the hospital was entering the whirlwind. During Robert Johnson's tenure, Grady, like hospitals across the United States, continued to confront dramatically rising costs for health care. During the recession of 1991, Grady saw a major increase in the number of indigent and uninsured patients. The spread of AIDS also affected Grady's finances—as it did other American hospitals.

In response, Johnson led Grady to increase its collection of payments from private patients and their insurance companies. He also pushed the hospital to more aggressively seek payment from federal insurance programs. At the same time, the percentage of Grady's operating budget paid for by the counties fell from 44% to 24%, a significant drop resulting from a combination of increased costs, more federal funding, and falling contributions from Fulton and DeKalb counties.

Johnson sought to make Grady more independent of the counties. While the county governments wanted to reduce their payments, they also wanted to exert more oversight over Grady's budget. He also had plenty of battles with county commissioners. Their political interference didn't make his life any easier. Although the Fulton-DeKalb Hospital Authority eventually conceded that the counties could have control over the hospital's budget, Johnson continued to object.

Johnson also wanted to change the internal management of the hospital, creating the positions of chief executive, chief operating officer, and chief financial officer. No longer would one person wear all those hats at the same time. Johnson also worked to modernize Grady's billing system in order to capture more revenue. In the process, Grady abandoned its long-standing practice of charging a flat fee for a room. Instead, it began to break down the bill, charging not just for the room but also for every service and medicine that the hospital provided to a patient.

Prior to coming to Atlanta in 1989, Robert Johnson had been a senior executive with several large institutions. He had been the Chief Executive Officer of the St. Louis Regional Health Care Corporation, the Chief Executive Officer of D.C. General Hospital in Washington D.C., and Chief Financial Officer of King County Hospital Center of Brooklyn, New York. After graduating with a Bachelor of Sciences degree from Tennessee State University, he earned a Master of Hospital Administration degree from the University of Michigan.

Robert Johnson left his post as Grady's executive director in February 1993 in order to take a position at Detroit Medical Center in his hometown.[86]

Donald Snell

Following the resignation of Robert Johnson, Don Snell became acting executive director of Grady. He understood that Grady had begun to embrace a different management philosophy during Johnson's reign. He bluntly contrasted the present with the past. Before Johnson arrived, he explained, "there was a philosophy that the hospital would spend whatever it took to take care of the population, and that there would be a minimal attempt to collect from the patients."[87] While his characterization was a caricature of the way things had been, Grady certainly became more aggressive in collecting fees from patients.

Snell emphasized Grady's effort to become self-sufficient. His vision was that in a few years, by 1998 to be exact, Grady would thrive without funding from its host counties.

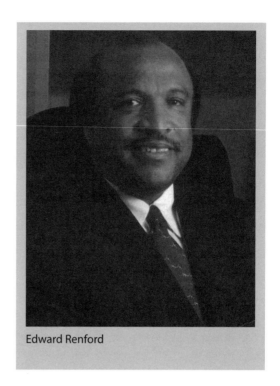
Edward Renford

Edward Renford

Edward Renford was appointed the CEO of Grady in April 1994, a position he would hold until his retirement in 2003. It would not be the first time he took on a challenging assignment.

In September 1989, the administrator of the Martin Luther King, Jr./Charles R. Drew Medical Center in Los Angeles, California, was fired because of severe deficiencies in the hospital. The problems were so severe that the institution was threatened with the withholding of $60 million in government funds. To turn the hospital around, Edward Renford was appointed Acting Administrator. Within three months, the deficiencies were overcome and public health funding was restored. Two months later, in February 1990, King/Drew received conditional accreditation. The conditions were later removed and the medical center was granted a three-year accreditation in December 1991. The dramatic turnaround attracted national attention for Mr. Renford.[88]

Grady had a $26 million debt when Renford arrived at the hospital in 1994; Grady was debt-free when he retired.

Attempting to improve access to health care for the poor, Mr. Renford oversaw Grady's opening of the nation's first health care center in a Kroger grocery store. In 1999, he initiated the Atlanta Regional Health Forum. (It involved 120 civic leaders in a study of ways to enhance access to the delivery of health care.)

As Mr. Renford retired on June 7, 2003, ending a thirty-year career in health care, his contributions to metropolitan Atlanta were recognized in a resolution passed by the Georgia House of Representatives. Mr. Renford had negotiated the shoals of politics and hospital administration for nine years, the longest tenure any CEO of Grady enjoyed since Bill Pinkston.[89]

Dr. Andrew Agwunobi

Born in Scotland and educated at the University of Jos in Nigeria, Dr. Andrew Agwunobi immigrated to the United States in 1992 and entered a pediatric training program at Howard University, which he finished in 1995. He practiced pediatrics in Gadsden, Alabama, from 1995 to 1997 and

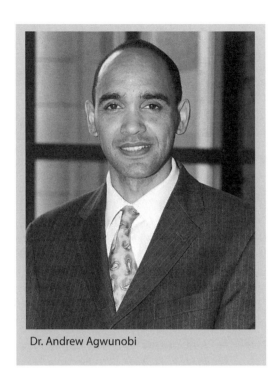

Dr. Andrew Agwunobi

then spent two years with the Harvard Vanguard Medical Associates, a 500+ physician multi-specialty group practice in Boston. From 1999 to 2001 he continued his education at Stanford University where he was awarded an MBA. After graduation, Dr. Agwunobi came to Atlanta and became the CEO of South Fulton Hospital where he remained for two years until being appointed the CEO of Grady Memorial Hospital in 2003. At thirty-seven years old, he was the youngest CEO in Grady's history. During his administration of Grady Memorial Hospital, Dr. Agwunobi began the negotiations to merge Hughes Spalding Children's Hospital with Children's Health Care of Atlanta (CHOA). As the Grady Health Systems continued to lose money ($10 million in 2005), Dr. Agwunobi was aggressive in limiting the use of Grady's resources to treating the indigent and uninsured residents of Fulton and DeKalb counties. He also focused on improving hospital efficiency and finances. After hiring the accounting firm of KPMG to study the financial health of the hospital's programs, Dr. Agwunobi decided to expand the institution's most profitable areas.[90]

He resigned from Grady after two years, in December 2005, in order to administer a network of Catholic hospitals in California. After leaving California, he worked for Wellcare in Florida for six months and then moved to AHCA (a government agency in Florida's Department of Health). Several years later "Dr. Andy," his wife, and their two daughters moved to Spokane, Washington, where he continued his career as a hospital administrator.

John Henry

Following Dr. Andy Agwunobi's departure to California, the board appointed John Henry as the interim CEO. The retired CEO of Emory Hospitals, Henry had been named Grady's Chief Operating Officer by Dr. Agwunobi. A former chairman of the Georgia Hospital Authority, Mr. Henry had won numerous awards in his career, including one from the Urban Land Institute for his oversight of the renovation and expansion of Emory Crawford Long Hospital.[91]

Michael L. Lomax

A native of California, Michael L. Lomax graduated magna cum laude and Phi Beta Kappa from Morehouse College in 1968. He earned an M.A. in literature from Columbia University and, in 1984, a Ph.D. in literature from Emory University. By the time he earned his doctorate he already had been elected to the Fulton County Commission. He had also been identified by *Time* magazine as a rising young black leader—one of five in the United States it identified in an article in 1981.[92]

Lomax became involved in politics during Maynard Jackson's campaign for mayor of Atlanta in 1973. At the time he was on leave from teaching in order to complete his dissertation. While doing that, Lomax started to write speeches for Jackson. After Mayor Jackson's election, Lomax served in the Jackson administration. He became a candidate himself in 1978, successfully running for a seat on the Fulton County Board of Commissioners. Three years later, in 1981, Lomax

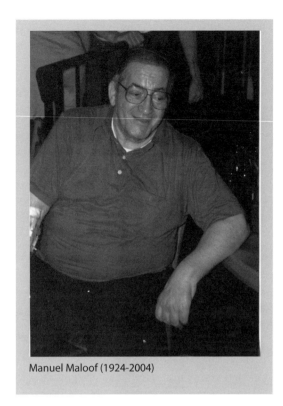

Manuel Maloof (1924-2004)

became the board's chairman—a post he held for twelve years. Hard working, Lomax continued his college teaching while serving as county commissioner. Strongly committed to the arts, in 1979 Lomax sponsored the legislation that created the Fulton County Arts Council. In 1988, he initiated the National Black Arts Festival in Atlanta and served as the festival's first chairman.[93]

After seeking—and getting—the support of former Mayor Jackson, Lomax decided to run for Mayor of Atlanta in 1989. Unfortunately for Lomax, Maynard Jackson decided he wanted his old job for himself. Undaunted, Lomax campaigned vigorously until running out of money shortly before the election.[94] Four years later Lomax resigned from the county commission to run for mayor again. After losing to Bill Campbell in a run-off, Lomax became president of the National Faculty, an organization linking scholars in higher education with elementary and high school teachers.

In 1997, Michael Lomax accepted an offer to become President of Dillard University, a historically black university in New Orleans. Urbane, erudite, and an effective administrator and fund-raiser, Lomax proved to be a successful university president. He left Dillard University in 2004 to become president and CEO of the United Negro College Fund.

Manuel Maloof

Manuel Maloof was born in Atlanta, the son of a Lebanese immigrant and a mother from Savannah, Georgia, of Lebanese descent. He graduated from Tech High School and then served in England during World War II. In 1956, he purchased Harry's Delicatessen on North Highland Avenue and renamed the business Manuel's Tavern. It would become one of the first bars in the Atlanta area to willingly integrate. He became a local folk hero after Paul Hemphill, a popular editorial writer for the *Atlanta Journal,* began featuring Manuel Maloof in some of his articles as a noteworthy philosophical bartender. His tavern became an important place for politicians, those elected and those wanting to be elected, to visit. Bill Clinton, Jimmy Carter, Andrew Young, Sam Nunn, Maynard Jackson, and Shirley Franklin are among the many politicians who would "drop in" for a conversation.

Entering politics himself, he won a seat on the DeKalb County Commission in 1974 and became its chairman in 1980. A recall attempt in 1982, prompted by popular anger about the county's reassessment of property values, failed for lack of enough signatures. In 1984, Maloof was elected to the new position of CEO for DeKalb County and served until 1992. During his time in office he expanded the roles of minorities and women in government. Through his efforts, the interchange of Interstate 85 and Interstate 285 was completed.

Manuel Maloof was blunt, caustic, colorful, confrontational, and honest. He was a leader and while leading was a major supporter of Grady Memorial Hospital. He died in 2004 from cardiac arrest, a complication of a long history of diabetes, at Emory University Hospital.[95]

Greater Grady Task Force

By the start of 2007, Grady's ongoing funding crisis had become so acute that the hospital appeared to be on its financial deathbed. In the face of a growing population in the metro area, increasing costs (which were in line with medical inflation in the United States), a decrease in funding from the counties, revisions to Medicaid reimbursement formulas, and other funding challenges, Grady's budget deficits simply were unsustainable. On top of other debts, the hospital owed $65 million to the Emory University School of Medicine and Morehouse School of Medicine.

In March, at the request of the hospital authority, the Metro Atlanta Chamber of Commerce created the Greater Grady Task Force to investigate the hospital's operations and finances and to recommend ways to strengthen the institution. The task force was chaired by two distinguished businessmen, A. D. "Pete" Correll, a former Chairman of Georgia-Pacific Corporation, and Michael B. Russell, the CEO of H. J. Russell & Company.

The fact that one was white and one was black may have been symbolically significant to some, but it would misread the evidence to suggest that Correll and Russell represented, respectively, White Atlanta and Black Atlanta. What they stood for was the business community's dedication to the area. Both men were experienced business leaders who were committed to metropolitan Atlanta, the disadvantaged, and Grady's mission. Donating time and expertise to advance the common good was part of what they were about.

They viewed Grady, in Michael Russell's words, as "a vital part of the fabric of this community." Pete Correll's assessment of Grady was blunt: "This hospital is too important to the community to let it go under."[96]

Grady's centrality to the larger community was enough of a reason to take on the immense challenge of saving the sinking ship and then turning it away from the shoals toward which it was headed.

The task force was composed of many distinguished civic leaders with deep business experience, including Tom Bell, the Chairman, President, and CEO of Cousins Properties, a national real estate investment trust, Ben Johnson, a distinguished civic leader and the managing partner of the law firm of Alston & Bird, Ronald Brown, the President and CEO of Atlanta Life, Bill Clement, the Chairman and CEO of DOBBS, RAM & Company, Tommy Dortch, the head of TWD, Inc., Jim Miller, the general counsel for Georgia Power, and Phil Humann, the CEO of SunTrust Banks, the successor company to Thomas Glenn's Trust Company of Georgia.

People who understood the interplay between government and the non-profit world also served on the task force: Carl Patton, the president of Georgia State University, Renee Glover, the head of the Atlanta Housing Authority, and Alana Shepherd, founder of the Shepherd Center, a leading rehabilitation hospital for people with brain or spinal cord injuries.

Other task force members were intimately acquainted with Grady: Robert L. Brown, the long-time chairman of the FDHA, Dr. Michael Johns, the CEO of Emory University's Woodruff Health Sciences Center, and John Maupin, President of Morehouse School of Medicine.

The two other members of the task force also brought important skills and relationships to the project. Guy Budinscak, the Managing Partner of Deloitte, a consulting firm, served ex officio because his firm was donating its expertise to the task force. As if to underscore the importance of the project to Atlanta's business leaders, Sam Williams, president of the Metro Atlanta Chamber of Commerce, also served on the task force.

Releasing its final report on July 13, 2007, the task force's most significant and dramatic recommendation centered on removing political influence from Grady's affairs. The solution was straightforward: change the hospital's governance.[97]

The hospital had been run by the FDHA since the 1940s. At the start of the twenty-first century, Grady was much more than a hospital. It was a health care system with hundreds of clinics at the hospital and nearly

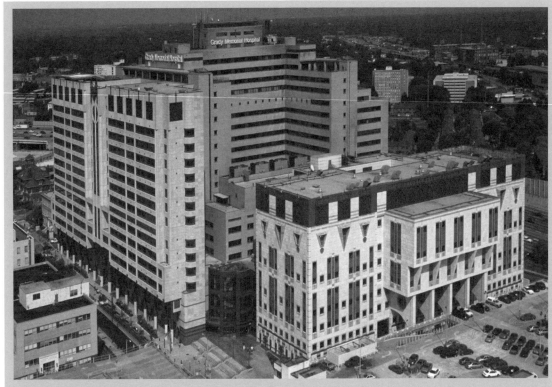

Grady Memorial Hospital, present day

a dozen satellite clinics in Fulton and DeKalb counties. The business of medicine and health care had changed dramatically since the era of World War II, and the task force believed that to turn Grady around, it needed a structure of governance to suit the times.

Just as Thomas Glenn saw to the creation of the Fulton-DeKalb Hospital Authority in the 1940s for a specific purpose—to get around restrictive bond referendum laws—so the task force also wanted a new governing structure to accomplish a single goal: Let Grady be Grady without political meddling from the outside.

As Michael Russell indicated, refiguring Grady's governance would be a big step in "winning back the confidence of the community."[98] Given Grady's precarious finances—it could run out of money before the end of the year—the hospital needed all the help it could get as fast as possible.

The task force suggested creating a new nonprofit corporation to provide governance of Grady and to oversee its operations. Fulton and DeKalb counties would continue to own the hospital through the FDHA. Crucially, the FDHA would still be able to float bonds. (Every other urban Georgia hospital authority, all of which were created after the FDHA, had already been converted to a nonprofit 501(c)3 model.)

In response, the Grady Coalition sprang back to life. It had been dormant since the successful battle against price hikes at Grady's pharmacy in the late 1990s. Veterans of the earlier fight, including Bert Skellie, a community activist and member of the Friends Meeting House, the Reverend Timothy McDonald III of the First Iconium Baptist Church and a leader in the Concerned Black Clergy, and Vincent Fort, a state senator and professor of history, were leaders in the revitalized group.

The Grady Coalition was skeptical of the Metro Atlanta Chamber's involvement. It was especially worried about Grady being turned over to private hands. The idea of privatizing Grady had been around for more than a century, ever since the idea was floated in the middle of a bitter debate about city taxes in 1903. More recently, an effort to privatize Grady had been narrowly averted during the 1990s. In 2007, some of the hospital's supporters saw the move toward a nonprofit corporation as effectively privatizing Grady.

Adamant about keeping public oversight of the taxpayer's hospital, the Grady Coalition worried about maintaining public accountability. It also was concerned that the non-profit corporation would reduce patient services and put jobs at risk. In addition to advocating for patients and saving jobs, more than anything else the coalition hoped to limit Emory's influence on the new board. Its mistrust of Emory ran deep, as did its wariness of the corporate orientation of the non-profit board's members.

Coalition leaders feared that the "privatization" of Grady through the nonprofit board might result in turning the hospital over to an out-of-state publicly traded corporation like HCA. The coalition's leaders wanted to protect the public trust from what it saw as rapacious capitalists more interested in profits than in people. There was also a fear that the private board would engineer a sale of Grady's assets. In short, the Grady Coalition, eager to speak for the powerless and to protect jobs, simply did not trust that Atlanta's civic leaders truly were focused on the needs of Grady or its people.[99] The mistrust was something which the task force simply had to work through.

The Greater Grady Task Force estimated that it would take an influx of $370 million over two years to turn around the hospital. Without that kind of additional money, it would be impossible to improve either Grady's finances or its service to patients. Grady required $120 million to pay its debt to the medical schools and address immediate needs; it would have to spend another $250 million to pay for improvements in equipment and services. In addition, the task force forecast Grady would, for the foreseeable future, have an operating deficit of $50 million per year. (Once more, the cost of uncompensated care was a major cause for the projected deficits.)[100]

How would Grady's funding change under the new governance? One fresh avenue was its ability to tap a few sources of funding unavailable to the FDHA. The other solutions, however, had been mentioned for decades. Most significantly, the task force suggested turning to the state of Georgia for help. It recommended that the state of Georgia increase its allowance for physicians in training, fund a statewide trauma network, and turn over more federal matching funds to hospitals that treat the indigent.

Even with more help from the state, serving only the poor and absorbing the cost of massive amounts of uncompensated care remained unsustainable. Besides additional aid from the state, Grady would need to attract more patients with commercially available insurance.

Out of all of the task force's recommendations, the strategy to immunize Grady from political interference was the most crucial. Supporters of a public hospital in Atlanta had understood the imperative that the institution be "free from politics" since before Grady was built. Only a few years into the twenty-first century, that dream was on the cusp of being realized.

The recommendation of the Greater Grady Task Force to turn Grady's governance over to an independent non-profit corporation with a civic-minded board of directors was effected in 2008.

In the hope of being freed from politics at last, Grady was ready to push forward into the twenty-first century.

Afterword
Into the Twenty-First Century

"Grady is the conscience of our area."

—Manuel Maloof, May 24, 1992

For over two centuries, Americans have supported the idea of public hospitals designed to serve the poor. Medical care for the poor began in North America in the form of almshouses. In those charitable institutions, people who were indigent, unable to care for themselves, or neglected or abandoned by their family or community could find a modicum of comfort and care. Toward the end of the nineteenth century, as the modern form of the American hospital began to take shape, health care for the poor moved to hospital facilities. Grady Memorial Hospital has been an important participant in that evolving tradition since its founding in 1892.

Whether it was the hookworm infections of Georgia's citizens in the early twentieth century or the AIDS epidemic in the latter part of the same century, Grady rose to the occasion to meet the needs of citizens in the Atlanta area and throughout the state of Georgia. Whether treating victims of violence in the community, those suffering workplace accidents, or the thousands of people critically injured in automobile accidents, in meeting the needs of its patients Grady's emergency room and Trauma Unit developed a national reputation for excellence during the past century. The Poison Control Center, located on the Grady campus, is the only one in Georgia. Each year it handles over 100,000 calls from people throughout the state. The Diabetes Clinic and Sickle Cell Clinic not only treat patients from around the state, but also train medical personnel who then return to their own communities to care for and improve the well-being of patients with these illnesses.

The Grady staff has met a range of exceptional events with the highest degree of professionalism. These include the results of natural disasters such as the tornado that struck Gainesville, Georgia, in 1937. It also includes man-made disasters such as the Winecoff Hotel fire, the tragedy of the John Hardy bootleg whiskey episode, and the bombing in downtown Atlanta's Centennial Park during the 1996 Olympic Games.

A police officer injured in the line of duty, a professional hockey player involved in a fatal auto accident, a millionaire businessman badly burned on his family farm, a beautiful model severely injured in an auto accident, and a fire-fighter with burns and smoke inhalation all have one thing in common—they were patients of Grady Memorial Hospital. The institution is not a hospital only for the poor—it serves all the citizens of Georgia.

Manuel Maloof, the late DeKalb County Commissioner, put the feeling of many Grady patients in blunt terms. In 1995, he told Dave Kindred, a columnist with the *Constitution*, what he had often said before: "If we ever abandon Atlanta, the last light we should turn out is Grady's."[1]

Acknowledgments

I am not a trained historian but rather I'm an individual who enjoys the reading and studying of past events and people. Consequently, this book would not have been possible without the assistance of numerous individuals and several organizations that offered photographs, suggestions, and information that would be incorporated into this book.

The first is my son Crawford who helped with the early research and was convinced that the Grady hospital story needed to be told. John Robitscher, formerly of the Henry Grady Foundation, encouraged my writing and provided a typist to read my sometimes illegible writing. The staff of the James G. Kenan Research Center located in the Atlanta History Center: Michael Rose, Paul Crater, Heather Culligan, Helen Matthews, Melanie Stephan, Laura Starratt and Sue VanHoef constantly pulled archival material. Their efforts were invaluable.

Matt Gove of Grady Memorial Hospital, Steve Davis of MAG Mutual Insurance Company, David Waldrop and Beverly Dickerson of the Medical Association of Atlanta, Donna Glass at the Medical Association of Georgia, and the Board of Atlanta Medical Heritage, led by Emory Schwall, and the Coca Cola Company, all contributed time or materials towards this book.

Mrs. Olivia Patton of All Saints Church, Taronda Spencer of Spelman College, Ansley Black of St. Joseph's Hospital of Atlanta, Karen Schindler, Nancy Watkins and Elizabeth Chase of Emory University all donated material and permissions to use their materials. A.D. "Pete" Correll spent his valuable time explaining the last four years of Grady. The librarian Brenda Curry-Wimberly and assistant librarian of Northside Hospital, Betty Blanchard, always made themselves available to gather articles from past medical journals.

Finally I would like to express my sincere appreciation to three special people. Esther Patrick for her patience and talents as she translated my written words onto the computer and had many wonderful suggestions. David Yntema, my editor, who added significantly to the information found in this book and whose countless hours of research and editing greatly improved the story of this wonderful hospital. Finally I want to express my deep appreciation to my wife Harriet for always being encouraging and supportive of this time-consuming project.

Thanks to all.

Selected Sources and Suggested Reading

Allen, Frederick. *Secret Formula: How Brilliant Marketing and Relentless Salesmanship Made Coca-Cola the Best Known Product in the World.* New York: Harper Business, 1994.

Atlanta: A City of the Modern South. Compiled by Workers of the Writers' Program of the Work Projects Administration in the State of Georgia. New York: Smith & Durrell, 1942.

Ayers, Edward L. *The Promise of the New South: Life After Reconstruction.* New York: Oxford University Press, 1992.

Bacote, Clarence A. *The Story of Atlanta University: A Century of Service, 1865-1965.* Atlanta: Atlanta University Press, 1969.

Bartley, Numan V. *The Creation of Modern Georgia.* Athens, Georgia: University of Georgia Press, 1983.

Bayor, Ronald H. *Race and The Shaping of Twentieth Century Atlanta.* Chapel Hill: The University of North Carolina Press, 1996.

Beardsley, Edward H. *A History of Neglect: Health Care for Blacks and Mill Workers in the Twentieth Century South.* Knoxville: University of Tennessee Press, 1987.

Bellamy, Verdelle B., ed. *History of Grady Memorial Hospital School of Nursing, 1917-1964.* Atlanta: Chi Eta Phi Sorority [1985].

Blackmon, Douglas A. *Slavery By Another Name: The Re-Enslavement of Black Americans from the Civil War to World War II.* New York: Doubleday, 2008.

Brandt, Allan M. *No Magic Bullet: A Social History of Venereal Disease in the United States Since 1880.* New York: Oxford University Press, 1985.

Burns, Rebecca. *Rage in the Gate City: The Story of the 1906 Atlanta Race Riot.* Cincinnati: Emmis Publishing, 2006.

Cash, W. J. *The Mind of the South.* New York: Alfred A. Knopf, 1931.

Clendenen, Lois with Nancy Yarn. *75 Years Between the Peachtrees: A History of Crawford W. Long Memorial Hospital of Emory University.* Atlanta: Susan Hunter, 1987.

Ditmer, John. *Black Georgia in the Progressive Era, 1900-1920.* Urbana: University of Illinois Press, 1977.

Dorsey, Allison. *To Build Our Lives Together: Community Formation in Black Atlanta, 1875-1906.* Athens: The University of Georgia Press, 2004.

Dowling, Harry F. *City Hospitals: The Undercare of the Underprivileged.* Cambridge: Harvard University Press, 1982.

Doyle, Don H. *New Men, New Cities, New South: Atlanta, Nashville, Charleston, Mobile, 1860-1910.* Chapel Hill: University of North Carolina Press, 1990.

Ellis, John H. *Yellow Fever and Public Health in the New South.* Lexington: University Press of Kentucky, 1992.

Etheridge, Elizabeth. *Sentinel For Health: A History of the Centers for Disease Control.* Berkeley: University of California Press, 1992.

Ettling, John. *The Germ of Laziness: Rockefeller Philanthropy and Public Health in the New South.* Cambridge: Harvard University Press, 1981.

Flexner, Abraham. *Medical Education in the United States and Canada: A Report to the Carnegie Foundation for the Advancement of Teaching*; Bulletin No. 4. New York: Carnegie Foundation for the Advancement of Teaching, 1910.

Fox, Daniel M. *Health Policies, Health Politics: The British and American Experience, 1911-1965.* Princeton: Princeton University Press, 1986.

Gamble, Vanessa Northington. *Making A Place for Ourselves: The Black Hospital Movement, 1920-1945.* New York: Oxford University Press, 1995.

Gentry, Jerry. *Grady Baby: A Year in the Life of Atlanta's Grady Hospital.* Jackson, Mississippi: University of Mississippi Press, 1999.

Godshalk, David Fort. *Veiled Visions: The 1906 Atlanta Race Riot and the Reshaping of American Race Relations.* Chapel Hill: University of North Carolina Press, 2005.

Gordon, Colin. *Dead on Arrival: The Politics of Health Care in Twentieth Century America.* Princeton: Princeton University Press.

Grantham, Dewey W. Jr. *Hoke Smith and the Politics of the New South.* Baton Rouge: Louisiana State University Press, 1958.

Gutman, Herbert G. *The Black Family in Slavery and Freedom, 1750-1925.* New York: Vintage Books, 1977.

Harris, Neil. *Building Lives: Constructing Rites and Passages.* New Haven: Yale University Press, 1999.

Hickey, Georgina. *Hope and Danger in the New South City: Working class Women and Urban Development in Atlanta, 1890-1940.* Athens, Georgia: University of Georgia Press, 2003.

Hines, Darlene Clark. *Black Women in White: Racial Conflict and Cooperation in the Nursing Profession 1890-1950.* Bloomington: Indiana University Press, 1989.

Howell, Joel D. *Technology in the Hospital: Transforming Patient Care in the Early Twentieth Century.* Baltimore: Johns Hopkins University Press, 1995.

Humphreys, Margaret. *Malaria: Poverty, Race, and Public Health in the United States.* Baltimore: Johns Hopkins University Press, 2001.

Hunter, Floyd. *Community Power Structure: A Study of Decision Makers.* Chapel Hill: University of North Carolina Press, 1953.

____. *Community Power Succession: Atlanta's Policy Makers Revisited.* Chapel Hill: University of North Carolina Press, 1980.

Hurst, J. Willis. *The Quest for Excellence: The History of the Department of Medicine at Emory University School of Medicine, 1834-1986.* Atlanta: Scholars Press, 1997.

Jackson, Kenneth T. *The Ku Klux Klan in the City, 1915-1930.* New York: Oxford University Press, 1967.

Jenkins, Herbert. *Keeping the Peace: A Police Chief Looks at His Job.* New York: Harper & Row, 1970.

Jennings, M. Kent. *Community Influentials: The Elites of Atlanta.* New York: Free Press of Glencoe, 1964.

Kean, Melissa. *Desegregating Private Higher Education in the South: Duke, Emory, Rice, Tulane, and Vanderbilt.* Baton Rouge: Louisiana State University Press, 2008.

Kruse, Kevin. *White Flight and the Making of Modern Conservativism.* Princeton: Princeton University Press, 2005.

Kuhn, Clifford. *Contesting the New South Order: The 1914-1915 Strike at Atlanta's Fulton Mill.* Chapel Hill and London: The University of North Carolina Press, 2001.

Kuhn, Clifford M., Harlan E. Joye, and E. Bernard West. *Living Atlanta: An Oral History of the City, 1914-1948.* Athens, Georgia: University of Georgia Press, 1990.

Ludmerer, Kenneth M. *Learning to Heal: The Development of American Medical Education.* New York: Basic Books, 1985.

McDowell, John Patrick. *The Social Gospel in the South: The Woman's Home Mission Movement in the Methodist Episcopal Church, South, 1886–1939.* Baton Rouge: Louisiana State University Press, 1982.

Martin, John D. Jr. and Garland D. Perdue. *The History of Surgery at Emory University School of Medicine.* Atlanta: The University, 1979.

Mays, Benjamin Elijah. *Born to Rebel: An Autobiography.* Athens, Georgia: University of Georgia Press, 1987.

Melosh, Barbara. *The Physician's Hand: Work, Culture, and Conflict in American Nursing.* Philadelphia: Temple University Press, 1982.

Morantz-Sanchez, Regina Markel. *Sympathy and Science: Women Physicians and American Medicine.* New York: Oxford University Press, 1985.

Norman, Elizabeth M. *We Band of Angels: The Untold Story of American Nurses Trapped on Bataan by the Japanese.* New York: Random House, 1999.

Norris, Jack C. *Gleanings From A Doctor's Eye.* Atlanta: Higgins-McArthur Company, Typographers and Printers, 1953.

Opdycke, Sandra. *No One Was Turned Away: The Role of Public Hospitals in New York City Since 1900.* New York: Oxford University Press, 1999.

Pomerantz, Gary M. *Where Peachtree Meets Sweet Auburn: A Saga of Race and Family.* New York: Penguin Books, 1996.

Preston, Howard L. *Automobile Age Atlanta: The Making of A Southern Metropolis, 1900-1935.* Athens: University of Georgia Press, 1979.

Rabinowitz, Howard N. *Race Relations in the Urban South, 1865-1890*. New York: Oxford University Press, 1978.

Rapport, Richard, M.D. *Physician: The Life of Paul Beeson*. Fort Lee, New Jersey: Barricade Books, 2001.

Reverby, Susan M. *Ordered to Care: The Dilemma of American Nursing, 1850-1945*. New York: Cambridge University Press, 1987.

Reynolds, P. Preston. *Watts Hospital of Durham, North Carolina, 1895-1976: Keeping the Doors Open*. Durham, North Carolina: Published by the North Carolina School of Science and Mathematics, 1991.

Roberts, Charles Stewart. *Life and Writings of Stewart R. Roberts, M.D.: Georgia's First Heart Specialist*. Spartanburg, South Carolina: The Reprint Company, 1993.

Rosenberg, Charles. *The Care of Strangers: The Rise of America's Hospital System*. New York: Basic Books, 1987.

Rothschild, Janice O. *As But A Day: The First Hundred Years, 1867-1967*. Atlanta: Hebrew Benevolent Congregation, 1967.

Russell, James Michael. *Atlanta 1847-1890: City Building in the Old South and the New*. Baton Rouge: Louisiana State University Press, 1988.

Schissel, Carla M. "The State Nurses Association in a Georgia Context, 1907-1946," Ph.D. dissertation, Emory University, 1979

Smith, Douglas. *The New Deal in the Urban South*. Baton Rouge: Louisiana State University Press, 1988.

Smith, John Robert. *The Church That Stayed: The Life and Times of Central Presbyterian Church in the Heart of Atlanta, 1858-1978*. Atlanta: Atlanta Historical Society, 1979.

Smith, William Rawson. *Villa Clare: The Purposeful Life and Timeless Art Collection of J. J. Haverty*. Macon, Georgia: Mercer University Press, 2006.

Spitzer, Lorrane Nelson and Jean B. Bergmark. *Grace Towns Hamilton and the Politics of Southern Change: An African American Woman's Struggle for Racial Equality*. Athens: University of Georgia Press, 1997.

Starr, Paul. *The Social Transformation of American Medicine*. New York: Basic Books, 1982.

Stevens, Rosemary. *In Sickness and in Wealth: American Hospitals in the Twentieth Century*. New York: Basic Books, 1989.

Stone, Clarence N. *Regime Politics: Governing Atlanta 1946-1986*. Lawrence, Kansas: University of Kansas Press, 1989.

Vogel, Morris. *The Invention of the Modern Hospital: Boston, 1870-1930*. Chicago: University of Chicago Press, 1980.

Wailoo, Keith. *Dying in the City of The Blues: Sickle Cell Anemia and the Politics of Race and Health*. Chapel Hill: The University of North Carolina Press, 2001.

Watts, Eugene, J. *The Social Basis of City Politics: Atlanta, 1865-1903*. Westport, Connecticut: Greenwood Press, 1978.

White, Walter. *A Man Called White: The Autobiography of Walter White*. New York, Viking, 1948.

Woodward, C. Vann. *Origins of the New South, 1877-1913*. Baton Rouge: Louisiana State University Press, 1951.

Woodford, Frank B., and Philip P. Mason. *Harper of Detroit: The Origin and Growth of a Great Metropolitan Hospital*. Detroit: Wayne State University Press, 1964.

Selected Articles

Beardsley, Edward H. "Goodbye to Jim Crow: The Desegregation of Southern Hospitals, 1945–70," *Bulletin of the History of Medicine*, 60:3 (1986), 367–86.

"Eugene Alston Stead, Jr., MD: A Conversation with J. Willis Hurst, MD," *The American Journal of Cardiology* 84 (September 15, 1999), 701-725.

Galishoff, Stuart. "Germs Know No Color Line: Black Health and Public Policy in Atlanta, 1900-1918, *Journal of the History of Medicine and Allied Sciences* 40:1 (January 1985), 22-41.

Hine, Darlene Clark. "The Ethel Johns Report: Black Women in the Nursing Profession, 1925," *The Journal of Negro History* 67:3 (Autumn 1982), 212-228.

Gamble, Vanessa Northington. "Black Autonomy versus White Control: Black Hospitals and the Dilemmas of White Philanthropy, 1920-1940," *Minerva*, 35:3 (September 1997) 247-267.

Lee, Richard V. "Changing Times: Reflections on a Professional Lifetime: An Interview with Paul Beeson," *Annals of Internal Medicine* 132 (January 4, 2000) 71-79.

Savitt, Todd L. "Entering a White Profession: Black Physicians in the New South, 1880–1920," *Bulletin of the History of Medicine,* 61:4 (1987), 507–40.

_____. "The Use of Blacks for Medical Experimentation and Demonstration in the Old South," *Journal of Southern History* 48:3 (August 1982), 331-348.

Shulman, Neil. "Prescription: Protest," *The Nation* (269:5) August 9-16, 1999.

Yancey, A. G. Sr. "Grady Memorial Hospital Centennial: History and Development, 1892-1992," *Journal of the Medical Association of Georgia* 81:11 (1992), 621-31.

Yancey, A. G. Sr. "Medical Education in Atlanta and Health Care of Black Minority and Low-Income People," *Journal of the National Medical Association* 80:4 (April 1988), 467-76.

Photo/Illustration Credits

Atlanta Medical Heritage: 4 all, 63, 64, 66, 85, 109;
Courtesy of St. Joseph's Hospital of Atlanta, Inc., copyright, 2010: 12, 13;
Courtesy of Spelman College: 15, 84;
The James Kenan Research Center at the Atlanta History Center: 18, 22, 24, 29, 31, 40, 43, 46, 60, 62, 68, 70, 72;
Medical Association of Atlanta: 42, 72, 74, 78, 130, 205, 215;
The Longino Family: 49;
Grady Memorial Hospital: 53, 54, 56, 61, 80, 83, 87, 88, 89, 90, 91, 92, 93, 96, 98, 103, 106, 110, 113, 121, 138 (top), 150, 154, 155, 156, 159 (bottom), 161, 163, 219, 248, 250, 262, 263, 266;
All Saints' Episcopal Church, Atlanta, Georgia: 77;
Georgia Baptist Hospital: 79 (top);
Piedmont Hospital: 79 (bottom), 82;
Taken from Annual Report, Fulton-DeKalb Hospital Authority: 83, 159 (bottom), 161, 163, 172;
Taken from Annual Report, Grady Memorial Hospital: 98, 107, 111, 123, 124;
Courtesey of Louis Sherman of The Albert Steiner Charitable Fund: 99, 100;
Emory University School of Medicine: 112
Courtesy of the Coca-Cola Company: 115, 139;
Courtesy of the Bartholomew Family: 127;
Courtesy of the Glenn Family: 129;
Courtesy of Oglethorpe University: 134;
Author's Collection: 138, 141;
Courtesy of the Roberts Family: 139 (bottom);
Photographic Collection, Special Collections and Archives, Georgia State University Library: 153;
Courtesy of Dr. Robert Shuler: 158, 159(top), 248;
Courtesy of the Wilson Family: 165;
Courtesy of King & Spalding: 171;
League of Women Voters of Atlanta: 173;
Courtesy of Morehouse College: 176;
Courtesy of the Ivan Allen, Jr., Family: 183;
Courtesy of Dr. Ann Bell Taylor: 184;
Mrs. Clinton Warner: 185;
Courtesy of Dr. Al Brann: 197;
Courtesy of Dr. Andre Nahmias: 198;
Courtesy of the Herman J. Russell Family: 209;
Courtesy of Dr. Edward Loughlin: 210;
Courtesy of Dr. Peter Symbas: 217;
Courtesy of Dr. Nanette Wenger: 218;
Courtesy of Lew and Barbara Regenstein: 223;
Bill Pinkston: 234;
Courtesy of Mrs. Marilyn Holmes: 237;
Courtesy of Robert Brown: 260;
Courtesy of the Clyde Shepherd Family: 261;
Courtesy of The Maloof Family: 264;

Endnotes

ABBREVIATIONS USED IN ENDNOTES:

AC	*Atlanta Constitution*
AD	*Atlanta Daily Constitution*
ADW	*Atlanta Daily World*
AHC	The James G. Kenan Research Center at the Atlanta History Center
AI	*The Atlanta Inquirer*
AJ	*Atlanta Journal*
AJC	*Atlanta Journal and Constitution*
FDHA	Fulton-DeKalb Hospital Authority
GMH	Grady Memorial Hospital
GMHC	Grady Memorial Hospital Collection, 1892-1980, MSS 429
Hamilton	Grace Towns Hamilton Collection
JAMA	*Journal of the American Medical Association*
MARBL	Manuscript, Archives, and Rare Book Library, Emory University
ROAO	Reports of Adminstrative Officers to the President of Emory University

Chapter 1

[1] Campbell Gibson, "Population of the Largest 100 Cities and Other Urban Places in the United States: 1790-1990," *Population Division Working Paper No. 27* (Washington D.C.: U.S. Bureau of the Census, 1998); Charles E. Rosenberg, *The Care of Strangers: The Rise of America's Hospital System* (New York: Basic Books, Inc., 1987).

[2] Laurel Thatcher Ulrich, *A Midwife's Tale: The Life of Martha Ballard, Based on Her Diary, 1785-1812* (New York: Alfred A. Knopf, 1990) vividly details the life and practice of a midwife in the United States during the early national period. For a detailed history of early medical practice in Georgia, see Gerald L. Cates, "A Medical History of Georgia: The First Hundred Years, 1733-1833" (Ph.D. dissertation, University of Georgia, 1976). On physicians and their marketing campaigns to attract patients in the early nineteenth century, see Cates, 155-157.

[3] Ullrich Bonnell Phillips, "An American State-Owned Railroad: The Western and Atlantic," *Yale Review* 15:3 (November 1906), 259-282; idem., *A History of Transportation in the Eastern Cotton Belt to 1860* (New York: The Columbia University Press, 1908).

[4] Daniel Walker Howe, *What God Hath Wrought: The Transformation of America, 1815-1848* (New York: Oxford University Press, 2007) gives context to the debates. Joseph S. Wood, "The Idea of a National Road," in Karl B. Raitz, ed., *The National Road* (Baltimore: The Johns Hopkins University Press, 1996), 93-122, explores the national purpose of the Cumberland Road. Carol Sheriff, *The Artificial River: The Erie Canal and the Paradox of Progress, 1817-1862* (New York: Hill & Wang, 1996) discusses how the rhetoric of "the common good" evolved in antebellum America in connection with internal improvements.

[5] In 1826, the state's Board of Public Works investigated building a series of canals to link the port of Savannah with the headwaters of the Coosa River near what is now Rome, Georgia. The cost, however, was prohibitive and the surveyor, Wilson Lumpkin, a future governor of Georgia, instead suggested the building of a railway (to be powered by teams of mules). See Phillips, "An American State-Owned Railroad," 262. For an overview of comparative economic advantages of canals and railroads at the time, see Alfred D. Chandler, Jr., *The Visible Hand: The Managerial Revolution in American Business* (Cambridge, Mass.: The Belknap Press of Harvard University Press, 1993), 81-87.

[6] Alfred D. Chandler, Jr., "Patterns of American Railroad Finance, 1830-1850," *Business History Review* 28:3 (September 1953), 248-263.

[7] Franklin Garrett, *Atlanta and Environs,* Volume 1*: A Chronicle of Its People and Events, 1820s-1870s* (New York: Lewis Historical Publishing Company, Inc., 1954), 189.

[8] Ibid., 218-219.

[9] U.S. Bureau of the Census, *Historical Statistics of the United States from Colonial Times to 1970,* (Washington D.C., 1976), 723-741.

[10] Philips, "An American State-Owned Railroad," 269-270; Royce Shingleton, *Richard Peters: Champion of the New South* (Macon: Mercer University Press, 1985), 13-25.

[11] Garrett, *Atlanta and Environs,* Volume 1, 216-217.

[12] Ibid., 355.

[13] Ibid., 375; William F. Norwood, *Medical Education in the United States Before the Civil War* (Philadelphia: University of Pennsylvania Press, 1944).

[14] F. Phinizy Calhoun, "The Founding and the Early History of the Atlanta Medical College," *Georgia Historical Quarterly* 9:1 (March 1925), 35-54. The college offered courses over the summer in an effort to keep southern students in the South and, more importantly, to provide a competitive alternative to "winter schools" in the north. See, for example, "Editorial and Miscellaneous," *Atlanta Medical and Surgical Journal* 2:5 (January 1857), 303-304 and "Editorial and Miscellaneous," *Atlanta Medical and Surgical Journal* 2:8 (April 1857), 502.

[15] Charles E. Rosenberg, *The Care of Strangers: The Rise of America's Hospital System* (New York: Basic Books), 193-200. Some medical schools were tied to charity hospitals. In smaller cities, however, medical schools tended "to create their own inpatient facilities." (Rosenberg, 199.) See also William G. Rothstein, *American Medical Schools and the Practice of Medicine: A History* (New York: Oxford University Press, 1987).

[16] Garrett, *Atlanta and Environs*, Volume I, 396, reproduces an advertisement for the infirmary of the Atlanta Medical College from the *Weekly Intelligencer*, October 12, 1855.

[17] Todd L. Savitt, "The Use of Blacks for Medical Experimentation and Demonstration in the Old South," *Journal of Southern History* 48:3 (August 1982), 334.

[18] Although sometimes indirectly challenged, the concept that even the indigent were entitled to medical care, on humanitarian grounds if nothing else, dominated the rhetoric of medical practitioners, philanthropists, and politicians in late nineteenth century Atlanta.

[19] Rosenberg, 157-158; Rosemary Stevens, *In Sickness and in Wealth: American Hospitals in the Twentieth Century* (New York: Basic Books, 1989).

[20] Ira M. Rutkow, *Bleeding Blue and Gray: Civil War Surgery and the Evolution of American Medicine* (New York: Random House, 2005).

[21] Louisa May Alcott's *Hospital Sketches: An Army Nurse's True Account of Her Experiences in the Civil War*, first published in 1863, was a popular account (and defense of) nursing in a Union hospital.

[22] Drew Gilpin Faust, *This Republic of Suffering: Death and the American Civil War* (New York: Knopf, 2008).

[23] Jack D. Welsh, *Two Confederate Hospitals and Their Patients: Atlanta to Opelika* (Macon: Mercer University Press, 2005), 5.

[24] Grigsby H. Wotton, Jr., "New City of the South: Atlanta, 1843-1873," (Ph.D. dissertation, The Johns Hopkins University, 1973), 116, reports an estimate that Atlanta had from 6,000 to 8,000 residents by June 1865; V. T. Barnwell, *Barnwell's Atlanta City Directory, and Stranger's Guide: Also a General Firemen's, Church, Masonic, and Odd Fellows' Record, Volume I, Compiled (Principally in January) for the Year 1867* (Atlanta: Intelligencer Book and Job Office, 1867), 16.

[25] Richard J. Hopkins, "Public Health in Atlanta: The Formative Years, 1865-1879," *Georgia Historical Quarterly* 53 (September 1969), 287-304.

[26] James Michael Russell, *Atlanta 1847-1890: City Building in the Old South and New* (Baton Rouge: Louisiana State University Press), 1988.

[27] City of Atlanta Records, Atlanta City Council Minutes, January 24, 1873, volume 7, page 411, AHC.

[28] "Atlanta Benevolent Home, Its History Briefly Sketched," AC, April 13, 1880, 4.

[29] Hopkins, "Public Health in Atlanta," 296; "We Must Have A Hospital," DC, January 23, 1876, 2.

[30] "Hospital Propositions," DC, January 30, 1876, 2.

[31] "City Hospitals: How They are Managed in Memphis and Worcester," DC, February 20, 1876, 3; "Hospitals" DC, February 20, 1876, 2.

[32] "A City Hospital," DC, April 2, 1876, 2.

[33] "The Hospital: Report of the Committee Appointed to Consider the Expediency of Establishing a City Hospital with Instructions if thought Advisable to Report and Ordinance on the Subject," DC, May 3, 1876, 1.

[34] "A City Hospital," DC, April 2, 1876, 2; "A City Hospital," DC, April 30, 1876, 2.

[35] John H. Ellis, "Businessmen and Public Health in the Urban South During the Nineteenth Century: New Orleans, Memphis, and Atlanta, [part one]" *Bulletin of the History of Medicine* 44:3 (May-June 1970), 197-212; idem., "Businessmen and Public Health in the Urban South During the Nineteenth Century: New Orleans, Memphis, and Atlanta, [part two]" *Bulletin of the History of Medicine* 44:4 (July-August, 1970), 346-371; Stuart Galishoff, "Germs Know No Color Line: Black Health and Public Policy in Atlanta 1900-1918," *Journal of the History of Medicine and Allied Sciences* 40:1 (1985), 22-41, discusses the attempt of business leaders to keep Atlanta's salubrious reputation during the Progressive Era.

[36] Margaret Humphreys, *Yellow Fever and the South* (New Brunswick: Rutgers University Press, 1992); Khaled J. Bloom, *The Mississippi Valley's Great Yellow Fever Epidemic* (Baton Rouge: Louisiana State University Press, 1993); Molly Caldwell Crosby, *The American Plague: The Untold Story of Yellow Fever, The Epidemic That Shaped Our History* (New York: The Berkley Publishing Group, 2006).

[37] Ellis, "Businessmen and Public Health [part two]," 348.

[38] "The Atlanta Hospital," DC, October 30, 1878, 1. The *Daily Constitution* claimed, "the healthy air of Atlanta is much cheaper and more pleasant than nurses and medicine."

[39] Ellis, "Businessmen and Public Health [part one]; John H. Ellis, *Yellow Fever and Public Health in the New South* (Lexington: The University Press of Kentucky, 1992), 125-145, discusses Atlanta's campaign for sanitary sewers, improved drainage, and other public health improvements in the decade after the Yellow Fever Epidemic of 1878.

[40] Ellis, *Yellow Fever and Public Health,* 125-145. See also, for example, "The Sanitary Interests of Atlanta," DC, January 15, 1881, 2.

[41] Hopkins, "Public Health in Atlanta" suggests the epidemic's role in prompting sanitary reforms in the city. New sanitary services like night soil removal, however, remained restricted to the central city.

[42] James Michael Russell, *Atlanta 1847-1890: City Building in the Old South and New* (Baton Rouge: Louisiana State University Press, 1988), 204-205.

[43] Ibid., 200-201.

[44] Ellis, *Yellow Fever and Public Health in the New South*, 137-138. For discussion of the assessment system and tax policies in American cities during the nineteenth century, among others see Robin Einhorn, *Property Rules: Political Economy in Chicago, 1833-1872* (Chicago: University of Chicago Press, 1991).

[45] Ellis, *Yellow Fever and Public Health*, 162.

[46] James M. Russell, "Politics, Municipal Services, and the Working Class in Atlanta, 1865-1890," *Georgia Historical Quarterly* 46:4 (Winter 1982), 467-491.

[47] This is captured eloquently in Ronald H. Bayor, *Race and the Shaping of Twentieth-Century Atlanta* (Chapel Hill: University of North Carolina Press, 1996), 9, where he writes, "Inadequate sanitation arrangements, unpaved streets, poor water supplies, insufficient transportation lines and fire services, deficient public health care and schools, and lack of park space prevailed in black neighborhoods through the late nineteenth century and into the twentieth and became an issue only when whites were affected in some way."

[48] The new medical schools were the Southern Medical College (1878), the Reformed Medical College of Georgia (1881), and the Georgia College of Eclectic Medicine and Surgery (1883).

[49] During fifteen years in existence it treated approximately 4,700 patients.

[50] The terms of transfer also limited how many people could belong to the same religious group. The women of

50 the benevolent home specified, "under no contingency shall there ever be more than two of any one sect or denomination on the board at one time." "The Benevolent Home, Passes Into the Hands of a New Board of Trustees," AC, February 2, 1881, 4.

51 "The Benevolent Home, Its Change in Management Yesterday," AC, February 5, 1881, 3.

52 "The City Hospital," AC, March 3, 1881, 4; "Report of H. H. Tucker, President Atlanta Hospital and Benevolent Home," AC, February 12, 1882, 7; H. H. Tucker, "For Charity's Sake," AC, January 19, 1883, 7.

53 H. H. Tucker, "The Benevolent Home," AC, January 4, 1887, 3.

54 Franklin Garrett, *Atlanta and Environs, Volume 2: A Chronicle of Its People and Events, 1880s-1930s* (New York: Lewis Historical Publishing Company, Inc., 1954), 8-9.

55 On the city's financial support for Atlanta's hospitals, including Ivy Street, see "Mayor Hillyer's Veto," AC, March 17, 1885, 7. On Ivy Street Hospital, see also, "Visiting the Hospital," AC, August 9, 1884, 7; Thomas S. Powell, "The Ivy Street Hospital," AC, August 31, 1884, 9; "Southern Medical College and Ivy Street Hospital," advertisement AC, October 1, 1884, 37; T. S. Powell, "To The Good People of Atlanta," AC, July 13, 1885.

56 Founded by Sophia B. Packard and Harriet E. Giles, The Atlanta Baptist Female Seminary opened its doors on April 11, 1881, in the basement of the Friendship Baptist Church. From the start it relied on financial support from northern donors. The school benefited greatly from the oil magnate John D. Rockefeller. He became an important financial supporter of the school after hearing an appeal for funds while attending church in Cleveland, Ohio. After visiting the school in 1884 with his family, he paid off the land mortgage and gave extra funds for new facilities. The school's name was then changed to Spelman Seminary in honor of Mrs. Lucy Spelman, Mr. Rockefeller's mother-in-law. The school changed its name to Spelman College in 1924.

57 "Franklin Hospital, Ground Purchased and an Organization to be Effected," AC, November 12, 1887, 4.

58 "Trained Nurses, Splendid Exhibition of Skill by Pupils from Spelman Seminary," AC, January 19, 1888, 8.

59 "The City's Sick," AC, July 17, 1888, 8.

60 City of Atlanta Records, Atlanta City Council Minutes, volume 11, page 602, July 16, 1888, AHC.

61 "The Proposed Hospital," AC, June 22, 1888, 7.

62 "King's Daughters, "The Origin of the Order and its Growth," AC, July 8, 1888, 4.

63 "King's Daughters Hospital, It Opens Today," AC, August 1, 1888, 8. Built only six years earlier at Pryor and Houston Streets, St. Luke's was Bishop Beckwith's cathedral until the early 1890s when the seat returned to St. Philips.

64 Ibid.; "The New Hospital Opens," AC, August 2, 1888, 7.

65 "A City Hospital, A Meeting," AC, February 16, 1888, 7; "For a City Hospital," AC, February 17, 1888, 5.

66 "Report of Relief Committee," *Annual Report of the Officers of the City of Atlanta for the year ending December 31, 1888, showing the condition of municipal affairs* (Atlanta: W. H. Scott, Book and Job Printers, 1889), 40.

67 "For a City Hospital," AC, February 17, 1888, 5.

68 "The Hospital Question," AC, March 4, 1888, 14.

69 Ibid.

70 "For a City Hospital," AC, February 17, 1888, 5.

71 "The Hospital Question," AC, March 4, 1888, 14.

72 "For a City Hospital," AC, February 17, 1888, 5.

73 Ibid.

74 "The New Hospital, What the Committee Proposes to Do In the Matter," AC, July 17, 1888, 8.

75 "Report of Relief Committee," *Annual Report of the Officers of the City of Atlanta for the year ending December 31, 1888, showing the condition of municipal affairs* (Atlanta: W. H. Scott, Book and Job Printers, 1889), 41-44; "A City Hospital, The Doctors Still Working on One," AC, December 24, 1888, 4.

76 "Report of Relief Committee," *Annual Report of the Officers of the City of Atlanta for the year ending December 31, 1889, showing the condition of municipal affairs* (Atlanta: W. H. Scott, Book and Job Printers, 1890), 34.

77 The social background of Atlanta's business leaders in the late nineteenth century is explored in James Michael Russell, *Atlanta 1847-1890: City Building in the Old South and New* (Baton Rouge: Louisiana State University Press, 1988), 146-168.

78 Stephen Hertzberg, "The Jews of Atlanta, 1865-1915," (Ph.D. dissertation, University of Chicago, 1975), 280.

Chapter 2

1 This chapter is indebted to two helpful biographies of Henry Grady. Harold E. Davis, *Henry Grady's New South: Atlanta, A Brave Beautiful City* (Tuscaloosa: University of Alabama Press, 1990) interprets Grady's life in the context of Atlanta's development. Raymond B. Nixon, *Henry W. Grady: Spokesman of the New South* (New York: Russell and Russell, 1943) remains valuable.

2 The ideas are explored in Paul M. Gaston, *The New South Creed: A Study in Southern Mythmaking* (New York: Alfred A. Knopf, 1970).

3 The scholarly literature on the New South is vast. C. Vann Woodward, *Origins of the New South, 1877-1913* (Baton Rouge: Louisiana State University Press, The Littlefield Fund for Southern History of the University of Texas, 1951) has been so influential that it earned its own birthday book fifty years after its debut: John B. Boles and Bethany L. Johnson, eds., *Origins of the New South Fifty Years Later: Continuing Influence of a Historical Classic* (Baton Rouge: Louisiana State University Press, 2003). Another rich and rewarding interpretation of the New South is Edward L. Ayers, *The Promise of the New South: Life After Reconstruction* (New York: Oxford University Press, 1992). For Atlanta, an important comparative study is Don H. Doyle, *New Men, New Cities, New South: Atlanta, Nashville, Charleston, Mobile, 1860-1910* (Chapel Hill: University of North Carolina Press, 1990).

[4] Sylvia Gailey Head and Elizabeth W. Etheridge, *The Neighborhood Mint: Dahlonega in the Age of Jackson* (Macon: Mercer University Press, 1986).

[5] H. David Williams, "Gambling Away the Inheritance: The Cherokee Nation and Georgia's Gold and Land Lotteries of 1832-33," *The Georgia Historical Quarterly* 73:3 (Fall 1989), 519-539.

[6] For interpretations of crucial events, see the essays in *The Georgia Historical Quarterly* 73:3 (Fall 1989) *a Special Issue Commemorating the Sesquicentennial of Cherokee Removal 1838-1839.* Also see Michael Morris, "Georgia and the Conversation Over Indian Removal," *The Georgia Historical Quarterly* 91:4 (Winter 2007), 403-423.

[7] Frank Luther Mott, *American Journalism, A History, 1690-1960* (New York: MacMillan, 1961), 454.

[8] The seventeenth amendment to the United States Constitution, ratified on May 31, 1913, provided for the direct election of senators, taking the power away from state legislatures.

[9] Woodward, *Origins of the New South*, 147.

[10] Ayers, *The Promise of the New South*, 87.

[11] J. F. Stover, *The Railroads of the South, 1865-1900: A Study in Finance and Control* (Chapel Hill: University of North Carolina Press, 1955). See also, Ron Chernow, *The House of Morgan: An American Banking Dynasty and the Rise of Modern Finance* (New York: Simon & Schuster, 1990).

[12] Henry Woodfin Grady, *The Complete Orations and Speeches of Henry W. Grady*, edited by Edwin DuBois Shurter (New York: Hinds, Noble & Eldredge, 1910), 7.

[13] Ibid., 14.

[14] Ibid., 221-232.

[15] Homeopathy was based on a theory of Dr. Samuel Hahnemann of Germany that a drug which produces certain symptoms in a normal person will cure a sick person with the same symptoms.

Chapter 3

[1] "To Grady's Memory, The Work of Erecting a Monument in Atlanta," AC, December 26, 1889, 4; "Chamber of Commerce, A Memorial Meeting Yesterday in Honor of Mr. Grady," AC, December 26, 1889, 1; "Christmas in Atlanta," AC, December 26, 1889, 5; George T. G. White, "The Grady Monument," AC, December 27, 1889, 1.

[2] "The Young Men at Work, Mr. Moore Makes a Suggestion," AC, January 3, 1890, 4.

[3] Ibid.

[4] "Report of Relief Committee," *Annual Report of the Officers of the City of Atlanta for the year ending December 31, 1888, showing the condition of municipal affairs* (Atlanta: W. H. Scott, Book and Job Printers, 1889), 40.

[5] "A City Hospital," AC, February 17, 1888, 4; "A City Hospital Needed," AC, January 6, 1889, 12; "A City Hospital," AC, January 23, 1889, 4.

[6] "H. W. Grady Hospital, The Special Committee of Five has a Meeting," AC, January 9, 1890, 2; "The Grady Hospital," AC, January 21, 1890, 8; "The City Council," AC, February 4, 1890, 1.

[7] "A Free City Hospital," AC, January 6, 1890, 4; "Mayor Glenn's Message," AC, January 7, 1890, 4; "A Hospital for Atlanta," AC, January 9, 1890, 4; "H. W. Grady Hospital," AC, January 9, 1890, 2.

[8] "It Will Be Built, The H. W. Grady Hospital an Assured Fact," AC, January 12, 1890, 23.

[9] "For the Afflicted," AC, February 6, 1890, 3.

[10] The $22,207 that W. A. Moore reportedly paid for the property at auction was about double what Joseph Hirsch had expected from the sale of the property. "Real Estate Sales," AC, May 21, 1890, 6.

[11] "For the Hospital," AC, February 14, 1890, 4.

[12] "The Grady Hospital, Contract for its Building was Made Yesterday," AC, October 22, 1890, 7; "The Grady Hospital, Contract for the Building Awarded Yesterday," AC, November 11, 1890, 1.

[13] This was apparently $5,000 below market value for the land. "The Grady Hospital, The Site Agreed Upon" AC, April 10, 1890, 4; "The Grady Hospital [editorial]," AC, April 10, 1890, 4. A little later the hospital would purchase the rest of the property on that block, raising the total cost for land acquisition to $16,000.

[14] "The Grady Hospital," *AC*, April 26, 1890, 14.

[15] Ibid.

[16] Ibid.

[17] "For the Afflicted," AC, February 6, 1890, 3. In February, the Grady hospital committee appeared to lean toward building separate hospitals for white and black citizens that probably would be located in different parts of the city.

[18] Ibid.

[19] Ibid.

[20] Ibid.

[21] Ibid.

[22] "Three Thousand Dollars," AC, September 22, 1890, 7.

[23] "The Grady Hospital," AC, November 2, 1890, 18.

[24] "Letters from the People," AC, November 7, 1890, 9.

[25] Among the other items placed inside the cornerstone during the ceremony were five Confederate $100 bank notes, two copies of the *Atlanta Constitution*, a copy of the city codes, and a photograph of the flowers that were laid on Henry Grady's casket. "The Corner Stone," AC, December 23, 1890, 2; "The Name of Grady," AC, December 24, 1890, 5. On the fascinating development of public ceremonies and rituals associated with the construction of American buildings, from groundbreaking to demolition, see Neil Harris, *Building Lives: Constructing Rites and Passages* (New Haven: Yale University Press, 1999), especially pages 19-31 for a discussion of cornerstone laying and the insertion of relics in cornerstones.

[26] A close friend of Henry Grady, Mr. Calhoun was the grandson of John C. Calhoun, the former Vice President, Secretary of War, and U.S. Senator.

[27] "The Name of Grady," AC, December 24, 1890, 5.

[28] For notices of relatively large gifts, see "The Hebrews and the Grady Hospital," AC, March 6, 1891, 4; "The Grady Hospital," AC, March 8, 1891, 22; "The Fund Still Grows," AC, March 11, 1891, 2.

[29] "Now All Together," AC, May 14, 1891, 5.

[30] On attempts raise funds from residents throughout the city, see "The Grady Hospital, The Work is Already Far Advanced," AC, March 1, 15; "The Grady Hospital," AC, March 1, 1891, 16; "The Grady Hospital," AC, April 9, 1891, 12. On the work stoppage when money ran out at the end of April 1890, see "Contractors Strike," AC, May 6, 1891, 5. On the struggle to raise money once the work stopped see "Atlanta and the Grady Hospital," AC, May 8, 1891, 4; "The Grady Hospital," AC, May 9, 1891, 1; "How to Complete the Hospital," AC, May 14, 1891, 4; "Now, All Together," AC, May 14, 1891, 5.

[31] "Raising Money," AC, November 24, 1891, 5; "For the Hospital," AC, March 10, 1892, 5.

[32] "Now All Together," AC, May 14, 1891, 5.

[33] "The Veto Stands," AC, October 6, 1891, 5; "Will Be Finished," AC, October 8, 1891, 5; "The City Council," AC, February 2, 1892, 1.

[34] Joseph Hirsch, "A Church's Good Work, The Church of the Redeemer Sends a Check To Grady Hospital," AC, May 4, 1892, 7; "It's the City's Now," AC, May 26, 1892, 5.

[35] "Engineers Leave," AC, May 29, 1892, 16; "A Fat Man's Game of Baseball," AC, May 31, 1892, 6.

[36] "For the Hospital," AC, March 11, 1892, 2. The members appointed by the Board of Trustees included Drs. James F. Alexander, J. S. Todd, Henry Bak, C. G. Giddings, R. B. Ridley, W. S. Kendrick, J. G. Earnest, Hunter P. Cooper, William S. Elkin, William P. Nicolson, W. S. Armstrong, Abner W. Calhoun, A. G. Hobbs, Virgil O. Hardin, and George H. Noble.

[37] "The Medical Board," AC, March 12, 1892, 5; "In the City Hall," AC, March 18, 1892, 7.

[38] Garrett, *Atlanta and Environs*, Volume 1, 808.

[39] Clifford M. Kuhn, *Contesting the New South Order: the 1914-1915 Strike at Atlanta's Fulton Mills* (Chapel Hill: The University of North Carolina Press, 2001), 8-11.

[40] Ibid., 10-11.

[41] Ibid., 15; Garrett, *Atlanta and Environs*, Volume 2, 170. On the links between Georgia Tech and New South ideology, see James E. Brittain and Robert C. McMath, "Engineers and the New South Creed: The Formation and Early Development of Georgia Tech," *Technology and Culture* 18:2 (April 1977), 175-201.

[42] The first settlement house in Atlanta, it was originally called the Methodist Home Settlement. The name was changed to Wesley House in 1906.

[43] For an overview of Methodist settlement houses in the South, see John R. Nelson, *Home Mission Fields of the Methodist Episcopal Church, South* ([Nashville]: Home Missions Department, Methodist Episcopal Church, South, 1909). Sarah Sloan Kreutziger, "Wesley's Legacy of Social Holiness: The Methodist Settlement Movement and American Social Reform," in Russell E. Richey, Dennis M. Campbell, and William B. Lawrence, eds., *Connectionalism: Ecclesiology, Mission, and Identity, United Methodism and American Culture* Volume 1 (New York: Abingdon Press, 1997), 137-175.

[44] Discussion of the strike is indebted to Kuhn, *Contesting the New South Order*, and Gary M. Fink, *The Fulton Bag and Cotton Mills Strike of 1914-1915: Espionage, Labor Conflict, and New South Industrial Relations* (Ithaca: ILR Press, 1993).

[45] Testimony of Emma Burton, U.S. Commission on Industrial Relations, EB 23, Fulton Bag and Cotton Mills Records 1897-1941, Box 8, Folder 33, Georgia Institute of Technology.

Chapter 4

[1] Now known as Georgia Hall, the building has undergone several minor modifications over the years.

[2] *The American Architect and Building News* 31:792 (February 28, 1891), 141.

[3] "Report of the Relief Committee," in *Annual Reports of the Committees of the Council, Officers and Departments of the City of Atlanta for the Year ending December 31, 1892* (Atlanta: Constitution Publishing Co., 1893), 55-56.

[4] Notably, during the nineteenth century it was the only medical school in Georgia that accepted women as students. One of them, Ms. Rosa Freudenthal, became Atlanta's first female medical graduate. The confusing sequence of names, movements, and merger in the Eclectic hospital's first half-century is summarized in Charles Edgeworth Jones, *Education in Georgia* (Washington D.C.: Government Printing Office, 1889), 127-128.

[5] "The Eclectic College," AC, March 13, 1892, 16; "From Our Notebooks," AC, March 16, 1892, 4; "In the City Hall," AC, March 18, 1892, 7; "Before the Council," AC, March 20, 1892, 23.

[6] The merger set the stage for a group of other doctors to establish yet another medical school, the new Atlanta School of Medicine (ASM), in 1905.

[7] Steven C. Wheatley, *The Politics of Philanthropy: Abraham Flexner and Medical Education* (Madison: University of Wisconsin Press, 1989) expertly analyzes Flexner's impact on medical education through the report for the Carnegie Foundation and during his later career with the Rockefeller foundations. Thomas Neville Bonner, *Iconoclast: Abraham Flexner and a Life in Learning* (Baltimore: Johns Hopkins University Press, 2002) is an outstanding study of Flexner's life and the major themes in his work.

[8] Abraham Flexner, *Medical Education in the United States and Canada* Bulletin No. 4 (New York: Carnegie Foundation for the Advancement of Teaching, 1910), 205.

[9] Ibid., 36.

[10] Ibid., 204.

[11] Ibid., 36-37.

[12] Ibid., 205.

[13] Ibid., 206-207.

[14] John S. Candler to W. B. Summerall, September 8, 1913, GMHC, AHC; Minutes, GMH Board of Trustees, August 26, 1913, GMHC, AHC; Minutes, Special Meeting GMH Board of Trustees, September 12, 1913, GMHC, AHC; Jno. W. White, et. al., to Board of Trustees of the Grady Hospital, September 25, 1913, GMHC, AHC; Minutes, GMH Board of Trustees, January 27, 1914, GMHC, AHC.

[15] Vanderbilt's story is elegantly summarized in George M. Marsden, *The Soul of the American University: From Protestant Establishment to Established Nonbelief* (New York: Oxford University Press, 1994), 276-280. A discussion of Vanderbilt's transition to independent status is in Paul Conkin, *Gone With The Ivy: A Biography of Vanderbilt University* (Knoxville: University of Tennessee Press, 1985). The history of Emory University's origins is told in Henry Morton Bullock, *A History of Emory University* (Nashville: Parthenon Press, 1936) and in Thomas H. English, *Emory University, 1915-1965, A Semi-centennial History* (Atlanta: Emory University Press, 1966).

[16] "It Opens Today," AC, June 2, 1892, 2.

[17] "Another Month," AC, November 30, 1892, 7.

[18] "With the New Year," AC, January 1, 1893, 19.

[19] "Dr. Kenan Resigns," AC, February 8, 1893, 7.

[20] "Dr. Kenan's Report," AC, February 11, 1893, 7; "A Clean Sweep," AC, March 1, 1893, 9.

[21] "The Grady Hospital," AC, January 3, 1894, 10.

[22] "He Wanted Trustees to Resign in a Body," AC, August 6, 1903, 1.

[23] "Pay Department May Have to Go," AC, September 6, 1903, B7; "Will Discuss the Hospital," AC, September 7, 1903, 7.

[24] "Would Lease the Hospital," AC, September 29, 1903, 4.

[25] The funding for Grady was only ten percent higher in 1903 than it had been eight years earlier when Joseph Hirsch threatened to close down the hospital unless the city increased funding for the institution.

[26] In 1900, Grady treated a total of 2,370 patients, of whom 234 were paying patients (212 white, 22 black). The average daily occupancy of the hospital was 79 (the building had 110 beds, 100 of which were designated for charity patients). The hospital's total expense that year was $32,965.40, but it generated $4,589.52 from paying patients, money that went directly to the city's treasury. Thus, the net cost to taxpayers came to $28,375.88 (a daily cost of $1.13 per patient). This cost, however, also included the expenses associated with the training school for nurses and the ambulance service's 2,140 runs.

[27] "Did Not Set Fracture," AC, August 12, 1903, 6; "Failed to Set Fractured Arm," AC, August 13, 1903, 3; "The Grady Hospital Service," AC, August 14, 1903, 6; "McWhirter Writes a Card," AC, September 3, 1903, 7.

[28] "The Grady Hospital Service," AC, August 14, 1903, 6.

[29] "Nurses in a Revolt Quit Grady Hospital," AC, March 8, 1905, 1; "The Grady Hospital Service," AC, March 8, 1905, 1.

[30] "Some Aftermath of Hospital Row," AC, March 14, 1905, A1.

[31] "Nurses Dismissed; Head Nurse Resigns," AC, March 9, 1905, 7.

[32] "Dr. Andrews Resigns; Nurses Back at Work," AC, March 11, 1905, 3.

[33] "Some Aftermath of Hospital Row," AC, March 14, 1905, A1.

[34] "Why the Nurses Were Dismissed," AC, March 9, 1905, 7.

[35] "Eskridge Now Says Another Wrote Card," AC, March 10, 1905, 1; "Dr. Andrews Resigns; Nurses Back at Work," AC, March 11, 1905, 3.

[36] "Doctors Dismissed; Resignations Held," AC, March 12, 1905, C1; "Hospital Quiet Following Storm," AC, March 13, 1905, 7.

[37] Smallpox vaccination was developed by Dr. Edward Jenner, a British physician, in 1796 using cowpox as a way to prevent smallpox. It was not unusual for 30% of smallpox victims to die during severe epidemics. After successful world-wide immunization programs, the World Health Organization in 1980 declared the world was free from this infectious agent.

[38] "New Grady Hospital Ranks With The Best in Country," AC, January 21, 1912, B5.

[39] Ibid.

[40] Ibid.

[41] Minutes, Special Meeting Board of Trustees, Grady Hospital, Friday, November 1, 1912, GMHC, AHC.

[42] "Atlanta Must Have Greater Grady Hospital If She Expects to Keep Up With the Progress of Other Twentieth Century Municipalities," AC, April 19, 1914, A4.

[43] Ibid.

[44] Ibid.

[45] "Bonds for Grady Favored by Labor," AC, August 15, 1915, 4.

[46] "Atlanta Must Have Greater Grady Hospital If She Expects to Keep Up With the Progress of Other Twentieth Century Municipalities," AC, April 19, 1914, A4.

[47] Ibid.

[48] "Million Dollar Medical Endowment Hinges on Greater Grady Hospital," AC, April 19, 1914, 1.

[49] "Preachers to Aid Grady Bond Issue," AC, April 30, 1914, 4.

[50] "Grady Bonds Receive Big Vote But Lose," AC, May 6, 1914, 1.

[51] Robert L. Foreman to F. J. Paxon, January 17, 1915, GMHC, AHC.

[52] "Atlanta's Best Institution: That is the Expression of the Atlanta Federation of Trades Concerning the Grady Hospital," *The Journal of Labor* 16:46 (August 13, 1915), 1.

[53] Ibid., 2.

[54] Ibid.

[55] Ibid.

[56] "Annual Report for 1916, Grady Memorial Hospital," 16.

[57] "Atlanta Scorched for Indifference to Grady Hospital," AC, December 30, 1916, 1.

[58] Douglas A. Blackmon, *Slavery by Another Name: The Re-enslavement of Black Americans from the Civil War to World War II* (New York: Doubleday, 2008), 338-346 discusses James English and the Chattahoochee Brick Company.

[59] "Council to Attend Funeral of Hirsch," AC, August 23, 1914, 13.

[60] Minutes, Medical Board of Grady Memorial Hospital, August 22, 1914, GMHC, AHC.

[61] "Preamble and Resolutions Passed by the Board of Trustees of Grady Hospital on the death of Honorable Joseph Hirsch," GMHC, AHC.

[62] "Sam Inman, 'Atlanta's First Citizen,' Dies," AC, January 13, 1915, 1; "Tributes Are Paid Memory of Inman," AC, January 14, 1915, 5; W. B. Candler, "A Tribute to S. M. Inman," AC, January 14, 1915, 4.

[63] R. O. Cotter, "A Report on the Progress of Ophthalmology and Rhinology," *Transactions of the Medical Association of Georgia* 41 (Macon: Medical Association of Georgia, 1890), 102; A. W. Calhoun, "Some Observations Upon Cataract Operations and After Treatment," *Transactions of the Medical Association of Georgia* 43 (Macon: Medical Association of Georgia, 1892), 259-269.

[64] Garrett, *Atlanta and Environs*, Volume 2, 429; Dr. Amos Fox and W. H. Harrison, "Dr. A. W. Calhoun, Noted Physician, Called by Death," AC, August 22, 1910, 1; "Abner W. Calhoun," AC, August 22, 1910, 4.

[65] In January 1987, the Calhoun Library together with the dental and nursing school libraries were incorporated into the library of the Woodruff Health Center. A conference room in the new center is dedicated to the memory of Abner W. Calhoun.

[66] Today, a marble bust of Dr. Noble stands in Atlanta's Academy of Medicine, next to a portrait of Dr. Abner Calhoun.

[67] "Annual Report of Wesley Memorial Hospital, April 16, 1928 to April 15, 1929," 1928-1929 ROAO, 146, MARBL.

[68] "The Grady Hospital Atlanta, Georgia: Training School for Nurses," pamphlet, GMHC, AHC.

[69] *Annual Reports of the Committees of Council, Officers and Departments of the City of Atlanta for the year ending December 31, 1904, Showing the Condition of Municipal Affairs* (Atlanta: The Byrd Printing Company, [1905]) 335.

[70] *Annual Reports of the Committees of Council, Officers and Departments of the City of Atlanta for the year ending December 31, 1899, Showing the Condition of Municipal Affairs* (Atlanta: Pease Printing Co., [1900]), 278.

[71] Minutes, GMH Board of Trustees, October 7, 1909, GMHC, AHC.

[72] Minutes, GMH Board of Trustees, February 22, 1910, GMHC, AHC; W. B. Summerall to GMH Board of Trustees, April 26, 1910, GMHC, AHC.

[73] "Special Communication No. 5 Series 1911," January 31, 1911, GMHC, AHC; Minutes, Annual Meeting of the Board of Trustees of the Grady Hospital, January 31, 1911, GMHC, AHC.

[74] Minutes, Special Meeting of [the] Board of Trustees of Grady Hospital, April 14, 1911, GMHC, AHC.

[75] "Statement for the Month of September 1911, The Grady Hospital" GMHC, AHC; Minutes, GMH Board of Trustees, September 26, 1911, GMHC, AHC.

[76] "Train Crashes Into Grady Ambulance Bearing Patient," AC, October 12, 1911, 10; W. B. Summerall to GMH Board of Trustees, October 31, 1911, GMHC, AHC.

[77] "The Ladies Meet," AC, July 21, 1894, 5; "To Aid the Hospital," AC, September 8, 1894, 8.

[78] "Money to Be Raised," AC, August 4, 1894, 8.

[79] "City Accepts the Children's Ward," AC, May 30, 1897, 12.

[80] "Woman and Society, Children's Ward Completed," AC, May 27, 1897, 9.

[81] "Woman and Society," AC, July 22, 1897, 6.

[82] Ibid.

[83] "Women Here and There," *The New York Times*, February 13, 1898, 16.

[84] "Women and Society," AC, March 3, 1897, 3; Mrs. Thaddeus Horton, "An Order of Old-Fashioned Women," *The Ladies' Home Journal* 42:8 (July 1906), 5-6, 38; "Women Here and There," *The New York Times*, February 13, 1898, 16.

[85] "For a Maternity Ward," AC, September 18, 1902, 8; "Bazaar Proves a Success," AC, December 3, 1902, 7; "Old-Fashioned Women," AC, November 6, 1903, 8; "Old-Fashioned Women," AC, April 24, 1904, B2; "Christening of New Ward," AC, June 23, 1904, 5.

[86] "Woman and Society, In the Interest of Grady Hospital," AC, August 10, 1897, 9.

[87] C. A. Smith, "Report of a Case of Ankylostomiasis," *American Medicine* 3:25 (June 21, 1902), 1062.

[88] The hookworm penetrates the skin after a person makes contact with contaminated soil. Usually it enters between a person's toes, leaving barefoot southerners walking outside susceptible to the parasite. The worms move their way through the body, eventually lodging in a person's intestinal lining. From there they attack the body, often living as long as five years. The female can lay up to 10,000 eggs per day, putting them right into the small intestine. The body then emits them with the feces. Thus, improved privy sanitation became extremely important in preventing the spread of hookworm infection. (Getting people to wear shoes while outdoors proved to be another extremely important means of hookworm prevention.) A severely infected individual can lose 200 cc. of blood per day, creating severe anemia.

[89] Alan I. Marcus, "The South's Native Foreigners: Hookworm as a Factor in Southern Distinctiveness," in Todd L. Savitt and James Harvey Young, eds., *Disease and Distinctiveness in the American South* (Knoxville: University of Tennessee Press, 1988), 79-99.

[90] C. A. Smith, "Uncinariasis or Hook-worm Disease in Georgia," *Transactions of the Medical Association of*

Georgia (Atlanta: Medical Association of Georgia, 1904), 171-187; idem., "Uncinariasis in the South: Further Observation," *Transactions of the Section on Pathology and Physiology of the American Medical Association at the Fifty-Fourth Annual Session Held at New Orleans* (Chicago: Press of American Medical Association, 1904), 135-149; idem., "Uncinariasis in the South, with special reference to mode of infection," JAMA 43:9 (August 27, 1904), 592-597.

[91] John Ettling, *The Germ of Laziness: Rockefeller Philanthropy and Public Health in the New South* (Cambridge, Mass.: Harvard University Press, 1981), 34-35.

[92] Ibid., 37-38.

[93] Alan I. Marcus, "Physicians Open a Can of Worms: American Nationality and Hookworm in the United States," *American Studies* 30:2 (Fall 1989), 103-121; on Smith's research on ground itch, see especially pages 113-114.

[94] Minutes of the Medical Staff of Grady Hospital, Meeting of Colored Unit Medical Staff, March 21, 1922, GMHC, AHC.

[95] The distinction was used in early debates about the creation of a public hospital for Atlanta. See, for example, "A City Hospital," AC, April 2, 1876, 2; "A City Hospital," AC, April 30, 1876, 2.

[96] "Draws His Probe for the Hospital," AC, August 28, 1897, 7.

[97] Ibid.

[98] "Neglect of Duty Charged to Grady Hospital," AC, January 30, 1907, 1.

[99] "Doctors at Outs About Hospital," AC, December 27, 1907, 4; "Are Colleges Behind Row?" AC, December 28, 1907, 3; "Says its College Against College," AC, December 29, 1907, 9; "The Hospital and Medical Colleges," AC, December 29, 1907, 9; "Hospital Row Still Goes On," AC, December 31, 1907, 3.

[100] On December 26, 1907.

[101] The discussion of the Atlanta Race Riot, a crucial event in shaping race relations in the city for generations, is informed by the interpretations of David Fort Godschalk, *Veiled Visions: The 1906 Atlanta Race Riot and the Reshaping of American Race Relations* (Chapel Hill: University of North Carolina Press, 2005) and Rebecca Burns, *Rage in the Gate City: The Story of the 1906 Atlanta Race Riot* (Cincinnati: Emmis Books, 2006). Allison Dorsey, *To Build Our Lives Together: Community Formation in Black Atlanta, 1875-1906* (Athens: University of Georgia Press, 2004) skillfully interprets Atlanta's African American communities in the decades before the race riot and offers a helpful understanding of the riot's roots and aftermath.

[102] C. Vann Woodward, *Tom Watson: Agrarian Rebel* (New York: Oxford University Press, 1963); Russell Korobkin, "The Politics of Disfranchisement in Georgia," *The Georgia Historical Quarterly* 74:1 (Spring 1990), 20-58. Data on black voter turnout in the south during the era is discussed in J. Morgan Kousser, *The Shaping of Southern Politics: Suffrage Restriction and the Shaping of the One-Party South, 1880-1910* (New Haven: Yale University Press, 1974). Also see Peter H. Argersinger, "The Southern Search for Order," *Reviews in American History* 3:2 (June 1975), 236-241.

[103] Cited in Dewey W. Grantham, Jr., "Georgia Politics and the Disfranchisement of the Negro," *The Georgia Historical Quarterly* 32:1 (March 1948), 7.

[104] Cited in Gregory Mixon, *The Atlanta Riot: Race, Class, and Violence in a New South City* (Gainesville: University Press of Florida, 2005), 1.

[105] Charles Crowe, "Racial Massacre in Atlanta September 22, 1906," *The Journal of Negro History* 54:2 (April 1969), 150-173, (the quotation is from page 153).

[106] Ibid., 162.

[107] Patricia D'Antonio, *American Nursing: A History of Knowledge, Authority, and the Meaning of Work* (Baltimore: The Johns Hopkins University Press, 2010), 111-113; Minutes, Medical Board of GMH, December 9, 1913, GMHC, AHC. The history of nursing in Georgia is difficult to understand without becoming indebted to the work of Carla M. Schissel.

[108] Minutes, Executive Committee, Grady Hospital White Unit, October 11, 1927, GMHC, AHC.

[109] Ibid.

[110] For an excellent analysis of black and white nursing at Grady, see D'Antonio, 106-130. The figure of $200 is from Sylvia Thomas, "Nurses Section," *Journal of the National Medical Association* 12:4 (October-December 1920), 71.

[111] Minutes, Grady Hospital Medical Board, May 13, 1920, GMHC, AHC.

[112] Steven Johnston to the GMH Board of Trustees, November 29, 1920, GMHC, AHC.

[113] [Joel Chandler Harris, ed.,] *History of the Emory Unit: Base Hospital 43, US Army Expeditionary Forces* (Atlanta: n.p., 1919).

[114] Ibid.

[115] Charles Pelot Summerall, *The Way of Duty, Honor, Country: The Memoir of General Charles Pelot Summerall*, edited and annotated by Timothy K. Nenninger (Lexington: The University Press of Kentucky, 2010).

[116] Carey Olmstead Shellman, "'One of the Lord's Democrats': Nellie Peters Black and the Practical Application of the Social Gospel in the New South, 1870-1919" (Ph.D. dissertation, University of Florida), 2007.

[117] "Over Fifty Blocks Destroyed By Flames, Fire Damage is Estimated At $5,000,000," AC, May 22, 1917, 1.

Chapter 5

[1] Eleanor Boykin, "Grady Hospital–Crippled for Lack of Funds," AC, February 9, 1919, D-3.

[2] "Grady Hospital $150,000 Drive Will Begin Soon," AC August 31, 1919, 1; "Medical Board Pleads for Grady," AC, September 11, 1919, 11; "Grady Hospital Calls Urgently For Help," September 21, 1919, 5.

[3] William Summerall to the Board of Trustees, Grady Hospital, May 31, 1910, GMHC, AHC.

[4] Minutes, GMH Board of Trustees, September 30, 1913, GMHC, AHC; Minutes, GMH Board of Trustees, October 28, 1913, GMHC, AHC; "Agreement Between Board of Trustees: Grady Hospital, and the Collegiate Members of the

Staff of the Grady Hospital: Atlanta" GMHC, AHC; Minutes, GMH Board of Trustees, November 25, 1913, GMHC, AHC.

[5] "That portion of the Medical Staff of Grady Hospital which is chosen from the city at large" to Board of Trustees of Grady Hospital in Minutes, GMH Board of Trustees, November, 1915, GMHC, AHC.

[6] Minutes, GMH Board of Trustees, February 24, 1914, GMHC, AHC. See also, D'Antonio, *American Nursing*, 113-115, and Darlene Clark Hine, *Black Women in White: Racial Conflict and Cooperation in the Nursing Profession, 1890-1950* (Bloomington: Indiana University Press, 1989).

[7] Minutes, GMH Board of Trustees, February 24, 1914, GMHC, AHC; Minutes, GMH Board of Trustees, November 24, 1914, GMHC, AHC.

[8] Darlene Clark Hine, "The Ethel Johns Report: Black Women in the Nursing Profession, 1925," *The Journal of Negro History* 67:3 (Autumn 1982), 212-228.

[9] Ethel Johns, "A Study of the Present Status of the Negro Woman in Nursing, 1925," cited in ibid., 215.

[10] Hine, "The Ethel Johns Report," 220-221.

[11] Ibid., 216.

[12] Ibid., 213.

[13] Ethel Johns, "A Study of the Present Status of the Negro Woman in Nursing, 1925," in ibid., 213.

[14] Eleanor Boykin, "Grady Hospital–Crippled For Lack of Funds," AC, February 9, 1919, D-3.

[15] Minutes, GMH Board of Trustees, December 27, 1910, GMHC, AHC; Committee on Hospital and Charities, Atlanta City Council, Annual Report, January 1, 1912, typescript, GMHC, AHC.

[16] Minutes, GMH Board of Trustees, September 24, 1912, GMHC, AHC; "Program of Competition for Nurses' Dormitory for Grady hospital, Atlanta, Georgia," GMHC, AHC.

[17] Minutes, Building Committee, Nurses Dormitory, GMH, February 25, 1913, GMHC, AHC; Minutes, Building Committee, Nurses Dormitory, GMH, April 1, 1913, GMHC, AHC.

[18] J. M. Hirsch, "Time to Act!" AC, September 9, 1914, 6; "Atlanta Scorched for Indifference to Grady Hospital," AC, December 30, 1916, 1.

[19] "Finances of City in Splendid Shape," AC, January 2, 1919, 1; "Committee Cuts Sum of $350,000 Off City Budget," AC, May 1919, 1; "Expenses of City Cut to the Bone to Meet Revenue," AC, May 6, 1919, 1.

[20] "Work on New Home For Grady Nurses Stopped; No Money," AC, July 16, 1919, 4.

[21] "Sum is Refused for Completion of Nurses' Home," AC, August 9, 1919, 9; "County Refuses Help for Grady New Dormitory," AC, August 31, 1919, 14.

[22] Eleanor Boykin, "Grady Hospital–Crippled for Lack of Funds," AC, February 9, 1919, D3, referred to the area immediately adjacent to the white nurses dormitory as "Darktown."

[23] "Asks Protection for Grady Nurses," AC, August 13, 1919, 4.

[24] Ibid. (This was the Reverend Ham's description of the nearby brothels.)

[25] Ibid.

[26] Isma Dooly, "Women Renew Pledges to Grady Hospital," AC, August 27, 1919, 11.

[27] Martha Giltner to Steve Johnston, July 5, 1919, GMHC, AHC.

[28] Garnett W. Quillian to Steve Johnston, May 24, 1919, GMHC, AHC.

[29] Ibid.

[30] "Grady Hospital $150,000 Drive Will Begin Soon," AC, August 31, 1919, 1.

[31] On Creel, among others see, Gregg Wolper, "The Origins of Public Diplomacy: Woodrow Wilson, George Creel, and the Committee on Public Information," (Ph.D. dissertation, University of Chicago, 1991).

[32] "J. R. Smith Will Direct Drive for Funds for Grady Hospital," AC, September 14, 1919, 11; "Drive for Grady to Open September 29," AC, September 19, 1919, 17; "Doctors Indorse Grady Campaign," AC, September 5, 1919, 1; "Women Will Aid Grady Campaign," AC, September 8, 1919, 5; "Grady Campaign Given Approval," AC, September 13, 1919, 7; "Council Indorses Grady Campaign," AC, September 16, 1919, 15; "Pastors Approve Grady Campaign," AC, September 17, 1919, 18.

[33] "Grady Campaign Depends on Tax," AC, September 29, 1919, 5; "Action on Emergency Tax By Council is Postponed Following Bitter Battle," AC, September 30, 1919, 1; "Proposed Public Campaign For Funds For Grady Called Off by Committee," AC, September 30, 1919, 9; "Emergency Tax Comes Up Today," AC, October 6, 1919, 1; "Emergency Tax Passes Council, Saving Hospital and City Schools," AC, October 7, 1919, 1.

[34] Steven R. Johnston, Monthly Report to the Board of Trustees, July 29, 1919, GMHC, AHC.

[35] Ibid.

[36] Ibid.

[37] Ibid.

[38] Minutes, City of Atlanta, Hospital and Charities Committee, June 4, 1925, GMHC, AHC.

[39] "Mrs. John C. Garner and Mrs. David L. Pittman both Claim Same Girl, Mrs. Garner Charging Babies Were Changed on Night of Birth," AC, January 30, 1920, 1; "How Babies Are Cared For at Grady," AC, January 31, 1920, 1; "Will Ask Courts To Make Decision on Baby Tangle," AC, January 31, 1920, 1; "Baby Case Goes to Court Today," AC, February 3, 1920, 4; Bessie Kempton, "'My Baby is Still Alive,' Asserts Mrs. J. C. Garner," AC, February 7, 1920, 1.

[40] "Women in Dispute Over Their Babies," AC, January 30, 1920, 10.

[41] "Fate Helps Solve Claims to Babies," *The Washington Post*, February 7, 1920, 1; "Unclaimed Babe to Rest Today in Church Yard," AC, February 8, 1920, 1.

[42] Loyd A. Wieheit, "Modern Solomon Must Soon Pass on Baby Tangle," AC, August 9, 1920, 12.

43 "System at Grady Termed 'Rotten,'" AC, October 13, 1920, 13.

44 "'Mixup' Case Girl Changes Parents," AC, August 5, 1936, 1, 9.

45 Ibid.; "4 Loving Parents Approve Decision on Future of Hospital 'Mixup Girl,'" AC, August 7, 1936, 11; "'Mix-Up' Girl Departs for Macon, Abandoning Stage 'Career' Contract," AC, August 9, 1936, 6C; "'Mix-Up Baby' of 20 Years Ago Weds and Gets Her Third Name," AC, November 5, 1939, 9B.

46 "Head of Nurses at Grady Quits," AC, July 20, 1921, 1; "Councilmen Back Board in Asking Nurse to Resign," AC, July 21, 1921, 1.

47 "Board Prepared to Hear Charge," AC, July 22, 1921, 12; "Nurses of Grady Hospital Are Now Preparing to Demand Investigation by City Councilmen," AC, July 23, 1921, 1; "Probe Promised by City Council Grady Committee," AC, July 24, 1921, 1.

48 "Two Reporters Caused Trouble Says Johnston," AC, July 27, 1921, 1.

49 This estimate from the time fits in with rates for sexually transmitted disease among African Americans in the South during the later 1920s, when the rate for syphilis alone ranged from 10% to 30%. See, Edward H. Beardsley, *A History of Neglect: Health Care for Blacks and Mill Workers in the Twentieth-Century South* (Knoxville: The University of Tennessee Press, 1987), 19.

50 Karen Jane Ferguson, *Black Politics in New Deal Atlanta* (Chapel Hill: University of North Carolina Press, 2003), 115.

51 These figures are for all ages from birth to age 55 and over. Five of the 49 girls who were under the age of fifteen tested positive on the Kahn test for syphilis; three of the 59 boys who were under fifteen years when tested also were positive. The sample for whites was slightly lower than for blacks, with 198 white women and 107 white men tested for syphilis versus 255 African American women and 218 African American men. Paul B. Beeson and Edward S. Miller, "Epidemiological Study of Lymphogranuloma Venereum, Employing the Complement-Fixation Test," *American Journal of Public Health* 34 (October 1944), 1077-1079.

52 Minutes, GMH Board of Trustees, June 24, 1919, GMHC, AHC.

53 "Steiner Leaves $500,000 to Grady," AC, February 23, 1919, 14; "Establishment of Cancer Hospital Here at Cost of $500,00 Offered City," AC, October 2, 1921, 1.

54 "Dr. Stone Holds Clinic on Cancer at Steiner Ward," AC, February 3, 1925, 16; "Cancer Authority Praises Steiner Clinic Facilities," AC, February 6, 1925, 7; Victor A. Triolo and Ilse L. Riegel, "The American Association for Cancer Research, 1907-1940, Historical Review," *Cancer Research* 21:2 (February 1961), 137-167; Victor A. Triolo and Michael B. Shimkin, "The American Cancer Society and Cancer Research Origins and Organization: 1913-1943," *Cancer Research* 29:9 (September 1969), 1615-1641.

55 Minutes, City of Atlanta, Hospital and Charities Committee, May 17, 1923, GMHC, AHC; "Donation of Elsas for Grady Accepted," AC, September 29, 1922, 4.

56 "South's Largest and Most Modern Clinic for Cancer Treatment, Gift of Late Albert D. Steiner, Will Be Opened Here Soon," AC, August 10, 1924, 4.

57 Minutes, City of Atlanta, Hospital and Charities Committee, October 21, 1921, GMHC, AHC.

58 Minutes, City of Atlanta, Hospital and Charities Committee, August 31, 1922, GMHC, AHC.

59 Minutes, Medical Board of White Unit, October 18, 1921, GMHC, AHC; "Nicolson Heads Graduate School; With Formal Opening of Outdoor Clinic at Grady," AC, October 28, 1923; "Physicians and Surgeons Graduate School to Open," AC, January 18, 1925, 5; "Another Forward Step," AC, January 18, 1925, C2.

60 "Grady Hospital Interns Asked to Quit Places," AC, August 31, 1925, 1; "Grady Internes to Serve Terms," AC, September 1, 1925, 1; "Fight Upon Grady Graduate School Regime Launched," AC, February 3, 1926, 1; "Committee to Decide Grady Fight Friday," AC, February 4, 1926; "New Committee Named For Grady," AC, February 17, 1926, 1.

61 Minutes, City of Atlanta, Hospital and Charities Committee, April 8, 1927, GMHC, AHC; "Grady Staff in Hot Debate on 'New Rules,'" AC, March 2, 1927, 1; "Grady Staff Row Settlement Seen," AC, March 3, 1927, 1; "Grady Rules Changed in Hot Session," AC, March 8, 1927, 1.

62 "New Grady Rules Fought By Staff," AC, April 9, 1927, 1; "New Grady Rules Foes Lose Again," AC, April 26, 1927, 1; "The Grady Hospital," AC, April 29, 1927, 6.

63 "Grady Hospital Called 'Disgrace' By Staff Doctors," AC, November 28, 1928, 1.

64 Ibid., 10.

65 "Grady Facilities Hit by Dr. Davison; Bond Issue Urged," AC, October 28, 1929, 1.

66 Ibid.

67 Ibid.

68 Ibid.

69 "X-Ray Room Explodes at Grady Hospital," AC, June 21, 1930, 1.

70 "Lethal Gas Peril Fails to Deter Hospital Heroes," AC, June 21, 1930, 1.

71 "Doctors Demand Full Renovation of Grady Unit," AC, June 23, 1930, 1-A

72 E. C. Thrash, "Member of Grady Staff Wants the Hospital Operated by Emory," AC, April 29, 1927, 6.

73 "Grady White Unit 'Politics' Scored By Steiner Chief," AC, November 19, 1930, 1.

74 Ibid.

75 Dr. L. Sage Hardin, "Divorce Grady Hospital Entirely From Outside Interests, Urges Hardin," AC, June 29, 1930, 13A.

76 Jesse O. Thomas, "Urban League," AC, November 3, 1929, 7.

77 Dr. L. Sage Hardin, "Divorce Grady Hospital Entirely From Outside Interests, Urges Hardin," AC, June 29, 1930, 13A.

[78] "$5,000,000 Issue for Grady Urged," AC, June 30, 1930, 1.

[79] James Adams Lester, *A History of the Georgia Baptist Convention 1822-1972* (n.p.: The Executive Committee, The Baptist Convention of the State of Georgia, 1972), 335, 387-388.

[80] "Control of Grady by Emory Opposed," AC, June 27, 1930, 8; "$5,000,000 Issue for Grady Urged," AC, June 30, 1930, 1.

[81] "$5,000,000 Issue for Grady Urged," AC, June 30, 1930, 1; "Time For Action," AC, July 1, 1930, 8.

[82] Walter White, *A Man Called White: The Autobiography of Walter White* (New York: Viking, 1948), 135-138.

[83] Minutes of the Medical Staff of Grady Hospital, Minutes of the Meeting of the Emory Division, Grady Hospital, March 10, 1925, GMHC, AHC; Minutes of the Medical Staff of Grady Hospital, Minutes of the Meeting of the Emory Division, Grady Hospital, April 13, 1925, GMHC, AHC.

[84] "Emory is Ready to Take Charge of Grady, Oppenheimer Says," AC, July 1, 1930, 6.

[85] "What Says–Everybody," AC, November 20, 1929, 10.

[86] "Probe of Huiet Charge Started," AC, November 21, 1929, 1.

[87] "Graft Reigns at City Hall, Grand Jury Charges; Councilmen Declare They Welcome Investigation," AC, January 5, 1930, 1; "Claiming City is Under 'Tweed' Rule, Boykin Asks Aid of Leading Citizens," AC, January 5, 1930, 1.

[88] "Conditions at Grady Flayed By Hutcheson," AC, March 21, 1930, 28.

[89] The anti-Catholic Hutcheson was prominent among the Ku Klux Klan as associate editor of the *Searchlight*, the unofficial newsletter of Georgia's KKK. (Hutcheson's law partner, Joe Wood, owned the *Searchlight*.) In 1920, Hutcheson was elected to the Atlanta School Board, joining his friend Walter A. Sims, a city councilman and prominent member of the KKK. James L. Key, the mayor of Atlanta, also served as a school board member *ex officio*. Quickly elected chair of a crucial board committee, Hutcheson organized a voting block with Mayor Key, Walter Sims, and another friend, William Gaines. Mayor Key, who left office in 1922, replaced by Councilman Sims, returned to the mayor's office in 1930, just months after Hutcheson sent his letter to Solicitor-General Boykin urging an investigation of Grady.

[90] "Conditions at Grady Flayed By Hutcheson," AC, March 21, 1930, 2B.

[91] "Dr. Thrash Scores Criticism of Grady," AC, March 26, 1930, 18.

[92] "Grand Jury Raps City Hospital System," AC, October 19, 1930, 9A.

[93] Ibid.

[94] Ibid.

[95] Ibid.

[96] Ibid.

[97] The timing was hardly auspicious, but the move had been set in motion months earlier when the Executive Committee of the Medical Staff at White Grady recommended that the Hospital and Charities Committee abolish the Department of Bronchoscopy. See, Minutes, Executive Committee of White Unit, June 10, 1930, GMHC, AHC.

[98] "Grand Jury Asks Johnston Ouster," AC, January 3, 1931, 1.

[99] Ibid.

[100] Ibid.

[101] "Key Urges Citizen Control of Grady, Mayor-Elect Would Make Hospital Charity Institution Alone, Asks Doctors' Aid," AC, November 7, 1930, 1.

[102] Ibid., 8.

[103] Ibid.

[104] Report of the Dean of the School of Medicine, 1927-1928 ROAO, 101-102, MARBL.

[105] Report of the Dean of the School of Medicine, 1928-1929 ROAO, 127, MARBL.

[106] Ibid.

[107] Report of the Dean of the School of Medicine, 1929-1930 ROAO, 113, MARBL.

[108] Report of the Dean of the School of Medicine, 1930-1931 ROAO, 146, MARBL.

[109] Minutes of the Medical Staff of Grady Hospital, The Meeting of the Staff, Colored Unit, April 13, 1926, GMHC, AHC.

[110] M. O. Bousfield, M.D., "Presidential Address, National Medical Association Annual Convention, August 14, 1934," *Journal of the National Medical Association* 26:4 (November 1934), 155. Dr. Bousfield also noted the irony of referring to Black Grady as "a Negro Hospital." He wrote, "The so-called unit of Grady Hospital in Atlanta receives only Negro patients, has colored nurses, under white supervision, white internes and a white visiting staff. There is not a Negro doctor anywhere. It is called a Negro hospital." ibid., 152.

[111] Ibid.

[112] W. Montague Cobb, "Relliford Stillmon Smith, M.D., 1889-1965," *Journal of the National Medical Association* 58:2 (March 1966), 146.

[113] Quoted in Bayor, *Race and the Shaping of Twentieth Century Atlanta*, 156.

[114] Ibid.

[115] Report of the Dean of the School of Medicine, 1930-1931 ROAO, 141, MARBL.

[116] Report of the Dean of the School of Medicine, 1931-1932 ROAO, 134-135, MARBL.

[117] "Emory and Grady in New Alliance Formed by Board," AC, August 19, 1931, 1; "An Object Lesson," AC, August 20, 1931, 8.

[118] Report of the Dean of the School of Medicine, 1931-1932 ROAO, 135, MARBL.

[119] Frederick Allen, *Secret Formula: How Brilliant Marketing and Relentless Salesmanship Made Coca-Cola the Best-Known Product in the World* (New York: Harper Business, 1994) offers a highly readable account of Samuel Candler Dobbs' role in the development of the Coca-Cola Company.

[120] Kathryn W. Kemp, *God's Capitalist: Asa Candler of Coca-Cola* (Macon, Ga.: Mercer University Press, 2002). See especially, pages 83-136, 171-190.

[121] Allen, *Secret Formula*, 84-91.

[122] Ibid., 94-101.

[123] "Mayor Defends Grady Chairman," AC, January 5, 1934, 9.

[124] "Speakers Laud Grady's Progress at Dinner Honoring Staff, Trustees," AC, February 12, 1936, 10.

[125] "Grady Expansion Plans Imperiled by Strife–Dobbs," AC, April 18, 1937, 1A.

[126] "Council to Vote on Grady Control," AC, April 19, 1937, 17.

[127] "Harmony Reigns at Grady Session," AC, April 15, 1937, 14.

[128] "Grady Expansion Plans Imperiled by Strife–Dobbs," AC, April 18, 1937, 1A.

[129] "Atlanta Medical Center in View," *New York Times*, April 18, 1937, 25.

[130] "Emory Purchases Land Near Grady for Development," AC, November 2, 1937, 1.

[131] "$2,500,000 Given for Development of University Center," AC, January 15, 1939, 1.

[132] William Randolph Smith, "Cardiorrhaphy in Acute Injuries, With Report of Two Cases and a Table of Reported Cases," *Annals of Surgery* 78:6 (December 1923), 696-710.

[133] *Annual Report of the Grady Memorial Hospital 1935*, 5-6.

[134] Garrett, *Atlanta and Environs*, Volume 2, 938.

[135] Minutes, Grady Memorial Hospital Board of Trustees, August 18, 1937, GMHC, AHC; Frank Drake, "Grady to Establish 'Blood Bank' Avoiding Delays in Transfusions," AC, August 19, 1937, 1.

[136] "Atlantans Hurry Gifts of Blood," AC, August 20, 1937, 1, 7; "'Vault' for 'Blood Bank' Arrives; Grady Ready for First Deposits," AC, September 29, 1937, 13; "Four Pints of Blood 'Deposited' By Four Donors to Hospital Bank," AC, October 7, 1937, 9; Grady Hospital, *Annual Report of the Trustees for 1937*, 7.

[137] Bernard Fantus, "The Therapy of the Cook County Hospital: Blood Preservation," *Journal of the American Medical Association*, 109:2 (July 10, 1937), 123-131; Louis K. Diamond, "History of Blood Banking in the United States," *Journal of the American Medical Association* 193:1 (July 5, 1965), 40-44.

[138] "A Review of the Complications Following the Administration of Sulfanilamides," *Journal of the Medical Association of Georgia* 27:21 (January 1938), 21-29.

[139] "Grady Tests Drug to Cure Pneumonia," AC, February 4, 1939, 1; "Grady Sees Victory Over Pneumonia," AC, March 19, 1939, 4A.

[140] Minutes, GMH Board of Trustees, April 14, 1931, GMHC, AHC.

[141] *Annual Report of the Trustees of Grady Hospital for the Year 1931*, [1-2].

[142] Ibid.

[143] *Annual Report of the Grady Memorial Hospital 1933*, 4-5.

[144] Ibid., 3.

[145] Ibid., 5.

[146] On state funding for New Deal programs in Georgia under Governor Talmadge see, Michael S. Holmes, *The New Deal in Georgia: An Administrative History* (Westport, Conn.: Greenwood Press, 1975), 321-336. On the New Deal in Atlanta, see Douglas Lee Fleming, "Atlanta, The Depression, and the New Deal," (Ph.D. dissertation, Emory University, 1984); Karen Jane Ferguson, *Black Politics in New Deal Atlanta* (Chapel Hill: The University of North Carolina Press, 2002); Georgina Hickey, *Hope and Danger in the New South City: Working-Class Women and Urban Development in Atlanta, 1890-1940* (Athens: University of Georgia Press, 2003), 207-215; Douglas L. Fleming, "The New Deal in Atlanta: A Review of the Major Problems," *The Atlanta Historical Journal* 30:1 (Spring 1986), 23-46.

[147] Holmes, *The New Deal in Georgia*, 22-23.

[148] "U. S. Expands Works Program in Georgia as Big Health Projects are Given Funds," AC December 10, 1933, 1A.

[149] "'That None Shall Die of Neglect,' Grady Becomes Noted U.S. Hospital," AC, March 22, 1936, 7K.

[150] "CWA Work Started at Grady Hospital," AC, December 14, 1933, 14; "120 CWA Workers at Grady Laid Off," AC, December 23, 1933, 1.

[151] "Grady Hospital To Furnish Funds Needed to Start WPA Projects," AC, July 17, 1935, 18.

[152] Jane Walker Herndon, "Ed Rivers and Georgia's 'Little New Deal,'" *Atlanta Historical Journal* 30:1 (Spring 1986), 97-105; Ferguson, *Black Politics in New Deal Atlanta*; Holmes, *The New Deal in Georgia*; Michael R. Grey, *New Deal Medicine: The Rural Health Programs of the Farm Security Administration* (Baltimore: Johns Hopkins University Press, 1999); Roger Biles, *The New Deal and the South* (Lexington: University Press of Kentucky, 1994).

[153] *Annual Report Grady Hospital 1939*, 18.

[154] Grady Hospital, *Annual Report of the Trustees for 1937*, 12, tells that black maternity and obstetrics patients stayed an average of 3.8 days while similar cases among whites stayed an average of 7.5 days.

[155] Harold H. Martin, *Atlanta and Environs: A Chronicle of Its People and Events: Years of Change and Challenge, 1940-1976* (Athens, Georgia: University of Georgia Press, 1987), 14.

[156] WPA Records Index Microfilm, Official Project Number 665-34-3-176, National Archives, Southeast Region, Morrow, Georgia.

[157] "WPA Gives Fulton Funds For Grady," AC, March 29, 1940, 5.

[158] "Malaria Increase Inspires Warning," AC, July 25, 1937, 6B.

[159] "Everhart Heads Grady Hospital," AC, September 25, 1918, 1; "Everhart Resigns Position as Head of Grady Hospital," AC, January 3, 1919, 6.

[160] Steven Johnston to GMH Board of Trustees, March 26, 1919, GMHC, AHC.

[161] Report of Steve Johnston to GMH Board of Trustees, September 20, 1919, GMHC, AHC; Minutes, GMH Board of Trustees, September 30, 1919, GMHC, AHC.

[162] "Franklin Takes Grady Post; To Give Public 'Square' Deal," AC, June 1, 1931, 1.

[163] "Franklin Tenders Resignation at Grady," AC, January 1, 1938, 1.

[164] Michael M. Davis and Mary Ross, "A County Hospital Health Center," *American Journal of Public Health and the Nation's Health* 22:8 (August 1932), 809-818.

[165] "New Grady Head Likes Hospital and Atlanta: Dr. James Moss Beeler Goes Through Busy First Day Here," AC, July 19, 1938, 2.

[166] "Council Abolishes Grady Board, Then Restores It," AC, January 4, 1938, 1; "Grady's Trustees to Fight Politics," AC, January 5, 1938, 10.

[167] "Council Abolishes Grady Board, Then Restores It," AC, January 4, 1938, 1.

[168] Ibid.

[169] Willard Neal, "A Big City Hospital's 75 Years," *Atlanta Journal and Constitution Magazine*, February 5, 1967, 27.

[170] William S. Goldsmith, "William Simpson Elkin, 1858-1944," *Annals of Surgery* 121:5 (May 1945), 767-768.

[171] J. D. Cantwell, "The Legacy of James Edgar Paullin, M.D.," *Journal of the Medical Association of Georgia* 79:10 (October 1990) 737-741; Mark E. Silverman and J. Willis Hurst, "James Edgar Paullin: Internist to Franklin Roosevelt, Oslerian, and Forgotten Leader of American Medicine," *Annals of Internal Medicine* 134:5 (March 6, 2001), 428-431.

[172] "Medical Society Seeks to Record Clinic Patients," AC, January 8, 1929, 10A.

[173] "Highlights of Survey By Dr. Thomas Reed," AC, February 6, 1938, 1A; "Reed Report Advises Merger of City-County Agencies," AC, February 6, 1938, 10.

[174] "Reed Report Advises Merger of City-County Agencies," AC, February 6, 1938, 10.

[175] Ibid.; "Doctors Indorse Reed's Survey," AC, March 20, 1938, 5.

[176] *Bulletin of the Fulton County Medical Society* 14:16 (August 15, 1940), 3.

[177] See the AC, August 26, 1940, 11.

[178] "Federation Campaigns for Bond Issue Passage," *The Journal of Labor,* August 23, 1940, 1.

[179] "Vast Fire Perils Grady, Razes 25 Homes," AC, March 28, 1938, 1; "Unnecessary Peril," March 31, 1938, 10; "Mayor Joins Doctors and Nurses to Help Calm Patients at Grady," AC, March 28, 1938, 2.

[180] "Financing Plan Lacks Majority by Slim Margin," AC, September 5, 1940, 1.

[181] "Hospital Authority Will Be Sought to Build Great Fulton, DeKalb Center," AC, January 12, 1941, 1A; "Five Million DeKalb-Fulton Hospital Asked," AC, February 6, 1941, 26; "Right to Set Up New Hospital Authority Given," AC, June 5, 1941, 3.

[182] "Authority Seeks Five Millions to Aid Grady," AC, August 12, 1941, 1.

[183] *The First Annual Report, Fulton-DeKalb Hospital Authority, 1946,* [9].

[184] "Grady Training Setup Stirs Ire of 120 Doctors," AC, October 30, 1943, 1; "Training Plan Stirs Protest," AC, October 31, 1943, 3-B; Report of the Dean of the School of Medicine, 1943-44 ROAO, 36-37, MARBL.

[185] "Negro Doctors Deliver White Babies in Ga.," *Chicago Defender* (National Edition), November 13, 1943, 20.

[186] "Grady Refuses Its Facilities to Oglethorpe," AC, November 5, 1943, 1; "Oglethorpe Quits Field of Medics; Shifts Pupils," AC, February 4, 1944, 15.

[187] Minutes, GMH Board of Trustees, June 1, 1920, GMHC, AHC.

[188] "Homosassa Club Sends Fish Supply to Grady Hospital," AC, January 24, 1920, 13.

[189] "Valuable Towels Will Be Auctioned for Grady Hospital," AC, April 15, 1921, 14; "Grady Collects Autographs" AJ, August 22, 1962, 34. An earlier report suggests that the towels found in Mrs. Lowry's garage may originally have been created for the hospital and nursery at the Cotton States and International Exposition and subsequently donated to Grady. See, "Woman and Society," AC, January 14, 1899, 9.

[190] "A Noble Will," AC, February 24, 1919, 4.

[191] Thomas L. Ross, M.D., "Memoirs of My Practice," *American Journal of Cardiology* 85:3 (February 1, 2000), 401.

[192] *Annual Report of the Grady Memorial Hospital 1933*, 7-8.

[193] Minutes of the Medical Staff of Grady Hospital, October 9, 1934, GMHC, AHC.

[194] William Rawson Smith, *Villa Clare: The Purposeful Life and Timeless Art Collection of J. J. Haverty* (Macon: Mercer University Press, 2006); "CWA Murals at Museum of Art Range From Missions to Tar Baby," AC, July 8, 1934, 11A, describes the coloring of the Farnsworth murals for Grady as "extremely delicate and soft." A photo of Mrs. Farnsworth with one of the Grady murals is published in the AC, July 29, 1934, N2.

[195] Atlanta claimed to have more murals coming out of the New Deal project than any other city in the South. See Holmes, *The New Deal in Georgia*, 178-179.

[196] "Telegraphic Dispatches," *Washington Post*, June 20, 1932, 2.

[197] "Hospital Authority Gets Steiner Ward for $15,000," AC, December 21, 1945, 14; *The First Annual Report, Fulton-DeKalb Hospital Authority, 1946,* [21-22].

Chapter 6

[1] "Two Georgia Nurses Found in Jap Camp," AC, February 6, 1945, 4; "Georgia Nurses Describe Santo Tomas Experiences," AC, February 26, 1945, 2; New York Life Ins. Co. v. White 190 F.2d 424 (1951).

² J. Willis Hurst, "Eugene Auston Stead, Jr., M.D.: A Conversation With J. Willis Hurst, M.D.," *The American Journal of Cardiology* 84 (September 15, 1999), 712.

³ William C. Roberts, "Stewart R. Roberts: An Ideal of Modern Medicine," *Annals of Internal Medicine* 70:5 (May 1, 1969), 1016; Charles Stewart Roberts, *Life and Writings of Stewart Roberts, M.D.: Georgia's First Heart Specialist* (Spartanburg, South Carolina: The Reprint Company Publishers, 1993).

⁴ John Laszlo and Francis A. Neelon, *The Doctors' Doctor: Eugene A. Stead, Jr., M.D.* (Durham, North Carolina: Carolina Academic Press, 2005); William Hollingsworth, *Taking Care: The Legacy of Soma Weiss, Eugene Stead, and Paul Beeson* (Chapel Hill: Professional Press, 1995).

⁵ Hurst, "Eugene Auston Stead, Jr.," 714.

⁶ J. V. Warren, E. A. Stead, Jr., A. J. Merrill, and E. S. Brannon, "The Treatment of Shock With Concentrated Serum Albumin: A Preliminary Report," *The Journal of Clinical Investigation* 23:4 (July 1944), 506-509; E. A. Stead, Jr., E. S. Brannon, A. J. Merrill, J. V. Warren, "Concentrated Human Albumin in the Treatment of Shock," *Archives of Internal Medicine* 77:5 (May 1946), 564-575.

⁷ Hurst, "Eugene Auston Stead," 720.

⁸ James V. Warren and Eugene A. Stead, Jr., "Fluid Dynamics in Chronic Congestive Heart Failure," *Archives of Internal Medicine* 73:2 (February 1944), 138-147.

⁹ Emmett S. Brannon, Stephen H. Weens, James V. Warren, "Atrial Septal Defect Study of Hemodynamics By the Technique of Right Heart Catheterization," *American Journal of the Medical Sciences* 210:4 (October 1945), 480-490.

¹⁰ Lorraine Nelson Spritzer and Jean B. Bergmark, *Grace Towns Hamilton and the Politics of Southern Change* (Athens: University of Georgia Press, 1997), 120; Grace Towns Hamilton to Alfred A. Weinstein, February 12, 1959, Hamilton, AHC.

¹¹ J. W. Hurst, "Robert Purves Grant," *Clinical Cardiology* 10:4 (April 1987), 286-287.

¹² Sharon R. Kaufman, *The Healer's Tale: Transforming Medicine and Culture* (Madison: University of Wisconsin Press, 1993), 70.

¹³ Paul B. Beeson, M.D., "Jaundice Occurring One to Four Months After Transfusion of Blood or Plasma: Report of Seven Cases," JAMA 121:17 (April 24, 1943), 1332-1334.

¹⁴ Alexander Fleming discovered the "miracle drug" accidentally in 1928 in London; it first came into widespread use during World War II. Dr. Beeson introduced the medicine at Grady after having prescribed it in the European war theatre. David Masters, *Miracle Drug: The Inner History of Penicillin* (London: Eyre & Spottiswoode, 1946) gives an engaging and highly readable account of the drug's development. Robert Bud, *Penicillin: Triumph and Tragedy* (New York: Oxford University Press, 2007) provides an excellent account of the development of the antibiotic and its use in the twentieth century.

¹⁵ Paul B. Beeson, "Temperature-Elevating Effect of a Substance Obtained from Polymorphonuclear leucocytes," in "Proceedings of the Fortieth Annual Meeting of the American Society for Clinical Investigation Held In Atlantic City, N.J., May 3, 1948," *The Journal of Clinical Investigation* 27:4 (July 1948), 524.

¹⁶ J. Willis Hurst, *The Quest For Excellence: The History of the Department of Medicine at Emory University School of Medicine* (Atlanta: Scholars Press, 1997).

¹⁷ Richard Rapport, M.D., *Physician: The Life of Paul Beeson* (Fort Lee, New Jersey: Barricade Books, Inc., 2001) ably captures Beeson's remarkable story.

¹⁸ Report of the Dean of the School of Medicine, 1936-1937 ROAO, 138, MARBL.

¹⁹ Ibid.

²⁰ Report of the Dean of the School of Medicine, 1938-1939 ROAO, 148, MARBL.

²¹ Report of the Dean of the School of Medicine, 1940-1941 ROAO, 142, MARBL.

²² Ibid.

²³ Ibid., 147.

²⁴ Ibid., 148.

²⁵ Report of the Dean of the School of Medicine, 1941-1942 ROAO, 50, MARBL; Report of the Dean of the School of Medicine, 1943-1944 ROAO, 35, MARBL.

²⁶ Report of the Dean of the School of Medicine, 1945-1946 ROAO, 21, MARBL.

²⁷ Originally named the Communicable Disease Center, in 1970 the name changed to the Center for Disease Control. Eleven years later it became the Centers for Disease Control, and was renamed in 1992 as the Centers for Disease Control and Prevention.

²⁸ Report of the Dean of the School of Medicine, 1944-1945 ROAO, 13, MARBL.

²⁹ Ibid., 16.

³⁰ Ibid., 14.

³¹ Ibid., 14-15.

³² Ibid., 15.

³³ Ibid., 17.

³⁴ Dean Stead estimated that it would only take two years for a clinic at Emory to become profitable and, if turned over to the medical school, would make the last two years of the medical school "more nearly self-supporting." Report of the Dean of the School of Medicine, 1944-45 ROAO, 18, MARBL.

³⁵ Ibid.

³⁶ Report of the Dean of the School of Medicine, 1945-1946 ROAO, 25, MARBL.

³⁷ The Emory University School of Medicine, A Report to the President, R. Hugh Wood to President Goodrich, September 9, 1953, 2, in 1952-1953 ROAO, MARBL.

³⁸ R.C. Mizell to R. Hugh Wood, unsigned draft, September 21, 1953, in 1952-1953 ROAO, MARBL.

³⁹ Ibid.

⁴⁰ "Basic Conflict Pits Clinic vs. Grady; Doctor vs. Policy," AJ, January 31, 1957, 1-2.

⁴¹ English, *Emory University, 1915-1965*, 158-160.

42 "Dr. Hurst Replaces Dr. Ferris at Grady," AJ, January 25, 1957, 6.

43 "Emory, Grady 'Differences' Patch Up Urged," AJ, January 24, 1957, 34.

44 Dean Arthur P. Richardson, "Annual Report to the President, January 1, 1957," 2, in 1955-56 ROAO, MARBL.

45 "Basic Conflict Pits Clinic vs. Grady; Doctor vs. Policy," AJ, January 31, 1957, 1.

46 Ibid.

47 "Emory Denies Care Affected By Change," AJ, January 28, 1957, 34.

48 Report of the Dean of the School of Medicine, 1956-1957 ROAO, 2, MARBL.

49 The figures for 1942 to 1957 are reported in "Emory Denies Care Affected By Change," AJ, January 28, 1957, 34.

50 English, *Emory University 1915-1965*, 159, reports that Dr. Caton had been told that his contract would not be renewed.

51 "Emory Shirks Duty at Grady–Medic," AJ, January 30, 1957, 4.

52 "Emory Denies Care Affected By Change," AJ, January 28, 1957, 34.

53 "Basic Conflict Pits Clinic vs. Grady; Doctor vs. Policy," AJ, January 31, 1957, 1. As cited in the article, Dr. Bloom's resignation letter read in part, "recent and past events would indicate that the ideals, principles, and educational goals for which I have been working are different from those currently employed in the school. The destruction of the clinical educational program and its full-time professorial staff without adequate consideration of the consequences to community health, patient and medical student welfare and research, in whose interest I have devoted my total efforts, leaves me no alternative but to decide that there is no future for one interested in medical education and research to pursue an academic career in this school."

54 "Dr. Hurst Replaces Dr. Ferris at Grady," AJ, January 25, 1957, 6.

55 "Public Can Inspect Grady on Saturday," AJ, January 19, 1958, 1-C; Edwina Davis, "Grady's Big 'Dream' Coming True–Soon," AJ, January 20, 1958, 12; Margaret Turner, "Grady Volunteers to Help Making Opening a Gala Day," AJ, January 23, 1958, 34; "New Monument to Progress," AJ, January 26, 1958, 6-E.

56 "Grady Hospital Opens New 26-Acre Building," AC, January 27, 1958, 1.

57 Ibid.

58 Ibid.

59 Ibid.

60 Report of the Dean of the School of Medicine, 1962-1963 ROAO, 1, MARBL.

61 *Grady News* 16:4 (April 1964), 1.

62 Hurst, "Eugene Auston Stead, Jr., M.D.," 713.

63 Ibid., 716.

64 Ibid., 719.

65 Report of the Dean of the School of Medicine, 1943-44 ROAO, 38.

66 Hurst, "Eugene Auston Stead, Jr., M.D.," 719.

67 Sam Heys and Allen B. Goodwin, *The Winecoff Fire: The Untold Story of America's Deadliest Hotel Fire* (Atlanta: Longstreet Press, 1993) vividly details the history of the tragedy and its aftermath.

68 "'Shucks I Was Scared,' Hero Interne Exclaims," AJ, December 9, 1946, 9.

69 Doris Lockerman, "City's Mass Sorrow Moves Into Sick Rooms of Tired Grady," AJ, December 9, 1946, 1.

70 Ibid.

71 This section is indebted to an extremely valuable history of this important federal agency, Elizabeth W. Etheridge, *Sentinel For Health: A History of the Centers for Disease Control* (Berkeley: University of California Press, 1992).

72 There were 308 black patients and 15 white patients; 210 males and 113 females.

73 "Poison Whiskey," AJ, October 24, 1951, 20; "12 Suspects Held as Poison Liquor Claims 27th Life," AC, October 24, 1951, 1; "Witnesses Identify 'Poison' Distributor," AJ, October 24, 1951, 1; "Ex-Convict Sought in Poison Cases," AC, October 25, 1951, 1; Keeler McCartney, "Webb Finds Source of Fatal Drink," AC, October 26, 1951, 1; "Hardy Arrested on Manslaughter Charge," AJ, October 25, 1951, 1. At Hardy's trial, Richard A. (Snooks) Weems, a runner for a wholesale customer for bootleg whiskey, testified, "Mr. Fats, he said there wasn't a damn thing wrong with it—cause he'd drink some of it himself." See, "Hardy Rented Barn, Used Broomstick To Mix Poison Brew, Witnesses Say," AC, December 12, 1951, 1; "Hardy's Fate Nears Jury; Death Asked," AC, December 13, 1951, 1.

74 Acidosis is a condition in which the normal balance between acids and alkalies that are found in the blood plasma is altered. Acidosis causes weakness, drowsiness, and coma. Severe acidosis is incompatible with life.

75 Curtis D. Benton, Jr., M.D., and F. Phinizy Calhoun, Jr., M.D., "The Ocular Effects of Methyl Alcohol Poisoning: Report of a Catastrophe Involving Three Hundred and Twenty Persons," *Transactions of the American Academy of Ophthalmology and Otolaryngology* 56 (November-December 1952), 875-885.

76 Ivan L. Bennett Jr., M.D., Freeman H. Cary, M.D., George L. Mitchell Jr., M.D., Manuel N. Cooper, M.D., "Methyl Alcohol Poisoning: An Account of the 1951 Atlanta Epidemic," *Journal of the Medical Association of Georgia*, 41 (1952) 48-51; idem., "Acute Methyl Alcohol Poisoning: A Review Based on Experiences in an Outbreak of 323 Cases," *Journal of Medicine* 32:4 (December 1953), 431-463. Among other research publications coming out of the incident is I. L. Bennett, Jr., T. C. Nation, and J. F. Oiley, "Pancreatitis in Methyl Alcohol Poisoning," *Journal of Laboratory and Clinical Medicine* 40 (September 1952), 405-409.

77 John W. Powell, "Poison Liquor Episode in Atlanta, Georgia," in *Conference on Field Studies of Reactions to Disasters, Held at the University of Chicago, January 29-30, 1952* (Chicago: National Opinion Research Center, 1953), 87-103.

⁷⁸ Alex Joiner, "Hardy Given Life Term as Brewer of Poison Potion," AC, December 14, 1951, 1. The conviction by the all-white jury was noted in the black press. See, for example, "Moonshine Murderer Gets Life Term," *Jet*, December 27, 1951, 28.

⁷⁹ General Memorandum, January 24, 1958, From Mrs. R.F. Schrader, Personnel Director, GMHC, AHC.

⁸⁰ Ibid.

⁸¹ *FDHA Annual Report, 1961*, 14-15.

⁸² "The Guild and Grady," AJ, August 8, 1958, 14; *FDHA Annual Report, 1964*, 12-13; *FDHA Annual Report, 1965*, 11-13; *Grady News* 23:3 (March-April 1971), 1; *FDHA Annual Report*, 1970, 40.

⁸³ *FDHA Annual Report, 1959*, 15; *FDHA Annual Report, 1965*, 11-13; *The Grady News* 17:11-12 (November-December, 1965), 1; *The Grady News* 17:1 (January 1965), 1; *The Grady News* 17:9-10 (September-October 1965), 1.

Chapter 7

¹ Alton Hornsby, Jr., and Alexa Benson Henderson, *The Atlanta Urban League, 1920-2000* (Lewiston, New York: Edwin Mellen Press, 2005).

² Atlanta Urban League, *A Report of Public School Facilities for Negroes in Atlanta, Georgia* (Atlanta: Atlanta Urban League, 1944).

³ Oral History Interview with Grace Towns Hamilton, July 19, 1974, Interview G-0026. Southern Oral History Program Collection, Southern Historical Collection, Wilson Library, University of North Carolina at Chapel Hill; Tomiko Brown-Nagin, *Courage to Dissent: Atlanta and the Long History of the Civil Rights Movement* (New York: Oxford University Press, 2011), 95-96; Lorraine Nelson Spritzer and Jean B. Bergmark, *Grace Towns Hamilton and the Politics of Southern Change* (Athens: The University of Georgia Press, 1997), 102-108.

⁴ *A Report on Hospital Care of the Negro Population of Atlanta, Georgia 1947* (Atlanta: The Atlanta Urban League [1948]). A helpful interpretation of the history of segregation and desegregation in American medical treatment is David Barton Smith, *Health Care Divided: Race and Healing a Nation* (Ann Arbor: University of Michigan Press, 1999).

⁵ *A Report on Hospital Care of the Negro Population of Atlanta, Georgia 1947*, 6.

⁶ Ibid., 7.

⁷ Mortality figures for 1938 are from Bayor, *Race and the Shaping of Twentieth-Century Atlanta*, 158.

⁸ *A Report on Hospital Care of the Negro Population of Atlanta, Georgia 1947*, 6.

⁹ Ibid., 20.

¹⁰ Ibid., 19-22.

¹¹ Ibid., 4.

¹² Ibid., 50-55.

¹³ Bayor, *Race and the Shaping of Twentieth-Century Atlanta*, 160.

¹⁴ Hughes Spalding to Frances Harriet Williams, October 20, 1958, Hamilton, AHC.

¹⁵ Hughes Spalding to G. Arthur Howell, January 8, 1948, Hamilton, AHC.

¹⁶ Frank Wilson to Hughes Spalding, July 9, 1949, Hamilton, AHC.

¹⁷ Louis T. Wright to Grace Towns Hamilton, April 21, 1948, Hamilton, AHC.

¹⁸ Spritzer and Bergmark, *Grace Towns Hamilton and the Politics of Southern Change*, 116.

¹⁹ Ibid., 119-120.

²⁰ Bayor, *Race and the Shaping of Twentieth-Century Atlanta*, 156.

²¹ William H. Sinkler to Charles R. Drew, February 11, 1947, Hamilton, AHC.

²² During the Great Depression the Fulton County Medical Society regularly made known its views about policies at the Gradys. It would become intimately involved in Grady's affairs again in the latter 1950s.

²³ *Bulletin of the Fulton County Medical Society*, May 15, 1948.

²⁴ Hughes Spalding to Advisory Board of Trustees, Negro Hospital, Fulton-DeKalb Hospital Authority, April 15, 1950, Hamilton, AHC.

²⁵ Spritzer and Bergmark, *Grace Towns Hamilton and the Politics of Southern Change*, 123.

²⁶ Hughes Spalding to Stephens Mitchell, December 23, 1949, Hamilton, AHC.

²⁷ Asa Yancey to Hughes Spalding, January 30, 1951, Hamilton, AHC.

²⁸ Spritzer and Bergmark, *Grace Towns Hamilton and the Politics of Southern Change*, 127-128.

²⁹ "New Hospital Dedication Today at 3 P.M.," ADW, June 22, 1952, Section 2, 1; William A. Fowlkes, Jr., "Atlantans Point With Pride to New Hospital," *The Pittsburgh Courier*, July 5, 1952. Clipping in Hamilton, AHC.

³⁰ "New Negro Hospital to Attract More Doctors," AC, August 10, 1952, 1.

³¹ Fowlkes, Jr., "Atlantans Point With Pride to New Hospital."

³² C. Christine Kelsey, "Crogman Pupil First To Enter New Hospital Here," ADW, July 8, 1952, 1.

³³ Fowlkes, Jr., "Atlantans Point With Pride to New Hospital."

³⁴ Minutes, Finance Committee, Advisory Board of Trustees, Hughes Spalding Pavilion, July 22, 1952, Hamilton, AHC; Minutes, Advisory Board of Trustees, October 28, 1952, Hamilton, AHC.

³⁵ George M. Coleman, "Adequate Hospital Facilities Still Unavailable in Atlanta," ADW, February 16, 1954, 1; idem., "Pavilion Still Beset With Controversial Problems," ADW, February 17, 1954, 1; idem., "Negro Doctors Still Limited in Professional Opportunities," ADW, February 18, 1954, 1.

[36] Samuel R. Poliakoff to Frank Wilson, June 26, 1953, Hamilton, AHC.

[37] "Auditor's Figures Not the Whole Story at Hughes Spalding," AI, August 21, 1960, 3.

[38] Charles R. Drew to Paul B. Beeson, January 20, 1947; R. Hugh Wood to Julia E. Baxter, October 14, 1947; R. Hugh Wood to W. Montague Cobb, January 7, 1948; Grace Towns Hamilton to W. Montague Cobb, January 22, 1948; Hugh Wood, James Paullin, and R. C. Mizell, "Proposed Relationship Between Emory University School of Medicine and the New Negro Hospital," [April 13, 1948]; all in Hamilton, AHC.

[39] Grace Towns Hamilton to W. B. Stubbs, November 19, 1949, Hamilton, AHC.

[40] Hughes Spalding to R. C. Mizell, July 20, 1948, Hamilton, AHC.

[41] W. Montague Cobb to Grace Towns Hamilton, May 18, 1951, Hamilton, AHC; Grace Towns Hamilton to Allen Gregg, September 7, 1951, Hamilton, AHC; Minutes of the Advisory Board of Trustees of the New Negro Hospital [October 2, 1951], Hamilton, AHC.

[42] Robert P. Grant to Paul Beeson, November 6, 1951, Hamilton, AHC.

[43] Spritzer and Bergmark, *Grace Towns Hamilton and the Politics of Southern Change*, 121.

[44] Ibid., 120-122, 128-129; Grace Towns Hamilton to Samuel Rothberg, August 12, 1960, Hamilton, AHC; Ira A. Ferguson to Bernard Hallman, June 2, 1959, Hamilton, AHC; Boisfeuillet Jones to Grace Towns Hamilton, September 16, 1959, Hamilton, AHC.

[45] Campbell Gibson and Kay Jung, "Historical Census Statistics on Population Totals By Race, 1790-1990, and By Hispanic Origin, 1970 to 1990, For Large Cities and Other Urban Places in the United States," Working Paper (Washington D.C.: U.S. Bureau of the Census, Population Division, 2005), [46].

[46] "Pavilion Suffered Neglect By Grady Administration, Advisory Board of Spalding Trustees Say, Little Hope Seen for Change of Status," ADW, February 18, 1962, 1.

[47] "Nurses to Take 'Drastic Action,'" AI, December 2, 1961, 1; "Nurses Win Pay Pledge At Spalding," AI, December 9, 1961, 1; "Nurses Are People Too," AI, December 9, 1961, 2.

[48] On the segregationist's self-understanding, see Kevin M. Kruse, *White Flight: Atlanta and the Making of Modern Conservatism* (Princeton: Princeton University Press, 2005), 9.

[49] Ibid., 126.

[50] Ibid., 128-130.

[51] Ibid.

[52] Ibid., 117-130.

[53] For a deft portrait of the student protests in Atlanta, see Nagin, *Courage to Dissent*, 133-174.

[54] Harry G. Lefever, *Undaunted by the Fight: Spelman College and the Civil Rights Movement, 1957-1967* (Macon, Georgia: Mercer University Press, 2005); James W. English, *The Prophet of Wheat Street, The Story of Reverend William Holmes Borders, A Man Who Refused to Fail* (Elgin, Illinois: David C. Cook Publishing Co., 1973).

[55] William H. Strong, "Bapt. Hosp. Denies Child First Aid," AI, May 20, 1961, 1.

[56] Ibid., 7.

[57] "*Inquirer* Seeks to End Atlanta Hospital Bias," AI, May 27, 1961, 1.

[58] Ibid.

[59] Ibid, 16.

[60] "Medical Association Continues Hospital Probe in Atlanta," AI, June 3, 1961, 1.

[61] "Hospital Apologizes Promises Care for All, Dr. Warner States Fight Just Begun; Aldermen Doubt Ordinance Authority," AI, June 10, 1961, 1.

[62] Ibid., 16.

[63] "Dr. Clinton E. Warner Chosen Man of the Year," AI, June 24, 1961, 1.

[64] "Grady Bars Negro Medics From Hospital Staff Duty," AI, July 29, 1961, 1.

[65] As this book neared completion, Dr. Roy C. Bell, Sr., died while visiting relatives in Williamsburg, Virginia, on July 1, 2011. Besides being a well-respected dentist in Atlanta from 1959 to 1979, Dr. Bell was a noted civil rights activist who contributed to the movement far beyond Atlanta. His service included work with the Southern Christian Leadership Conference. In addition to his leadership in the fight to desegregate Grady, Dr. Bell pushed to end segregation in the Georgia Dental Association and the American Dental Association.

[66] "Group to Air Medical Care for City Negroes," AI, July 22, 1961, 1.

[67] "Dr. Bell to Get National Support," AI, August 19, 1961, 1.

[68] Ibid., 20.

[69] Ibid., 1.

[70] Margaret Long, "Desegregation is Here, –But, Suspended in Air," AI, September 2, 1961, 8.

[71] Ibid.

[72] "Grady Under Fire: Health, Race Issues Aired at Oct. 2 Meet," AI, September 30, 1961, 1.

[73] "Ask Quick Action on Grady Bias," AI, October 7, 1961, 1.

[74] Ibid.

[75] "Hospital is Picketed in Segregation Plaint," AI, November 18, 1961, 1.

[76] Ibid.

[77] "Hospital Jim Crow Clause Under Fire, Senator Javits and *Inquirer*," AI, November 25, 1961, 1.

[78] "Negroes Picket Grady Anew," AC, February 7, 1962, 9; Keeler McCartney, "23 Arrested at Grady; Capitol Case is Heard," AC, February 14, 1962, 1; Pete Greenlea, "23 Fined In Grady Hospital Incident," ADW, February 15, 1962, 1; "Pay $17 Fines or Go To Jail, Court Tells 23 Grady Pickets," AC, February 15, 1962, 8.

[79] "Some Rights and Wrongs at Grady," AC, February 7, 1962, 4.

[80] "Grady Waiting Room Loses Bias for Short Time," ADW, February 15, 1962, 1.

[81] "Dr. Yancey Elected to Grady Staff," ADW, March 6, 1962, 1.

[82] "Dr. Yancey's Appointment to Grady Hospital Staff a Move in the Right Direction," ADW, March 8, 1962, 6.

[83] Pete Greenlea, "Grady Problem Can Be Resolved By Good Will, Appreciation of Equal Rights, Grand Jury Told," ADW, March 7, 1962, 1.

[84] Ibid.

[85] Ibid.

[86] "Accepting Yancey One Step Forward, Bell Declares," ADW, March 7, 1962, 1; "Yancey Appointed, Grady Battle Sizzles," AI, March 10, 1962, 1.

[87] "Edwina Davis, "Maid Left Savings: People 'Looked Up' to Grady Benefactor," AJ, March 9, 1961, 6.

[88] "All Big Guns on Grady Racial Bias," AI, March 10, 1962, 8.

[89] Pete Greenlea, "J. B. Blayton Named to Bond Commission," ADW, March 8, 1962, 1.

[90] Ibid.

[91] "Dr. Bell Blasts Negro Leaders," AI, May 19, 1962, 3.

[92] "8 Sue Grady Over Race Bias," AI, June 23, 1962, 1.

[93] Jerry Gentry, *Grady Baby: A Year in the Life of Atlanta's Grady Hospital*, (Jackson, Mississippi: University of Mississippi Press, 1999), 202-247; Brown-Nagin, *Courage to Dissent*, 205.

[94] Cynthia Griggs Fleming, *Soon We Will Not Cry: The Liberation of Ruby Doris Smith Robertson* (Lanham, Md.: Rowan and Littlefield, Inc., 1998); Lefever, *Undaunted by the Fight*, 149-150.

[95] "Sue Hospital Over Bias," *Chicago Defender*, June 21, 1962, 2.

[96] Ivan Allen's testimony is quoted in Kruse, *White Flight*, 206.

[97] Bell v. Georgia Dental Association, 231 F. Supp. 299—Dist. Court, ND Georgia 1964.

[98] "Grady Hospital Desegregated, Patients Re-Grouped Quietly A Month Before Deadline," AC, June 2, 1965, 6.

[99] Author Interview, Bill Pinkston, April 23, 2009.

[100] Jill Quadagno, "Promoting Civil Rights Through the Welfare State: How Medicare Integrated Southern Hospitals," *Social Problems* 47:1 (February 2000), 68-89; E. H. Beardsley, "Goodbye to Jim Crow: The Desegregation of Southern Hospitals, 1945-1970," *Bulletin of the History of Medicine* 60 (Fall 1986), 367-386.

[101] "Grady Accepts Its First Negro Woman Physician," ADW, April 20, 1962, 1.

[102] "Atlanta Medical Society Relaxes Race Rules," *Journal of the National Medical Association* 54:5 (September 1962), 628-629.

Chapter 8

[1] John D. Thompson, M.D., "'A look at the Sunny Side': A Report for the Decade 1961-1971 on the Activities of the Department of Gynecology and Obstetrics, Emory University School of Medicine, Grady Memorial Hospital, Atlanta, Georgia," Hamilton, AHC; A. S. Llorens, J. H. Grinder, J. D. Thompson, "Maternal Mortality at Grady Memorial Hospital: A 13 Year Survey," *American Journal of Obstetrics and Gynecology* 87 (October 1, 1963), 386-393.

[2] W. N. Long, "A Description of the High Risk Pregnancy Project at Grady Memorial Hospital," *Journal of the Medical Association of Georgia* 55:12 (December 1966), 497-499.

[3] *The Grady News* 17:3 (March, 1965), 1.

[4] Ibid.

[5] Thompson, "'A Look at the Sunny Side,'" 14-15.

[6] *Grady-HSP News*, October 1971, 3. In 1926, Dr. Emmett Colvin became the first person to finish Grady's residency in Gynecology and Obstetrics. By 1971, 123 physicians had completed the residency program at Grady.

[7] Robert A. Hatcher to Grace Towns Hamilton, October 5, 1973, Hamilton, AHC.

[8] Sharon Johnson, "A Woman's Voice in Medicine," *New York Times*, May 13, 1984, A53.

[9] "Brann Wants World's Mothers and Children Healthy," *Emory Report* 50:1 (August 25, 1997).

[10] Richard J. Whitley, M.D., Andre J. Nahmias, M.D., *et. al.*, "Vidarabine Therapy of Neonatal Herpes Simplex Virus Infection," *Pediatrics* 66:4 (October 1980), 495-501.

[11] Richard J. Whitley, M.D., *et. al.,* "Vidarabine Versus Acyclovir Therapy in Herpes Simplex Encephalitis," *New England Journal of Medicine* 314:3 (January 16, 1986), 144-149.

[12] Author Interview, Andre J. Nahmias, M.D., June 21, 2011.

Chapter 9

[1] "Impact of Governmental Programs on Public Hospitals–Directions for the Future. Conference Report," *Public Health Reports* 83:1 (January 1968), 53-60; Alice Tetelman, "Public Hospitals–Critical or Recovering?" *Health Services Reports*, 88:4 (April 1973), 296-297.

[2] *FDHA Annual Report, 1967*, 3.

[3] *FDHA Annual Report, 1970*, 29.

[4] *Hospital-Based Emergency Care: At the Breaking Point*, (Washington D.C.: Institute of Medicine, 2006).

[4] *FDHA Annual Report, 1970*, 36.

[5] *FDHA Annual Report, 1987*, 11.

[6] "$26 Million Eyed in Grady Growth," AJ, January 27, 1970, 1.

[7] Cresap, McCormick and Paget, Inc., "Grady Memorial Hospital and Emory University School of Medicine: A Long-Range Plan for Future Development," September 29, 1969, Hamilton, AHC.

[8] Ibid.; "$26 Million Eyed in Grady Growth," AJ, January 27, 1970, 1.

[9] *The Grady News* 22:2 (February-March 1970), 1.

[10] "Nation's First Regional Kidney Center Opens," *The Grady News* 22:5 (August-September 1970), 1; Christene Bledsoe, "State Help Urged by Kidney Center," AJ, January 22, 1969, 6A; Phil Garner, "Governor Pledges Kidney Unit Fund," AJ, February 17, 1969, B6; "Kidneys Via Computer," AJC, January 25, 1970, E1.

[11] "They Talk a Lot But…" AJ, October 21, 1970, 1.

[12] "Fact Sheet, Grady Memorial Hospital, 1975" (author's collection).

[13] Ibid.

[14] *Annual Report of the Grady Memorial Hospital 1933*, 7.

[15] June J. Isaf and Maria T. Alogna, "Better Use of Resources Equals Better Health for Diabetics," *American Journal of Nursing* 77:11 (November 1977), 1792-1796.

[16] Dr. Davidson discontinued the use of oral hypoglycemic drugs at Grady after the current medical literature indicated that those agents did little good and probably led to early death for some patients.

[17] John K. Davidson, ed., *Clinical Diabetes Mellitus: A Problem-Oriented Approach* (New York: Thieme, 1986).

[18] "John K. Davidson III," AJC, December 19, 2008, C10.

[19] Christena Bledsoe, "Hospital's Huge: That's Part of the Trouble," AJ, October 18, 1970, A1.

[20] While daily inventory logs for the hospital's supply closets are unavailable, the views that nurses in Black Grady had fewer available resources than those in White Grady was repeated frequently in the black press. By 1962, more than three-fifths of the hospital's patients were crowded into the black wards with the reported number of black patients at Grady ranging from two-thirds to four-fifths. See, for example, "Grady Hospital to be Relieved of Some Of Its Handicaps," ADW, February 4, 1962, 4, and Pete Greenlea, "J. B. Blayton Named to Bond Commission," ADW, March 8, 1962, 1.

[21] On the concept of "suburban secession," see, Kruse, *White Flight*, 234 ff.

[22] Kruse, *White Flight*, 243-246.

[23] John York, "Fulton Official Urges State to Run Grady," AJ, July 20, 1970, A2.

[24] Ibid.

[25] *Report of the National Advisory Commission on Civil Disorders,* (New York: Bantam Books, 1968), 1.

[26] Frederick Allen, "State Funding of Grady is Sought By Fulton Panel" AC, January 4, 1973, A8.

[27] Cresap, McCormick and Paget, Inc., "Grady Memorial Hospital and Emory University School of Medicine," IV-20, Hamilton, AHC.

[28] Gene Stephens, "Grady Status Periled, Accreditation is Challenged," AC, March 20, 1970, A3.

[29] "Success is a Quiet Word, Atlanta's Herman J. Russell," AI, April 15, 1961, 8.

[30] Reportedly the chamber, unaware of his race, sent H. J. Russell an invitation by accident, and he became a member of the chamber simply by filling out the membership form and attaching the required dues. There are reasons to doubt this official tale. Under the chamber's rules, for H. J. Russell to become a member, someone belonging to the chamber had to have nominated him. For his part, H. J. Russell was coy about which white business leader might have been his sponsor. He told *The Atlanta Inquirer* that he wasn't sure who might have nominated him, simply saying, "a number of my business associates are presently members of the Chamber of Commerce." See, "Local Chamber of Commerce Accepts First Negro Member," AI, November 24, 1962, 1.

[31] Wright, Jackson, Brown, Williams & Stephens, Inc., "Grady Hospital: Inside and Out," 83, Hamilton, AHC.

[32] Ibid.; *The Grady News* 22:5 (August-September, 1970), 1.

[33] Jim Gray and Celestine Sibley, "Rep. Hamilton Loses Hospital Authority Post," AC, February 20, 1975, A1; "An Outrage," AC, February 21, 1975, A4.

[34] Jim Gray and Celestine Sibley, "Rep. Hamilton Loses Hospital Authority Post," AC, February 20, 1975, A1.

[35] "Fulton Delegates Call Hearing, Rep. Hamilton Lauded," AC, February 21, 1975, A11.

[36] "'Grady Was His Focus in Life': Surgeon, Mentor Served on Hospital Board 21 Years," AJC, March 22, 2011, B6.

[37] "Mrs. Yancey, Mrs. Wilson Head Hosp. Campaign's Women's Group," ADW, February 7, 1959, 1. ("Mrs. Yancey stated…As it is now, my husband spends many hours a week driving to and from the downtown hospital.")

[38] Meeting an urgent need, the clinic grew to include a four-bed ward, an operating room, and outpatient rooms; it attracted black and white volunteer physicians, Catholic and non-Catholic, who saw patients each weekday. By 1958, the laity and diocese began developing a hospital in southwest Atlanta. Amanda Fuhr Cooke, "A Study of the Development of the Catholic Colored Clinic, October 1944-January 1947," M.S.W. Thesis, Atlanta University, 1947; "Catholic Colored Clinic, Atlanta, Georgia," *The Medical Missionary,* September-October 1955, 115.

[39] "Holy Family Hospital and Center $3-Million Project," ADW, June 12, 1958, 1; "Hospital Campaign Steering Committee Formulates Plans," ADW, February 10, 1959, 1; "Mrs. Yancey, Mrs. Wilson Head Hosp. Campaign's Women's Group," ADW, February 7, 1959, 1; "Holy Family Hospital Fund Drive Opens," ADW, March 4, 1959, 1.

[40] Gene Stephens, "Grady Status Periled, Accreditation Status Threatened," AC, March 20, 1970, A3.

[41] Ibid.

[42] Ibid.

[43] *Physician Manpower in Georgia: Report of the Task Force for Physician Manpower to the Georgia Comprehensive Health Planning Council* (Atlanta: Georgia State Department of Public Health, Office of Comprehensive Planning, 1969), 9.

[44] Ibid., 14.

[45] Ibid.

46 "Black Medical Renaissance in Atlanta," *Ebony* 34:2 (December 1978), 104.

47 H. M. Gloster, "New Medical School at Morehouse?" *Journal of the National Medical Association* 66:2 (March 1974), 167-170; Louis Sullivan, "The Education of Black Health Professionals," *Phylon* 38:2 (2nd Quarter, 1977), 191-192.

48 Louis W. Sullivan, "Statement Announcing Receipt of Provisional Accreditation by the School of Medicine at Morehouse College, April 24, 1978," *Journal of the National Medical Association* 70:11 (November 1978), 867-868.

49 Louis W. Sullivan, "The Morehouse School of Medicine: A State of Mind, of Mission, and of Commitment," *Journal of the National Medical Association* 75:8 (August 1983), 837.

50 "Morehouse and Medicine," AC, July 28, 1974, 16-A; Nancy Lewis, "Morehouse Gets Med School Grant," AC, July 28, 1974, 5-B; Hugh M. Gloster, "Progress of the Morehouse College Medical Education Program," *Journal of the National Medical Association* 66:6 (November 1974), 530-531.

51 Robert A. Holmes, "The Georgia Legislative Black Caucus: An Analysis of a Racial Legislative Subgroup," *Journal of Black Studies* 30:6 (July 2000), 776-777.

52 Sullivan, "Statement Announcing Receipt of Provisional Accreditation by the School of Medicine at Morehouse College, April 24, 1978," 867-868.

53 "Fact Sheet, Grady Memorial Hospital, 1975" (author's collection).

54 Alexis Scott Reeves, "Grady Burn Team Was Ready for Patients," AC, April 5, 1977, A6.

55 Jerry Schwartz and Craig R. Hume, "67 Are Killed and 29 Hurt As Jet Crashes in Paulding," AC, April 5, 1977, 1; Alexis Scott Reeves, "Grady Burn Team Was Ready for Patients," AC, April 5, 1977, A6; Robert Lamb, "Kennestone Gets Flood of Victims," AC, April 5, 1977, A6.

56 Alexis Scott Reeves, "Grady Burn Team Was Ready for Patients," AC, April 5, 1977, A6.

57 Arthur P. Liang, et. al., "Risk of Breast, Uterine Corpus, and Ovarian Cancer in Women Receiving Medroxyprogesterone Injections," JAMA 249:21 (June 3, 1983), 2909-2912.

58 Howard W. Ory, et. al., "Mortality Among Young Black Women Using Contraceptives," JAMA 251:8 (February 24, 1984), 1044-1048.

59 The book was republished in 1978 and retitled in later editions as *Trauma to the Heart and Great Vessels*.

60 P. N. Symbas, "Autotransfusion from Hemothorax: Experimental and Clinical Studies," *The Journal of Trauma* 12:8 (August 1972), 689-695.

61 "Dr. Nanette Kass Wenger" *http://www.nih.gov/changingthefaceofmedicine/physicians/biography_330.html* accessed March 11, 2011.

62 Patricia Guthrie, "A Place of Their Own: Grady Hospital's Sickle Cell Center Sets the Standard for Treatment of Care," AJC, October 31, 2000, D1; "Persistence Pays Off for Sickle Cell Activist," AJC, October 31, 2000, D5.

63 Holmes, "The Georgia Legislative Black Caucus," 768-790.

64 Guthrie, "A Place of Their Own," D1.

65 Keith Wailoo, *Dying in the City of the Blues: Sickle Cell Anemia and the Politics of Race and Health* (Chapel Hill: University of North Carolina Press, 2001) analyzes the politics associated with the disease in the United States during the 20th Century.

66 "Where You Live," AJC, June 7, 2000, B2; Alicia Lurry, "Scholarship & Research: Pain Assessment Now Fits in Doctor's Palm," *Emory Report*, November 13, 2000.

67 Minutes, Hughes Spalding Pavilion Study Committee, April 15, 1980, Hamilton, AHC.

68 Hughes Spalding Pavilion Study Committee Report [1980], Attachment C, Hamilton, AHC.

69 Hughes Spalding Pavilion Study Committee Report [1980], Appendix H, Hamilton, AHC; Hughes Spalding Pavilion Study Committee Report [1980], Attachment C, Hamilton, AHC.

70 Hughes Spalding Pavilion Study Committee Report [1980], Attachment C, Hamilton, AHC.

71 Ibid.

72 Minutes, Hughes Spalding Pavilion Study Committee, March 18, 1980, Hamilton, AHC; Minutes, Hughes Spalding Pavilion Study Committee, April 15, 1980, Hamilton, AHC.

73 *Family Circle*, April 27, 1982; *Ladies Home Journal*, November, 1982.

74 John Pekkanen, "Our No. 1 Medical Need," *Reader's Digest*, July 1985, 100-106.

75 Tetelman, "Public Hospitals—Critical or Recovering," 296.

76 J. W. Pinkston, Jr., "Statement to the Health Subcommittee of the House Committee on Ways and Means on the Hospital Financing Crisis Confronting Many Public and Private Non-Profit Hospitals, February 29, 1980." Typescript, GMHC, AHC.

77 Ibid.

78 Ibid.

79 "Fulton Commission Asks Ga. to Give Grady $29 Million," ADW, October 3, 1978, 5.

80 "Fulton Tax Bills List Grady Hospital Funding," ADW, July 26, 1979, 10.

81 This developed out of a call from Fulton County Commissioner Michael Lomax for a county-wide investigation into Grady's long-term finances. See, "Fulton to See Tax Hike, Grady Cutbacks," AC, May 4, 1979, C1.

82 George Rodrigue, "Grady May Face Revenue Woes In '80, Study Finds," AC, October 26, 1979, C1.

83 "Experts Say Emory-Grady Ties Unbalanced in School's Favor," AC, October 11, 1979, C2.

84 See, for example, "More Pay For Employees At Grady OK'd," ADW, May 29, 1977, 2; "$75 Million Budget Proposed for Grady," ADW, November 30, 1978, 2.

85 Pinkston, "Statement to the Health Subcommittee…."

86 Ibid.

87 Kevin Sack, "Grady Budget Cut; Most Workers Won't Get Raises," AC, January 26, 1982, A10.

88 "Board of Trustees Report," *FDHA Annual Report, 1982*, 6-7.

89 *FDHA Annual Report, 1982*, 15.

90 Asa G. Yancey, M.D., "Medical Director's Report," *FDHA Annual Report, 1982*, 18.

91 "Authority Supports Proposed Sales Tax," *GMH-HSCH Together* 2:8 (October 1982), 1; J. W. Pinkston, Jr., "Thoughts of the Executive Director," *GMH-HSCH Together* 2:8 (October 1982), 2.

92 "Morehouse Granted Access to Grady Memorial Hospital," ADW, March 6, 1984, 1.

93 Renee D. Turner, "Fulton OKs 30-year Contract With Grady for Care to Poor," AC, June 21, 1984, 4-D.

94 "AIDS Testing Available for High Risk Groups in GA," ADW, December 9, 1986, 1; "Grady Hospital Says They Will Test Pregnant Women for AIDS Virus," ADW, July 5, 1987, 1; "Commissioners Suggest Hughes Spalding Become AIDS Treatment Center," ADW, August 23, 1987, 1.

95 "Rape Crisis Center Plans Taking Shape in DeKalb; Community Task Force Working to Open Facility in Two Years," AC, January 4, 1988, 1A; "Rape Crisis Center to Open in Decatur," AC, May 18, 1989, 4A; "DeKalb Rape Hotline to Start But Clinic is Still Up in the Air," AC, October 30, 1989, 1C; "Rape Clinic Opens in DeKalb, Medical Center Sets Up Program," AC July 20, 1990, 6E.

96 "Grady Hospital: Renovate or Start Over?" AC, September 19, 1987, B1; "Young Voices Support For New Grady Hospital, Domed Stadium," AC, October 1, 1987, E4; "Grady Officials Favor Renovation Instead of Constructing A New Hospital," AC, December 21, 1987, B1.

97 "Grady Officials Propose $295 Million Renovation," AC, March 17, 1988, A1.

98 Cynthia Tucker, "It's Past Time for Hughes Spalding to Find New Role," AC, March 26, 1988, A19; Mike King, "Racial Conflicts Threatening Grady's Renovation, Future," AC, April 21, 1988, A1; "Grady Needs Renovating No Matter What," AC, April 15, 1988, A18; Jeff Dickerson, "It's Time For Commission To Do Its Job For Grady," AC, April 8, 1988, A18; Gary C. Richter, "Letter to the Editor," AC, April 12, 1988, A18.

99 Cynthia Tucker, "Commissioners Take Wrong Tack on Grady Funds," AC, April 23, 1988, A21.

100 "Fulton Warns Grady to Resolve Gripes or Imperil Renovation," AC, April 7, 1988, A1; "Fulton Funds Grady Planning, Withholds Commitment on Renovation," AC, May 13, 1988, A14.

101 "Officials Vote to Close Hughes Spalding Hospital," ADW, September 4, 1988, 1; "Spalding Closing Concerns Community," ADW, September 6, 1988, 1.

102 David Corvette, "Fulton, DeKalb Asked for $7.3 Million to Help Grady Serve Poor," AC, June 23, 1988, C4.

103 Mike King, "Racial Conflicts Threatening Grady's Renovation, Future," AC, April 21, 1988, A1.

104 Scott Bronstein, "Board Votes to Close Hughes Spalding, Use It For Grady Overflow," AC, September 2, 1988, A21; Eugene Morris, "Board's Plan to Close Hughes Spalding Stirs Ires of Doctors, Union," AJC, September 4, 1988, C2.

105 Mike King, "Racial Conflicts Threatening Grady's Renovation, Future," AC, April 21, 1988, A1.

106 Hal Straus, "Grady Study Cites Need to Improve; Hospital Board, Facilities, Treatment Draw Criticism," AC, December 2, 1988, A17.

107 Personal Communication with Dr. Loughlin.

108 S. E. McNagny and R. M. Parker, "High Prevalence of Recent Cocaine Use and the Unreliability of Patient Self-Reporting in an Inner-City Walk-In Clinic," JAMA 267:8 (February 26, 1992), 1106-1108; M. E. Sprauve, M. K. Lindsay, S. Herbert, & W. Graves, "Adverse Perinatal Outcome in Patients Who Use Crack Cocaine," *Obstetrics and Gynecology* 89:5 (Part 1) (May 1997), 674-678.

109 W. R. Sexson and D. Carson, "Cocaine, Birth Weight, and Lack of Prenatal Care in Special Care Nursery Admissions," *Pediatric Research* 25 (1989), 230A; William R. Sexson, "Cocaine: A Neonatal Perspective," *The International Journal of the Addictions* 28:7 (1993), 585-598; "Crack: The City's Plague," AJC, January 3, 1992, A1; "Pumpkin, Crack Baby Who Moved City, 'Still Doesn't Have a Home,'" AJC March 26, 1992, A13; "A Big Hand for Baby Pumpkin," AJC, November 28, 1991, A1; "The Crack Epidemic, Saving Not One Life, But Two, Project Prevent: Grady Program Treats Pregnant Women Addicted to Cocaine," AJC, November 28, 1991, E1; "A Pound of Despair," AJC, October 26, 1991, A1; Jeff Dickerson, "Crack Babies Cost Us More Than $504 Million," AJC, September 20, 1991, A18; Claran S. Phibbs, David A. Batemen, and Rachel M. Schwartz, "The Neonatal Costs of Maternal Cocaine Use," JAMA 266:11 (September 18, 1991), 1521-1526.

110 Sidney H. Newman, Mildred B. Beck and Sarah Lewit, "Abortion, Obtained and Denied: Research Approaches," *Studies in Family Planning* 1:53 (May 1970), 7.

111 David Beasley, "Georgia Abortion Bills Planned," AC, July 4, 1989, A1; David K. Secrest and Sam Hopkins, "Miller, Murphy Cautious on Abortion," AC, July 8, 1989, C1; David Beasley, "Grady Caught in Abortion Fight," AJC, July 23, 1989, B1; Lorri Denise Booker and Bill Rankin, "Anti-Abortion March Targets Grady Clinic," AJC, October 1, 1989, C1; Margaret L. Usdansky and Lorri Denise Booker, "The 1990 Legislative Session–Abortion Issue Wanes as Lawmakers Approach Election Year," AC, December 25, 1989, E1.

112 Author Interview, Bill Pinkston, April 28, 2009.

113 "Grady Chief Pinkston Retiring After Quarter-Century's Tenure," AC, October 29, 1989, C1; Celestine Sibley, "Grady Babies Still in Good Hands," AC, December 3, 1989, M1.

114 Douglas B. Kendrick, et. al., *Blood Program in World War II* (Washington D.C.: Office of the Surgeon General, Department of the Army, 1964); "Douglas Kendrick, Army Surgeon, 87," *New York Times,* September 6, 1994, B6.

115 "The President-Elect," *Journal of the National Medical Association* 26:4 (November 1934), 176; John A Kenney, "The Negro's Contribution to Surgery," *Journal of the National Medical Association* 33:5 (September 1941), 208.

[116] "Two Morehouse Alums Mark 70th Anniversary," AJC, July 12, 2007, E7; "Carolyn D. 'Marge' Yancey: Educator, Civic Volunteer," AJC, November 17, 2010, B9; Asa G. Yancey, Sr., "The Surgical Program of a Veterans Administration Hospital," *Journal of the National Medical Association* 47:2 (March 1955), 77-87; Asa G. Yancey and Herbert F. Ryan, "The Surgical Residency Programs of the Tuskegee VA Hospital and The Hughes Spalding Pavilion, Atlanta," *Journal of the National Medical Association* 54:2 (March 1962), 166-173.

[117] John Head, "Role Model in Two Eras," AC, October 31, 1995, A12; Doug Cumming, "Hamilton Holmes Dies, Integrated UGA," AC, October 25, 1995, C1.

[118] "Volunteers Take Needed Project," *The Grady News* 21:2 (February 1969), 1.

[119] "Robert Regenstein, 83, Chairman of Atlanta retailers, Grady board," AJC, March 14, 1998, D10.

[120] Mary B. Mallison, "Editorial: Unsinkable Nurses," *The American Journal of Nursing* 88:10 (October 1988), 1317.

Chapter 10

[1] Rashi Fein, Ph.D., "What is Wrong With the Language of Medicine?" *New England Journal of Medicine* 306:14 (April 8, 1982), 863-864.

[2] Ibid.

[3] National Research Council, *Hospital-Based Emergency Care: At the Breaking Point* (Washington D.C.: The National Academies Press, 2007).

[4] David Pendered, "Bill Would Pressure Grady Hospital; Threatened With Loss of Funds Without New Adviser," AJC, January 18, 1997, C1; Susan Meyers Laccetti, "Grady Study Must Benefit Taxpayers," AJ, November 13, 1997, A22.

[5] Susan Meyers Laccetti, "Grady Study Must Benefit Taxpayers," AJ, November 13, 1997, A22.

[6] Kathey Alexander, "Gingrich Urges Local Privatization; He Calls For Study, Citing Grady as Possible Candidate," AJ, March 27, 1995, A1.

[7] Chuck Bell, "County's Property Reappraisal Raises Fear of Boost in Taxes," AJC, June 28, 1990, H4; Brian McGreevy, "Notices of New Tax Valuations to Hit Mail," AJC, January 24, 1991, H1; Mark Sherman, "Atlanta-Fulton Appraisals to Increase 30%," AC, January 24, 1991, D1; Chuck Bell, "Tax-Bite May Not Be As Bad As Anticipated," AJC, January 31, 1991, H9; Barbara Ann Moore, "Bad News, Tax Values Mailed Out," AJC, Febraury 14, 1991, K3; Mark Sherman, "Atlanta-Fulton Appraisals Hike Land Values 50%," AC, March 17, 1991, C1.

[8] Mark Sherman, "Angry Fulton, City Taxpayers Get Busy Signals," AJC, March 21, 1991, F6; "Taxes Hit Home, Property Owners Complain," AC, March 29, 1991, E4; Mark Sherman and David Corvette, "Tax Revolt on Pryor Street," AJC, April 18, 1991, D3; Dick Williams, "Voters Should Build on Fulton County's Tax Revolt," AJC, April 20, 1991, A19; "The Fulton Tax Revolt," AC, April 27, 1991, B3; "Appraisers Accuse Foes of Slander," AC, November 23, 1991, B3.

[9] David Corvette, "Lomax: Palm Trees Are 'Indoor Park' Paid For By Feds," AC, May 23, 1991, E3; Dick Williams, "Lomax Problems Began With $8,500 Palm Trees," AJ, February 8, 1991, A19; Dick Williams, "Lomax Talks Substance, Symbols Could Undo Him," AJ, May 11, 1991, A15.

[10] Eddie Lee Brewster, "Taxpayers Voice Anger at Public Hearing Here," ADW, April 21, 1991, 1.

[11] Dick Williams, "Lomax Talks Substance, Symbols Could Undo Him," AJ, May 11, 1991, A15.

[12] Ibid.

[13] "Grady Was Main Reason for Tax Boost, Lomax Says," AJC, May 23, 1991, H5.

[14] Joe Earle, "Tax Protesters Seek to Broaden Support Net for Grady Hospital," AC, August 1, 1991, H11.

[15] Ibid.

[16] Brian McGreevy, "Group Seeking Lomax Recall Comntinues With Meetings," AJC, September 19, 1991, K2; Ken Foskett, "North Fulton Taxpayers Blast Grady," AC, January 9, 1992, E2.

[17] Dick Williams, "Recall Drive Falls Short But Sends Loud Message," AJC, November 23, 1991, A19.

[18] "Fulton's Lomax Facing Crisis Moment," AC, April 14, 1991, G1.

[19] Brown-Nagin, *Courage to Dissent*, 243-244; Kruse, White Flight, 223 ff.

[20] David Corvette, "Lomax: Palm Trees Are 'Indoor Park' Paid For By Feds," AC, May 23, 1991, E3.

[21] Dick Williams, "Lomax Reacts To Protests By Choosing to Race-Bait," AJC, May 28, 1991, A13.

[22] David Corvette, "Focus: Hospital Renovation," AC, October 29, 1991, B3; "The Cost of Grady's Facelift," AC, November 5, 1991, A18; "Pay Attention to LOGTAX," AJ, October 30, 1991, A8.

[23] Ken Foskett, "Proposed Budget for Grady Increases Almost 10 Percent," AJ, November 26, 1991, B1.

[24] Richard Whitt, "Minority Deals Raise Grady Price," AC, May 21, 1991, D1; Ken Foskett, "Angry Lomax Delays Filling Grady Positions," AC, December 19, 1991, D6; Ken Foskett, "Hospital Authority Chairman is Ousted," AC, January 9, 1992, E2; Ken Foskett, "Grady Board Implements Ethics, Purchasing Policies," AC, January 28, 1992, C2.

[25] "Grady Budget Hearing Tonight Amid Sour Relations," AJC, January 8, 1992, C3; "North Fulton Taxpayers Blast Grady," AJC, January 9, 1992, E2.

[26] Ken Foskett, "Hospital Authority Chairman is Ousted," AJC, January 9, 1992, E2.

[27] Frank L. Wilson, "Letters to the Editor," AJ, January 24, 1992, A8.

[28] Ken Foskett, "North Fulton Taxpayers Blast Grady," AJC, January 9, 1992, E2.

[29] Ken Foskett, "Employees, Taxpayers Blast Grady," AJC, January 16, 1992, E9.

[30] Ken Foskett, "Grady Budget Hearing Tonight Amid Sour Relations," AJC, January 8, 1992, C3.

[31] Ken Foskett, "'The Right Thing': No Fulton Tax Hike," AJC, January 23, 1992, D2.

[32] Robert L. Brown, "Fulton-DeKalb Hospital Authority Role Vital in Grady's Funding," AJ, November 3, 1992, A21.

[33] Ken Foskett, "Fulton, DeKalb Halt Funds For Grady," AC, May 21, 1992, E3.

[34] "End Budget Flap Before Grady is Hurt," AC, May 26, 1992, A8.

[35] Ken Foskett, "Grady Executive Warns of Dire Cuts in Services, Staff," AC, May 29, 1992, D1; "Accountability is the Issue in Budget Battle at Grady," AJ, June 1, 1992, A12; "Counties, Grady Must Declare Truce," AC, June 2, 1992, A10.

[36] Ken Foskett, "Accord Reached in 2-Month Grady Budget Dispute," AC, June 23, 1992, D4.

[37] Richard Whitt, "A Poor Prognosis–Plagued By Problems, The Grady Hospital Renovation is Falling Behind Schedule and Running Over Budget," AJC, April 16, 1991, D1.

[38] Ibid.

[39] Richard Whitt, "Minority Deals Raise Grady Price; 3 White Companies to Get Extra $49,800 to Divvy Up Renovation," AC, May 21, 1991, D1.

[40] Ibid.

[41] Richard Whitt, "A Poor Prognosis–Plagued By Problems, The Grady Hospital Renovation is Falling Behind Schedule and Running Over Budget," AJC, April 16, 1991, D1; Ken Foskett, "Delays at Grady Irk DeKalb Officials," AJC, April 26, 1991, D3.

[42] Ken Foskett, "A New Emergency Room at Grady; Hospital Dedicates $7.2 Million Facility, Defends Level of Care, AC, June 26, 1992, G1.

[43] Ken Foskett, "AIDS Clinic Seeks Room To Breathe," AC, May 27, 1992, B1; Ken Foskett, "2 Emergency Room Patients at Grady Die After Neglect," AC, June 25, 1992, A1.

[44] Holly Morris, "70 Activists Demonstrate Outside Grady, Call for Expanded Disease Clinic," AJC, June 1, 1991, C6; "Support Grady's AIDS Clinic Plans," AJC, July 5, 1992, C6.

[45] Norma Wagner, "DeKalb Withdraws Support for Relocating AIDS Clinic," AC, June 24, 1992, D3; Ken Foskett, "AIDS Clinic Proposal Falls Short in Fulton; Commissioners Cite Disputes With Grady," AJC, July 2, 1992, E3.

[46] Ken Foskett, "AIDS Clinic Seeks Room To Breathe," AC, May 27, 1992, B1; Ken Foskett, "Fulton Agrees to Midtown AIDS Clinic; Grady Still Needs DeKalb's OK to Buy Property," AC, July 16, 1992, C2.

[47] "Elton John Helps Open Grady Clinic; Facility for AIDS Patients Overcame Early Obstacles," AJC, October 15, 1993, H2.

[48] "Grady Clinic For AIDS Patients Opens Doors, Even Critics Offer Praise For Facility," AJC, August 10, 1993, C3; Holly Morris and Anne Rochelle, "AIDS Services: State-of-the-Art Care More Readily Available; Facility Gets High Marks for Privacy, Treatment," AC, October 14, 1993, B1.

[49] Morris and Rochelle, "AIDS Services: State-of-the-Art Care More Readily Available," B1.

[50] S. Nesheim, S. Henderson, M. Lindsay, J. Zuberi, V. Grimes, et. al., "Prenatal HIV Testing and Antiretroviral Prophylaxis at an Urban Hospital, Atlanta, Georgia, 1997-2000," *Centers for Disease Control and Prevention Morbidity and Mortality Weekly Report*, January 2, 2004, 1245-1248.

[51] Ellen Whitford, "Hughes Spalding Comes Back to Life for Poor Kids," AJC, May 20, 1993, N4.

[52] "Children's Healthcare to Manage Grady Unit," AJC, December 16, 2005, F4.

[53] H. Kenneth Walker, et. al, ""Georgia to Georgia Initiative," *British Medical Journal* 331:7510 (July 21, 2005), 237.

[54] Anita Sharpe, "Cash on Delivery: How 'Medicaid Moms' Became A Hot Market for Health Industry; Doctors and Hospitals Chase Poor Pregnant Women and Fat Reimbursements," *Wall Street Journal*, May 1, 1997, A1.

[55] Shelley Emling, "Competing for the Health-Care Dollar, Public Hospital Prepares to Become Self-Sufficient," AC, April 21, 1993, B1; Helene Cooper, "If Poor Can Choose, Will They Pick Urban Hospitals?" *Wall Street Journal*, November 2, 1993, B1.

[56] Ken Foskett, "The People's Diagnosis May Bring Cure To Grady's Ills," AJC, January 2, 1993, B5.

[57] Carrie Teegarden, "Grady Reinventing Itself: Charity Hospital Must Compete to Become Functional Facility With a Future," AJC, April 28, 1996, G4; Devid Pendered," Grady to Shut Down HMO Program," AC, September 28, 1999, E1.

[58] David Pendered, "Grady's Critical Condition," AJC, September 11, 1994, G1.

[59] Ibid.

[60] David Pendered, "Grady Staff Cuts May Be In Offing," AJC, August 13, 1994, G1.

[61] David Pendered, "Grady's Critical Condition–Battle Brewing over Hospital Funding Care–Critics Find Support in Unexpected Corners," AJC, September 11, 1994, G1.

[62] Ibid.

[63] David Pendered, "Grady to Shut Down HMO Program; Prompted By State Action, Trustees Vote to End Both Medicaid and Managed Care Plans," AC, September 28, 1999, E1.

[64] David Pendered, "Grady Holds off $10 fee; Near Riot: Raucous Meeting Ends with 30-day Delay on Prescription Drug Price Increase," AJC, March 23, 1999, A1.

[65] Ibid.

[66] David Pendered, "Grady Slashes Free Services to Economize," AC, March 15, 1999, C1.

[67] David Pendered, "Grady Coalition's Efforts Show Results," AC, December 16, 1999, D7; David Pendered, "Activists Want Charges Dropped," AC, September 25, 1999, E2.

[68] David Pendered, "Grady Holds off $10 fee; Near Riot: Raucous Meeting Ends with 30-day Delay on Prescription Drug Price Increase," AJC, March 23, 1999, A1.

[69] Andy Miller, "Board Approves Plan to Give Grady More Than $50 Million," AC, October 14, 1999, F3; David Pendered, "Grady: Fulton Reneging," AJC, January 18, 2000, B1.

70 Rhonda Cook, "Senate Ex-Leader Indicted," AJC, June 24, 2004, A1; John McCosh, "Walker's Dealings Draw New Scrutiny," AJC, August 10, 2002, H6.

71 James Salzer, "Augusta Legislator Convicted of Fraud," AJC, June 4, 2005, A1; idem., "Federal Prison Awaits Walker; Ex-Legislator Gets 10 Years for Fraud," AJC, November 30, 2005, A1; Jay Bookman, "Sen. Walker Gets What He Courted," AJC, December 12, 2005, A13.

72 James Salzer, "Walker's Daughter Admits to Tax Fraud," AJC, July 13, 2005, D1; idem., "Walker's Daughter Gets Probation, Fine," AJC, December 20, 2005, C3.

73 The data for county contributions are taken from the FDHA's *Annual Reports* for Grady Hospital for the years 1995 through 2005.

74 Inflation is calculated from data on the Federal Reserve Bank of St. Louis (FRED) website, *http://www.research.stlouisfed.org/fred2/categories/32419*

75 Percentages are calculated from data in the FDHA's *Annual Report* for the years 1995 through 2005.

76 Dick Williams, "A $37 Million Soaking," *Atlanta Business Chronicle*, August 31, 2007, 26A.

77 Patricia Guthrie, "New Cancer Center Dedicated at Grady," AJC, March 4, 2003, D12; Giannina Smith, "Beating Back Breast Cancer for Minorities," *Atlanta Business Chronicle*, May 24, 2010.

78 Arthur L. Kellerman, "Crisis in the Emergency Department," *New England Journal of Medicine* 355:13 (September 28, 2006), 1300-1303.

79 Ibid.; National Research Council, *Emergency Medical Services: At the Crossroads* (Washington D.C.: The National Academies Press, 2007); idem., *Hospital-Based Emergency Care: At the Breaking Point* (Washington D.C.: The National Academies Press, 2007).

80 National Research Council, *Hospital-Based Emergency Care*, 37-80.

81 Ron Martz, "Grady Teaches Iraq-Bound GIs Lessons on Saving Lives," AJC, July 19, 2004, A1.

82 Yolanda Rodriguez, "New Grady Clinic Tries to Put Spanish Speakers at Ease," AJC, May 20, 2002, A1; Allison Shirreffs, "Dr. Genao's Labor of Love: Aiding Latinos at Grady," *Atlanta Business Chronicle*, May 14, 2004.

83 Patricia Guthrie, "Georgia Taxpayers Foot Bill for Crisis Care for Illegals," AJC, December 4, 2005, E13; Yolanda Rodriguez, "New Grady Clinic Tries to Put Spanish Speakers at Ease," AJC, May 20, 2002, A1.

84 Ernest Holsendolph, "Hospital Board Chief Dedicated to Improvement," AJC, September 3, 1993, D1.

85 Martha Ezzard, "Grady's Shpeherd Not Easy to Replace," AJC, December 31, 2000, B3; "William Shepherd, Jr.," AC, June 19, 2010, B7.

86 "Hospital Official From St. Louis to Head Grady," AC, August 24, 1989, C1; "4-Year Renovation Awaits New Grady Chief," AC, August 25, 1989, D2; Ken Foskett, "Grady Hospital Chief to Quit February 26," AC, January 21, 1993, F2; "Grady's Tough Act to Follow," AC, January 25, 1993, A10.

87 Shelley Emling, "Competing for the Health-Care Dollar, Public Hospital Prepares to Become Self-Sufficient," AC, April 21, 1993, B1.

88 David Pendered, "L.A. Medical Center Chief Named New Grady CEO," AC, February 26, 1994, D4.

89 "Last Day Arrives For Grady CEO," AJC, June 7, 2003, H1.

90 "Grady Health System Names CEO," AJC, April 26, 2003, G2; "Next Chief of Grady Prepares For Change," AJC, April 30, 2003, B8; "Medicine is CEO's Mission," AJC, June 9, 2003, B1; "Children's Healthcare to Manage Grady Unit," AJC, December 16, 2005, F4; "Grady CEO Resigns," AJC, November 15, 2005, A1.

91 Patricia Guthrie, "Grady Awaits Aid With '05 Debt at $12.5 Million," AJC, February 23, 2006, F3; Andy Miller, "Grady Spends Big Bucks to Solve Budget Crisis," AJC, December 14, 1996, A1.

92 Gary M. Pomerantz, *Where Peachtree Meets Sweet Auburn: A Saga of Race and Family* (New York: Scribner, 1996), 499-500.

93 Helen C. Smith, "Black Arts Leader Finds You Can Go Home," AJ, March 4, 1987, B1; idem., "Arts Notes: Fulton County To Sponsor National Black Arts Festival," AJC, November 17, 1986, B2; idem., "Black Arts Festival Exceeds Its Organizers' Expectations, AC, August 9, 1988, E1.

94 Pomerantz, 504-505.

95 Ben Smith, Tom Bennett, "Manuel Maloof: 1924-2004: Atlanta Legend Caustic, Beloved," AJC, August 8, 2004, A1.

96 Metro Atlanta Chamber of Commerce, "Greater Grady Task Force Members Named," Press Release, April 9, 2007; Metro Atlanta Chamber of Commerce, "Greater Grady Task Force Final Recommendations," Press Release, June 25, 2007.

97 Metro Atlanta Chamber of Commerce, "Greater Grady Task Force 'Ready and Willing' to Recruit Leaders to Serve on Nonprofit Board if Asked," Press Release, July 13, 2007.

98 Ibid.

99 Jonathan Springston, "Citizens Fight Privatization of Grady Hospital," *Atlanta Progressive News*, September 1, 2007; Craig Schneider and Gayle White, "Is Race on Table in Grady Choice?" AJC, December 15, 2007, A1.

100 Mike King, "Saving Grady: How to Nurse the State's Largest Public Hospital Back to Health," AJC, July 1, 2007, B6; Mike King, "Moving Beyond the Trauma Unit," AJC, July 29, 2007, B6; Shaila Dewan and Kevin Sack, "A Safety-Net Hospital Falls Into Financial Crisis," *The New York Times*, January 8, 2008, 1A.

101 "Grady Hospital Admits McNugget of an Idea: The fast-food restaurant," AJC, May 4, 1991, A1.

102 Jim Stewart, "Emergency Room, There's No Such Thing as a Good Weekend at Grady," AC, November 12, 1973; Jane Hansen, "Grady's New Facilities Mark End Of Era," AC, June 27, 1992, D1.

103 David Corvette, "Fulton Considers Handing Crestview Nursing Home to Grady," AJ, July 20, 1989, B3; Ann Hardie, "Answering the Cries From Crestview Nursing Home," AC, November 23, 1993, C1.

[104] Ibid.; "Nursing Home Patients Face Filth, Neglect," AC, October 7, 1993, D1; "Nursing Home Should Be Salvaged," AC, October 9, 1993, A14; "A New Day at Crestview," AC, December 25, 1990, D1; "Fulton Considers Handing Crestview Nursing Home to Grady," AC, July 20, 1989, B6.

Afterword

[1] David Kindred, "Barkeep, Politician, Regular Guy: Maloof Lived Dreams of Immigrant Dad," AC, September 6, 1995, C3.

Index

A

Abercrombie, T. F., 124
Abernathy, Ralph David, 184, 188
abortion, 195, 233–234
Academy of Medicine, 64, 66
ACCA. *See* Atlanta Committee for Cooperative Action
acyclovir, 198
Adair, Mrs. A. O., 11
Adams, Jacob, 196
Addams, Jane, 61, 77
Agnes Scott College, 63, 119, 260
Agwunobi, Andrew, 262–263
AIDS. *See* HIV/AIDS
Aids Coalition to Unleash Power (ACT-UP), 249–250
Alaska Railroad, 141
Albert Steiner Charitable Fund, 99, 100
Alexander, James F., 13
Alford, C., 198
Allen, Ivan E., 94
Allen, Ivan, Jr., 183, 192
All Saints Episcopal Church (Atlanta), 214
Alston & Bird, 171, 265
Alston, Mrs. Philip, 155
Alston, Philip H., Jr., 208
Alston, Robert, 25
American Academy of Orthopaedic Surgeons, 211
American Academy of Pediatrics, 197
American Association for Cancer Research, 100
American Cancer Society, 100
American College of Obstetricians and Gynecologists, 197
American College of Surgeons, 102, 131
American Diabetes Association, 205
American Gastroenterologic Association, 73
American Heart Association, 138, 140, 156, 158, 219
American Hospital Association, 110
American Medical Association (AMA), 45, 73, 132, 152, 173, 185, 238
American Medical Women's Association, 218
American Red Cross, 84, 146, 256
American Society for Clinical Investigation, 142
American Society for the Control of Cancer, 100
American Trust and Banking Company, 60
Amster, Ludwig, 79, 82
Amster, Mrs. Ludwig, 79
Amster's Sanatorium, 79
Andrews, Charles R., 51
Andrews, E. E. (Shorty), 160
Andrews, Ludie, 84–85

Aoki, F. Y., 198
APM Management Consultants, 239
Appeal for Human Rights, 183
Archives of Grady Municipal Hospital, White Unit, 102
Archives of Internal Medicine, 140
A Report on Hospital Care of the Negro Population of Atlanta, Georgia, 169–171
Arkwright, Mrs. Preston, 71
Arkwright, Preston, 136, 148
Armstrong, William, 39
Arnold, Virginia, 84
Arthur Andersen and Company, 200
Arthur Young & Associates, 231
Art Institute of Chicago, 53
Ashford, Bailey, 74
Atkins, Samuel, 221
Atlanta Artificial Kidney Center, 202
Atlanta Association of Independent Insurance Agents, 165
Atlanta Athletic Club, 132
Atlanta Benevolent Home, 8, 9, 11, 12, 18, 32, 33, 35, 63
Atlanta Board of Education, 62, 64, 169, 176, 196, 236–237
Atlanta Brewing and Ice Company, 99
Atlanta Chamber of Commerce, 94, 116, 134, 183, 186, 192, 208, 224. *See also* Metro Atlanta Chamber of Commerce.
Atlanta Christian Council, 184
Atlanta College of Physicians and Surgeons, 42, 43–44, 45, 64, 76, 89, 131
Atlanta Committee for Cooperative Action (ACCA), 184, 185, 208
Atlanta Constitution, 25, 27, 29, 186
Atlanta Council on Human Relations, 186
Atlanta Daily Constitution, 9, 10
Atlanta Evening News, 80
Atlanta Federal Savings & Loan Association, 167
Atlanta Federation of Trades, 57, 129, 134
Atlanta-Fulton County Stadium, 79, 208
Atlanta, Ga.:
 bond referendum (1910), 53
 bond referendum (1914), 55–56, 57, 86, 105
 bond referendum (1915), 58
 bond referendum (1929), 103
 bond referendum (1940), 134–135, 158
 bond referendum (1962), 182
 Centennial Olympic Park, bombing of, 258
 citizens' hospital committee (1888), 19, 33

299

Atlanta, Ga. (continued):
  citizens' hospital committee (1890), 32, 38
  city council, 8, 19, 30, 32, 36, 38, 60, 75–76, 87, 92, 117, 165
    committee on hospitals and charities, 98, 101–102, 103, 109, 127
    finance committee, 48
    hospital committee (1873), 8
    hospital committee (1876), 8–9
    relief committee, 15, 16, 30, 41
  civic leaders in, 10, 11, 12, 20, 30, 34, 38, 57, 86, 172, 173–174
  Confederate Soldiers Home, 28, 63
  firefighters, 36, 104
  origins of, 4–5
  ward physician system in, 16–17
  Yellow Fever Hospital, 10
Atlanta Georgian, 80
Atlanta Graduate School of Physicians and Surgeons, 101–103
Atlanta Hadassah, 218
Atlanta Hebrew Benevolent Congregation, 99
Atlanta Hospital, 13
Atlanta Housing Authority, 265
Atlanta Inquirer, 184, 187, 189, 190
Atlanta Journal, 10, 178, 186
Atlanta Life, 265
Atlanta Medical Association, 174, 176, 186, 188, 212, 214, 221
Atlanta Medical College (1854), 4, 6, 8, 9, 33, 41–42
Atlanta Medical College (1913), 43, 45, 46, 64, 75, 83, 88, 131
Atlanta Medical Society, 184, 185
Atlanta Opera House, 71
Atlanta Paper Company, 114
Atlanta Retail Merchants Association, 95, 223
Atlanta Savings Bank, 60
Atlanta School of Medicine, 43, 44, 45, 64, 76, 78, 83
Atlanta Society of Medicine, 39, 65, 77
Atlanta South Central Community Mental Health Center, 202
Atlanta Surgical Infirmary, 11
Atlanta Terminal Company, 60
Atlanta University, 183–184
Atlanta University Center, 174, 213, 214
Atlanta Urban League, 104–105, 141, 169–171, 174, 175, 181, 213
Atlanta West Point Railway Company, 60
Atlantic Coast Line, 26
Atlantic Steel Company, 92, 130
Augusta Medical College, 4, 5
Avon Foundation For Women, 258

B

Baird, James B., 51
Ball, Thomas, 57
Banting, Frederick Grant, 204
Baptist Tabernacle Church (Third Baptist Church, Atlanta), 82, 93, 105, 106
Barnes, Roy, 255, 258
Barnes, W. Harry, 236
Bartholomew, Rudolph A., 127–128
Battle Hill Sanitarium, 127, 135
Bayer Corporation, 120
Baylor University Hospital, 128
Bay State Club, 27
Bearden, W. Horace, 187, 216
Beavers, James, 93
Beckwith, John, 16
Beecher, Henry Ward, 7
Beeler, J. Moss, 129–130, 165
Beeson, Paul, 141–142, 143, 144, 157, 174, 178, 179
Bell, Charles, 181
Bellevue Hospital (New York), 51, 64, 143
Bell, George, 97
Bell, Roy C., 184, 184–187, 188, 190
Bell, Tom, 265
Bennett, Ivan, Jr., 160
Benton, Curtis, 160
Bergmark, Jean B., 172, 173
Berman, Joseph F., 116
Best, Charles H., 204
Bethesda Naval Hospital, 158
Biggers, Stephen Terry, 5
Biggins, J. Veronica, 255
Bird and Howell (law firm), 171. *See also* Alston & Bird
Bird, F. M. "Buster," 171
Black, Charles, 186, 189
Black, George, 77
Black, Mary Ellen (Nellie) Peters, 16, 69, 77, 95
Blackmon, Douglas A., 61
Blackstock, George, 81
Blair Kern & Adams (architectural firm), 92
Blalock, Tully, 152
Bloom, Walter, 156–157
Blount, Annie, 160
Blount, John, 160
Blue Cross and Blue Shield, 177
B'nai B'rith, 62
Bobby Jones Golf Course, 181
Body, Phillip, 142
Boland, Kells, 11
Bolster, Paul, 224
Booker T. Washington High School, 90
Borders, William Holmes, 183
Borders, William Holmes, Jr., 208

Boston City Hospital, 138
Boston Merchants Association, 27
Bothwell, L. J., 14
Boykin, Eleanor, 92
Boykin, John A., 108
Boy Scouts of America, 95
Brandon, Mrs. Morris, 71
Brann, Alfred, Jr., 196, 197–198
Brannon, Emmett, 139, 140
Brawley, Otis, 258
Brewster, Tomlinson Fort, 47–48, 50–51, 76
Bridges, Anna Y., 52
Broughton, Len, 105–107
Brown, Calvin A., Jr., 213
Brown, Charlie, 209
Brown, Julius, 32
Brown, Louis C., 213
Brown, Murray, 178
Brown, Robert L., 245, 255–256, 260, 265
Brown, Ronald, 265
Brown v. the Board of Education of Topeka, Kansas, 181, 190
Broyles, Mrs. Arnold, 94
Bryant, George M., 57
Budinscak, Guy, 265
Buff, Julian H., 110
Bullock, Rufus B. B., 32
Burkhalter, Mark, 241, 242
Burnham, Daniel H., 14
Burton, Emma, 37
Busbee, George, 214
Bush, George H. W., 252
Business Week, 222
Butler, Henry Rutherford, 114
Butler, Nicholas Murray, 77
Butler Street YMCA, 184, 209

C

Cale, Elsworth, 180
Calhoun, Abner W., 13, 16, 32, 38, 39, 42, 63–64, 76
Calhoun, Andrew, 63
Calhoun, King & Spalding, 36
Calhoun, Patrick, 36
Calhoun, Phinizy, 145, 160
Calhoun, Susan, 63
Calhoun, William L., 19
Call, L. P., 120
Calloway, Fletcher Maye, 84
Campbell, Bill, 264
Camp, Milton, 75–76
Candler, Asa, 45, 92, 94, 115, 131
Candler, Howard, 115
Candler, Scott, 260

Candler, Warren, 45, 115
Capital City Bank, 31
Capital City Club, 69
Carnegie, Andrew, 27, 42, 43
Carnegie Foundation, 42, 45
Carroll, Sister Mary Cecilia, 13
Carter, Jimmy, 194, 207, 264
Cary, Freeman, 160
Case Western Reserve University, 196
Cates, Goodwyn (Shag), 209
Catholic Colored Clinic, 173, 211. *See also* Holy Family Hospital
Caton, William, 151, 156
Centers for Disease Control and Prevention (CDC), 145, 198
Central Georgia Company (railway), 60
Central Ivy Street Hospital, 13, 15, 17
Central of Georgia (railway), 4
Central Presbyterian Church, 48, 52, 162, 251
Centre College, 131
Chamberlain, Roderick L., 174
Chance, Ira, 120
Charleston, S.C.:
    earthquake of 1886, 25
Chattahoochee Brick Company, 32, 60–61, 61, 73
Chenopodium, 74
Chesire, M. A., 98–99
Chicago Defender, 136, 191
Children's Healthcare of Atlanta, 251
Cincinnati General Hospital, 110, 128
Citizens and Southern Bank, 207, 223
Citizens Bank Company, 167
Citizens Trust Bank, 167, 260
Citizens Trust Company, 208
City Federation of Women's Organizations, 93, 94
Civil Rights Act of 1964, 192, 193, 242–243
Civil War, 6, 7–8, 21, 24, 33, 60, 61, 63
    Army of Northern Virginia, 49, 60, 63
    Battle of Petersburg, Virginia, 24
    First Battle of Manassas, 52
Clark, Septima, 190
Clayton County, 257
Clement, Bill, 265
Clement, Rufus, 174, 183-184
Cleveland, Grover, 27, 46, 78
Cleveland, R. H., 104
Clinton, Bill, 252, 259, 264
COAHR. *See* Committee On Appeal for Human Rights
Cobb County, 181, 206
Cobb, Mrs. Thomas R. R., 71
Cobb, W. Montague, 179
Coca-Cola Company, 45, 92, 115–116, 139, 148, 166
Colby, James, 204
Cole-Layer-Trumble Company, 240

Coleman, Allen R., 187
Coleman Industrial Contractors of Atlanta, 247
Coles, Mrs. A. P., 93
Columbia Psychoanalytic Clinic, 164
Columbia University, 77, 101, 164
Committee On Appeal for Human Rights (COAHR), 183, 186, 187, 189, 190
Concerned Black Clergy, 255, 266
convicts, 60–61, 72–73, 96
Cook County Hospital, 120, 128
Cooper, A. B., Sr., 189
Cooper, Hunter P., 19, 32, 38, 39, 71, 131
Cooper, Manuel, 160
Cornell University School of Medicine, 140
Correll, A. D. "Pete", 265
Cotton, Dorothy, 190
Cotton States and International Exposition (1895), 46
Council of Jewish Women, 167
Council of Urban Health Providers, 222
Council on Medical Education, 113
Courier (Rome), 24
Cournand, André F., 143
Cousins Properties, 265
Cox, Harvey, 107, 117, 118
Cramer, Ann, 255
Crawford Long Memorial Hospital, 84, 130, 149, 170, 173 207, 211, 221
Creel, George, 94
Cresap, McCormick and Paget, 201, 207, 212
Crestview Nursing Home, 243, 253
Currie, Marie, 101
Currier, Charles E., 92
Curtis, Howard Candler, 85
cytokines, 142

D

Dahlonega, Ga., 23
Dalton, Mildred, 137
D'Alvigny, Noel, 4, 6
D'Arcy, William, 115
Darling Brothers, 32, 36
Darnell, Emma, 249
Daughtry, Estelle, 67, 68
Davidson, John K. III, 204-205
Davidson, John S., 35–36
Davis, Edward C., 84
Davis-Fisher Sanatorium, 84
Davis, Murphy, 255
Davison, T. C., 101–102, 102
Decatur Cooperative Ministry, 228
DeKalb County, Ga., 134-135, 144-145, 149, 224, 227-228, 242, 254, 257, 261, 263

DeKalb County Commission, 135, 150, 222, 224, 226, 231, 236, 241, 243, 245-246, 247, 248, 249, 255, 264
DeKalb Rape Crisis Center, 228
DeLaurentis, Susan, 198
Delmonico's, 26
Deloitte, 265
Depot Medroxyprogesterone, 217
Derr, John, 65
desegregation
   Atlanta public schools, 181, 187
   Grady Memorial Hospital, 169-190
   golf courses, 181, 193
   parks, 182, 193
Detroit General Hospital, 237
Dickerson, Durice, 121
Dillard University, 264
Divine, K.C., 16
Dobbs, Mrs. Samuel Candler, 94
DOBBS, RAM & Company, 265
Dobbs, Samuel Candler, 112, 115–117, 231
Dodson, Henry, 209
Donaldson, Henry R., 101–102
Dooly, Isma, 55–56
Dortch, Tommy, 265
Doyle, Alexander, 29
DPM-Heery, 247
Drew, A. Farnsworth, 123
Drew, Charles, 175, 178
DuBois, W. E. B., 61
Duke University, 138, 140
Durham, Plato T., 45
Durham, W. M., 16, 19
Duvall, W. O., 167–168
Dwelle's Infirmary, 173

E

East Atlanta Land Company, 33
Eberhart, Charles, 228
Eckman, James, 219, 220
Ecole des Beaux-Arts, 101
Economic Opportunity Atlanta (EOA), 202, 206
Egan, Mike, 209
Egleston Children's Health Care System (hospital), 173, 197, 251
Eisenhower, Dwight D., 148
Elizabeth Glaser Pediatric AIDS Foundation, 198
Elkin-Cooper Sanatorium, 131
Elkin, Dan C., 112–113
Elkin, William S., 39, 45, 46, 51, 71, 89, 130–131
Elks Club, 120
Ellijay, Ga., 23
Ellis, John H., 11

Ellis, Mrs. William, 71
Elsas, Jacob, 31, 32, 37, 38, 59, 101–102
Elsas, May and Company, 31
Elsas, Mrs. Ben, 94
Emory Clinic, The, 149-150, 151–152, 156
Emory College, 45
Emory Regional Perinatal Center, 196
Emory University, 45, 66, 89–90, 119, 130, 144, 148
   desegregation, resistance to, 179
   donors, 150
   and Oglethorpe University, 136
   Candler School of Theology, 45, 63–64
   Hughes Spalding Pavilion, and, 179–180
   Rollins School of Public Health, 258
   Woodruff Health Sciences Center, 265
Emory University Board of Trustees, 151
Emory University Hospital, 144–145, 145, 149, 152, 170, 173, 207. *See also* Wesley Memorial Hospital
Emory University School of Law, 46
Emory University School of Medicine, 44, 45, 46, 64, 74, 85, 101, 103, 105, 109, 131, 136, 138, 144, 177, 181, 204
   Abner Calhoun, M.D. Medical Library, 64
   Black Grady, and, 89
   black patients, and, 112
   Emory Clinic, and, 149
   desegregation of, 173, 212, 237
   Division of Neonatal-Perinatal Medicine, 197
   planning committees at, 144–145, 148, 149
   research growth at, 155
   White Grady, and, 107, 112, 114
Empire Real Estate Board, 185
English, Emily Alexander, 60
English, James W., 10, 32, 38, 59, 60, 72, 81
EOA. *See* Economic Opportunity Atlanta
Erwin, Thomas C., 99
Eskridge, F. Lewis, 51
Eskridge, Frank, 101–102, 104, 135
Etheridge, Elizabeth W., 148
Ettling, John, 73
Everhart, Lawrence, 127
Ewing, James, 100

F

Fambro, Lillie Mae, 84
Family Circle, 222
Fantus, Bernard, 120
Farris, Milton, 207, 249
FDHA. *See* Fulton-DeKalb Hospital Authority
Federal Reserve Bank of Atlanta, 130
Feebeck, Annie Bess, 82–83, 91, 98, 137
Fein, Rashi, 239

Fensch, Albert, 46–47
Ferguson, Ira, 137
Ferris, Eugene, 151, 156, 157, 158
Field, Mrs. Julian, 71
Fike, R. H. "Rube," 102, 104
Finley, Ada, 67, 68
First Congregational Church (Atlanta), 81, 167
First Iconium Baptist Church (Atlanta), 266
First Methodist Church (Atlanta), 27
Fischer, Luther C., 130, 149
Flexner, Abraham, 42–44, 86, 154
Foreman, Mrs. Robert, 71
Foreman, Robert L., 57
Forssmann, Werner, 143
Fort McPherson, 47, 83
Fort Stewart, 259
Fort, Vincent, 266
Fourth National Bank, 14, 60, 99
Franklin Hospital, 14–15, 34
Franklin, John B. 117–118, 128, 129
Franklin, Shirley, 264
Fraser, Carlyle, 185
Free Kindergarten Association (Atlanta), 77
Freeman, Malcolm, 195, 196
Friedewald, William, 142
Fuller, Drew, 227
Fulton Bag and Cotton Mills Company, 31, 37
Fulton Cotton Spinning Company, 31
Fulton County, Ga., 144, 149, 150, 206-207, 222, 223, 224, 236, 240-245, 254, 259, 261, 263, 266
Fulton County Commission, 167, 185–186, 188, 207-209, 210, 224, 225, 226, 227, 228, 229-231, 241, 243-244, 245, 246, 248, 249, 255, 257, 263
Fulton County Medical Society, 94, 109, 111, 113, 128, 131, 133–134, 134, 135, 140, 152, 154, 156, 157, 174, 185, 190, 191, 213
   and Emory University, 152–153
Fulton-DeKalb Hospital Authority 134-135, 147, 152, 158, 161, 165–167, 167, 171, 174, 179, 182, 185, 186, 191, 201, 202, 207-210, 212, 220-222, 226-227, 229-231, 237, 243-245, 254-255, 260, 261, 265-267. *See also* Metro Hospital Authority
Fulton, Robert, 254
Funk, Wells, and Dimon, 210

G

Gabram-Mendola, Sheryl, 258
Gainesville tornado (1937), 120
Gaines, W. J., 14
Gardner, Eugene Clarence, 32, 33–34
Gardner, Payne, and Gardner, 32
Garlington, Mrs. J. P., Jr., 167
Garner, Mary Elizabeth, 97–98

Garner, Mrs. John, 97–98
Gaston, James, 75
Gate City Drugstore, 167
Gayles, Joseph N., 213
Genao, Inginia, 259
General Education Board, 119
General Electric Company, 139
General Memorial Hospital for Cancer (New York), 100
Genuine Parts Company, 185
George, C. J., 47
Georgetown University, 166, 171
George Washington University School of Medicine, 197
Georgia Baptist Convention, 79, 105, 183
Georgia Baptist Hospital, 79, 82, 105, 127, 128, 170, 173, 183–184, 207, 211
Georgia Cancer Center for Excellence at Grady, 258
Georgia College of Eclectic Medicine and Surgery, 42, 45
Georgia Comprehensive Health Planning Council, 212
Georgia Dental Association, 193
Georgia Dental Society, 191
Georgia Department of Public Health, 202
Georgia Federation of Women's Clubs, 77
Georgia Hospital Association, 83, 128
Georgia Institute of Technology, 28, 31, 63, 77, 157, 252
Georgia Legislative Black Caucus, 214, 219
Georgia National Bank, 7
Georgia-Pacific Corporation, 265
Georgia Power Company, 130, 148, 260, 265
Georgia Railroad, 5
Georgia Railway and Electric Company, 50, 64, 130
Georgia, Republic of, 197, 252
Georgia State Federation of Labor, 57
Georgia State Medical Association, 213
Georgia State Nurses Association, 83
Georgia, State of, 67, 83–84
    Legislature (General Assembly), 4, 5, 48, 135, 207, 209–210, 219, 223, 229
    Maternal and Infant Care Council, 194
    physician shortages in, 212–213
    State Board of Regents, 166
Georgia State University, 220, 252, 265
Georgia Task Force on AIDS, 227
Geronimo, 47
Gholston, Ada, 188
Gibson, James O., 186
Giddings, Glenville, 145, 148
Gilbert, Joshua, 4, 5
Gill, H. L., 47
Giltner, Martha, 93
Ginder, David, 142
Gingrich, Newt, 239, 241

Glaser, Elizabeth, 198
Glenn, John Thomas, 30, 32, 36, 59
Glenn, Thomas K., 116, 119, 129–130, 135, 145, 165, 231, 266
Glenn, Wadley R., 130
Gloster, Hugh, 213
Glover, Renee, 265
Goddard, John, 155
Goddard, Mrs. John, 155
Golden, Abner, 139
Goldsmith, William, 78
Gone With the Wind, 4, 6, 142
Gordon, John B., 25
Gordon, W. W., 4
Grady, Ann Elizabeth Gartrell, 24–25, 36
Grady Coalition, 254–255, 266-267
Grady Health Foundation, 255
Grady, Henry (born 1788), 23
Grady, Henry Woodfin, 14, 16, 19, 21–28, 29, 30, 35, 36, 38, 62, 63, 78, 92, 136
   and New South 25, 26–27, 31, 32
Grady Hospital Aid Association, 55, 69, 71, 72
Grady, John W., 23
Grady, Jonathan, 23
Grady, Julia King (Mrs. Henry Woodfin Grady), 25, 36, 69
Grady, Leah King, 23
Grady Memorial Hospital
   African American patients at, 34, 46, 51, 55, 56
   African American physicians at, 170, 173–174, 184, 187
     teaching clinics for, 113–115, 178
   ambulance service, 57, 59, 67–69, 72
   anesthesiology department, 164–166
   Atlanta Regional Nephrology Center, 201
   Avon Cancer Center, 257
   Black Grady, 55, 55–56, 57, 88–89, 90, 91, 101, 103, 106–107, 107–108, 162, 179, 190
     fire at, 104
   board of trustees (1892), 39, 48, 51, 59–60, 59–63, 98, 105
   board of trustees (1931), 112
   building dedication (1892), 38, 40
   building dedication (1958), 162
   burn unit, 216, 232
   Butler Street Building, 54, 58
   cardiology at, 120, 143, 218–219
   children's ward, 48, 70, 87
   claims processing at, 200
   clinics at, 201–204
   computers at, 200–201, 202
   contagious disease hospital, 98–99
   cornerstone laying ceremony (1891), 35–36
   corruption probe, 109-112

Grady Memorial Hospital (continued)
  design of, 33–34, 40–41, 53–54
  diabetes clinic (1930s), 120
  diabetes patients at, 204–205
  Diabetes Treatment Center, 203, 245
  Elsas Clinic, 101
  Emergency Room, 249, 258–259
  Emory University, and, 107, 144, 145, 146, 147, 149–151, 151, 156, 157, 162, 166, 210, 225, 226–227, 230
  endowment funds at, 19
  Family Planning Program, 195, 196, 220, 256
  Family Planning Project, 164
  Feebeck Hall, 137
  foster grandparents, 256
  gastroenterology department, 164
  Glenn Building, 157
  Grady Rooters, 249
  Great Depression at, 122-124
  Greater Grady, idea of, 57, 86, 87, 94, 117–119, 145
  Grey Ladies, 146
  Gynecological Cancer Program, 164
  gynecology-obstetrics department, 162, 178, 184, 194–198
  hematology department, 164
  Hemophilia Clinic, 201
  Hirsch Hall, 92–94, 99, 167
  HIV/AIDS, and, 227, 248–249, 251
  Infectious Disease Clinic, 248–250
  innovation at, 119–120, 120–122
  International Medical Center, 259
  Interpregnancy Care Program, 197
  investigations of, 75–77, 108–110
  John Newton Goddard Memorial Chapel, 155
  kidney transplants, 202
  labor unrest at, 95–97
  Ladies Aid Society of Grady Hospital, 93, 95
  laundry workers at, 96
  Lindbergh Women and Children's Health Care Center, 259
  Loughlin Radiation and Oncology Center, 211
  Maternal and Infant Care Project, 164, 194–195
  maternity ward (colored), 56, 57
  maternity ward (white), 48, 67, 71
  medical board, 39, 48, 51, 62–63, 84, 94
  medical education and, 40, 41–42, 44, 66, 164, 165
  medical experimentation, 61
  medical records department, 200
  mission of, 50, 162, 165, 199, 223, 253
  Muscular Dystrophy Clinic, 201
  neonatology, 180
  Nephrology Center, 201–202
  neurology department, 164
  new central building (1958), 158-160, 161–163, 165

Grady Memorial Hospital (continued)
  Night General Admission Clinic, 202
  nursing at, 6, 14, 47, 88, 90–94, 98, 107, 114, 125, 126, 134, 137, 179, 229, 232-233, 236, 260
    and housing, 41, 47, 55, 57, 58, 67, 72, 91, 92–95, 137, 186,
    and salaries, 47, 48, 94, 125, 225
    diabetes, 203–204
    schools. *See* Grady Memorial Hospital, nursing schools at
    shortages, 88, 94, 97, 166, 179, 235, 254, 258
    working conditions, 47, 51, 82-84, 93, 126, 167, 179
  nursing schools at, 48, 51–52, 67–69, 82–84, 85, 88, 90-92, 98, 103, 162, 188, 220
  obstetrics department. *See* gynecology-obstetrics department
  origins of, 32–33
  outpatient pharmacy
    fee hike (1982), 225-226
    fee hike (1999), 254-255
  pathology department, 164
  patient satisfaction, 205–206
  pediatric AIDS clinic at, 198
  pediatric intensive care unit, 203
  picketing of, 186, 187
  Poison Control Center, 203
  privatization, 49–51, 239, 254, 266–267
  Psychiatric Day Center, 201
  Psychiatric Emergency Clinic, 202
  psychiatry department, 164
  racial desegregation, 56, 169–190
  radiology department, 162–164
  Rape Crisis Center, 216, 228
  renovation of, 210, 228–230, 239–240, 243, 247
    and Hughes Spalding Pavilion, 229
  research at, 41, 65, 67, 72–75, 106, 112, 117, 119, 120-121, 138-143, 144, 145, 149, 152, 155–156, 157, 160, 164, 165, 195-198, 217–218, 220, 250, 257–259
  rodents at, 104, 107
  School of Medical Technology, 162, 173, 180
  School of Radiologic Technology, 162, 173, 180
  Sickle Cell Center, 219–220
  Social Service Department, 126–127, 160
  surgery at, 48, 113, 119, 217–218
  Thyroid Clinic, 256
  Trauma Center, 222, 235, 247
  uncompensated care, and, 200, 223–224, 248, 250, 252, 253, 255, 257, 258, 259
  volunteers at, 71–73, 82, 94, 100, 120, 146, 147, 154-155, 157, 162, 167, 203, 211, 214, 216, 232, 256
  White Grady, 55, 58, 83, 89, 91, 102, 102–103, 135, 190
  and Emory University School of Medicine, 107

Grady, William Sammons, 23
Grant, James P., 173
Grant, Lemuel P., 33
Grant, Robert P., 140–141, 179
Grant, Ulysses S., 63, 100
Great Atlanta Fire (1919), 81
Greater Atlanta Council on Human Relations, 186
Greater Grady Task Force, 265–266
Greater Travelers Rest Baptist Church (Atlanta), 214
Greeley, Horace, 7
Green, Alice G., 213
Greenberg, Jack, 185, 191
Griffin, Marvin, 162
Gwinnett County, 181, 206

H

Hall, H. Lee, 164
Hallinan, Paul, 211, 237
Hallman, Bernard, 157, 213
Hamilton, Grace Towns, 141, 169–176, 179, 186, 207–208, 209, 210, 221
Ham, John Wyley, 93, 95
Hardin, L. Sage, 48, 104–105
Hardin, Mrs. Allen S., 167
Hardy, John "Fats," 160
Harlem Hospital (New York), 123
Harper, Berrutha, 219
Harper, Kerry, 219
Harris, Arthur, 114
Harris, Claire, 84
Harris, James B., 176
Harris, Joe Frank, 214, 226
Harris Memorial Hospital, 173, 177
Harrison's Principles of Internal Medicine, 144
Hartsfield, William B., 128, 129–130, 162, 181
Harvard Field Hospital Unit, 141
Harvard University Medical School, 139, 218
Haverty, James J., 123
Hatcher, Charles, 227
Hatcher, Robert A., 196
Hawkins, John, 224
Heard, James, 81
Heart of Atlanta Hotel v. United States, 243
Hebrew Orphans Home, 31, 62
Heidt, John, 35
Hemphill, Mrs. W. A., 69
Hemphill, Paul, 264
Henry, John, 263
Hentz, Adler, and Shutze (architects), 137
Hentz, Reid and Adler (architects), 101
Hermann Hospital (Houston, Texas), 128
Herring, Virginia, 214
Hewes, G. Lemuel, 255

Hickam, John, 139
Hightower, Michael, 254
Hill, Benjamin H., 26, 29
Hill-Burton Act. *See* The Hospital Survey and Construction Act
Hill, Heyward, 186
Hill, Monique Walker, 257
Hillyer, George, 48–51
Hines, Darlene Clark, 91
Hines, Joseph, 117–118, 128, 129, 135
Hirsch, Joseph, 30, 32, 36, 38, 48, 51, 59, 61, 76, 92
  heirs of, 92, 95
Hirsch, Joseph H., 100
Hirsch, Morris, 61
HIV/AIDS, 198, 227–228, 233, 234, 248, 250–251
H. J. Russell & Company, 247, 265
H. M. Patterson Funeral Home, 69
Hobbs, A. G., 16
Holland, Bernard, 164
Hollowell, Donald Lee, 191
Holmes, Alfred "Tup," 181
Holmes, Hamilton E., 181, 237
Holmes, Hamilton M., 181
Holmes, Oliver, 181
Holmes, Robert, 224
Holmes v. Atlanta, 181
Holton, John, 180
Holy Family Hospital, 211–212. *See also* Southwest Hospital and Medical Center
Holy Innocents Mission, 77
Homer G. Philips Hospital (St. Louis), 174
hookworm, 72–74, 125
Hooper, Frank, 193
Hooper, Joseph, 146
Hope, John, 61
Howard, John, 151, 156–157
Howard University College of Medicine, 190
Howe, Julia Ward, 95
Howell, Albert, 32
Howell, Clark, 78–79, 108
Howell, Evan P., 25, 57, 78
Howell, Mrs. Clark, 69
Hughes Spalding Children's Hospital, 251, 263
Hughes Spalding Pavilion, 165, 166, 167, 185, 200, 220
  advisory board, 177, 179
  closing, 207, 208, 229–231
  dedication, 175–176
  development, 174–177
  naming, 175
  nursing, 179
  obstetrics at, 221
  physicians at, 212
  physician training at, 179, 208
  use of, 211–212

Humann, Phil, 265
Hunter, Floyd, 139
Hunter-Gault, Charlayne, 237
Hunter Street YMCA, 167
Hurst, J. Willis, 139, 157–158, 204
Hurt, Charles D., 75
Hurt, Joel, 33, 36
Hurt, John, 50
Hutcheson, Carl F., 108–109
Hynds, John A., 100

I

Igaravidez, Pedro Gutierrez, 74
infant mortality, 196, 197
Ingram, John F. Jr., 207
Inman, Hugh T., 32, 48
Inman, Mrs. Henry, 71
Inman, Mrs. Samuel, 69, 70
Inman, Samuel, 11, 14, 16, 19, 30, 32, 36, 38, 59, 63–64
Interdenominational Theological Center, 186
Interleukin-1, 142
International Cotton Exposition (1881), 28
International Society on Thrombosis and Haemostasis, 141

J

Jackson, Maynard, 214, 263, 264
Jackson, William 'Uncle Jack', 117
Jacobs, Thornwell, 134, 136
Javits, Jacob, 187
Jefferson Medical College, 47, 64
Jerusalem House, 250
Jewish Children's Service, 218
Jim Crow, 56, 78–79, 170-171, 172, 176, 180, 183, 191, 211
John D. Archbold Memorial Hospital (Thomasville, Ga.), 128
John, Elton, 250–251
Johns, Ethel, 91–93
Johns, Michael, 265
Johnson, Ben, 265
Johnson, "Doch," 84
Johnson, Lyndon Baines, 158, 193, 202, 206
Johnson, Robert B., 245, 246–247, 260–261, 261–262
Johnston, Richard H., 209
Johnston, Steve, 84, 93, 96–97, 98–99, 104, 111, 127
Joint Commission on Accreditation of Hospitals, 207, 212
Jones, Bird & Howell. *See* Bird and Howell
Jones, Bobby, 171
Jones, Boisfeuillet, 151
Jones, Herman D., 136
Jones, James, 104

Journal of the American Medical Association (JAMA), 120, 131, 142, 217
Joyner, Gordon, 244
Judaism, 11, 20, 37, 62, 167
Junior League of Atlanta, 167, 256
J. Walter Thompson (advertising agency), 169

K

Kantz, E. C., 77
Kellerman, Arthur, 258
Kelsey, Mrs. Frank III, 167
Kenan, Augustus Holmes, 47
Kenan, Thomas, 47
Kendrick, Douglas, 201, 212, 235–236
Kendrick, William, 42
Kennedy, Don (Officer Don), 167, 203
Kennedy, John F., 184, 187
Kennestone Hospital, 216
Kentucky School of Medicine, 105
Kerner Commission, 206–207
Kerner, Otto, 206
Key, James L., 94, 109, 111, 115, 120, 122
Keyserling, Harry, 227
Kilgore, Thomas, 213
Kimball, Allen, 41, 69, 72
King and Walker (architectural firm), 53
King, Martin Luther, Jr., 184, 188, 206, 209, 237
King, Martin Luther, Sr., 188
King's Daughters Hospital, 15, 19, 30, 69
King & Spalding, 166, 255
King, Walter, 74
Kirkwood, Ga., 69
Klein, Luella, 195–197
Knott, James J., 13
Kruse, Kevin, 182
Ku Klux Klan, 108
Kurt Salmon Associates, 222
Kurtz, Wilbur G., 123

L

Ladies Home Journal, 222
La Grange College, 130
Landford, Tom, 96
Lanier, Mary Day, 95
Lee, Robert E., 8, 60, 63
LeMaistre, Charles, 157
Lemoine, Anne, 216
Lewis H. Beck Foundation, 119
Lewis, Hezekiah, 188
Liebman, Frank, 100
Lister, Joseph, 65–66
Lockwood, Belva, 95
Logan, Joseph P., 13, 14, 16, 19

Logue, R. Bruce, 157, 158
Lomax, Michael, 211, 228, 229, 231, 240–241, 243–244, 254, 263
Longino, Thomas D., 16, 48, 76–77
Long, Margaret, 186–187
Long, Newton, 194
Loring, Ed, 255
Loughlin, Edward C., Jr., 210, 226–227, 229, 231, 243, 244
Louisville and Nashville Railroad, 26
Lower Our Grady Tax Coalition (LOGTAX), 241–243
Lowe, Tom, 211, 244
Lowry, Mrs. Robert J., 69, 93, 94, 95
Lowry, Robert J., 30, 32, 38, 59, 186
Lowry, Robert W., 7
Lula Grove Hospital and Training School for Colored Nurses, 83
Lyle, George, 109

M

MacAllister, Ann, 216
Macleod, John, 204
MacVicar Infirmary, 84
Maddox, Jr., Mrs. Robert, 71
Maddox, Lester, 183
malaria, 126, 148
Maloof, Manuel, 230, 231, 238, 245, 254, 264, 268
Manning, Gwendolyn Cooper, 189
Manuel's Tavern, 264
Marcus, Sidney, 209–210, 224
Marietta, Ga., 5
Marist High School, 166
Marquardt, Louie P., 57
Marsh, John, 142
Martin, Jim, 248
Martin, John D., 119
Marx, David, 94
Maryville College, 63
Massachusetts General Hospital, 157
Massachusetts Institute of Technology, 31, 53
Massee, Joseph, 140
Maupin, John, 265
Mayflower Garden Club, 167
May, Isaac, 31
Mays, Benjamin Elijah, 174, 175–176, 177, 182, 196, 213
McCord, Bert, 138
McCord, J. R., 136
McDonald's (Corporation), 245
McDonald, Timothy III, 255, 266
McGill University, 141
McGinty, A. Park, 120
McGroarty, Margaret A., 51–52
McKenzie, Sam Phillips, 187–188
McKinley, William, 82
McLendon's Medical Clinic, 173
McRae, Floyd, 42, 51, 79, 82
McWhirter, James, 50
Meador, James J., 52
Mears, Sue Ellen, 228
Medicaid, 193, 199, 200–201, 221, 223, 224–226, 233, 234, 236, 253, 254–255, 259, 265
  eligibility rules, 225
  reform of, 252
Medical Association of Atlanta, 211, 227
Medical Association of Georgia, 65, 191
Medical College of Georgia, 5, 157
Medical College of Oglethorpe University, 135
Medicare, 193, 199, 201, 207, 221–223, 252, 253, 259
Meharry Medical College, 178, 185, 189
Meltsner, Michael, 191
mental health, 165
Mercado, Flavia, 259
Mercer University, 132, 214
Merrill, Arthur, 139, 142
Methodist Episcopal Church, South, 37, 45, 106
Metro Atlanta Chamber of Commerce, 260, 265
Metro Hospital Authority, 135–136
Middleton, John, 190
Miles, Ruby Mae, 176
Milledge, John, 32
Milledge, Mrs. John, 11
Miller, Ed, 139
Miller, James, 162
Miller, Jim, 265
Miller, Mrs. James, 162
Millican, G. Everett, 104, 107, 184
Milton, Lorimer D., 167
Minkowski, Oskar, 204
minority contracting, 244–245, 247
Mitchell, George, Jr., 160
Mitchell, Margaret, 4, 142, 175
Mizell, Robert C., 145, 149
M & J Hirsch Company, 62
Moore and Marsh Company, 29
Moore, Mrs. William, 71
Moore, William A., 29–30, 32, 59
Moore, William W., Jr., 213
Moore, Wilmer, 45
Morehouse College, 61, 84, 167, 174, 176, 182, 187, 213, 263
Morehouse School of Medicine, 212–214, 229, 252, 265
  and Grady, 227–228
  Department of Health, Education, and Welfare, grant from, 213
  Emory University, agreement with, 230
  Hughes Spalding Pavilion, and, 230

Morgan, J. Pierpont, 26
Morris Brown College, 208
Morrison, Ursel Warren, 203
Mortgage Guarantee Building, 146
Mountin, Joseph W., 148
Murphy, Tom, 219, 226

N

NAACP. *See* National Association for the Advancement of Colored People
NAACP Legal Defense and Educational Fund, 191
Nabrit, James M. III, 191
Nahmias, Andre, 197–198
Nash, Frances, 137
Nash, Homer E., 114
National Association for the Advancement of Colored People, 105, 107, 186
National Association of Colored Physicians, Dentists and Pharmacists, 114
National Bank of the Republic (New York), 7
National Black Arts Festival, 264
National Council of La Raza, 259
National Dental Association, 185
National Distinguished Clinician Award, 220
National Heart Institute, 141, 179
National Institutes of Health, 141, 213, 252
National Medical Association, 114, 185, 214, 237
National Municipal League, 133
National Research Council, 143
National Surgical Institute, 11
National Urban League, 169
Neal, Thomas B., 59
Nelson, Levi B., 14
Nelson, Lillian, 98
Nelson, Mrs. Levi B., 16
New Deal, 99
   and Grady hospital, 124–127
     Civil Works Administration (CWA), 124
     Federal Emergency Relief Administration (FERA), 125–126
     Tennessee Valley Authority (TVA), 124–125
     Works Progress Administration (WPA), 124, 125, 148
Newell, Alfred, 87
New England Journal of Medicine, 239
New England Society of New York, 26
New South, The, 21, 25, 30, 31, 65, 73–74, 78–79, 85, 86, 162
New York Cancer Hospital, 100
New York Herald, 25
New York Sun, 73
New York Times, 118
Nicolson, William Perrin, 16, 19, 39, 42, 51, 76

Nightingale, Florence, 7
Nobel Prize for Peace, 237
Nobel Prize in Physiology or Medicine, 143, 204
Noble, George, 64
Norris, Jack C., 116
Norris, Thomas E., 213
North Carolina A&T University, 183
Northen, Charles, 69
Northern District Dental Society, 191, 193
North Georgia Dental Association, 184
North Georgia Dental Society, 188
Northside Hospital, 245
Norwood, Irving C., 73
Nunnally, Charles T., 87, 99
Nunn, Sam, 264
nursing. *See* Grady Memorial Hospital, nursing at

O

Oakland Cemetery, 4, 5, 27, 31, 52, 61, 64
O'Brien, Camille Louise, 85
Odd Fellows, 62
Oglesby, Stuart R., 162
Oglethorpe University, 63
O'Grady, William, 23
Ohio State University, 140
Olmsted, John C., 16
Olmsted, Mrs. John C., 16
Open Door Community, 255
Oppenheimer, Russell, 107, 112–114, 131–132, 136, 139, 144, 145
Order of Old-Fashioned Women, 71–72
Orme, Frances H., 19, 27
Orr, W. W., 94
Osler, William, 138
Owensby, Newdigate, 83
Oxford University, 142

P

Palmer, James D., 189, 212
Parker, Lella, 67, 68
Park, Roswell, 100
Parsons, Frank, 61, 136
Pasteur, Louis, 65
patient consent, 61
Patterson, Adah, 67
Patterson, Fred, 69
Patton, Carl, 265
Paullin, James Edgar, 102, 132, 136, 145
Paxon, Frederick, 45
Peachtree Golf Club, 182
Peachtree Orthopedic Clinic, 210, 211
penicillin, 142
Perlino, Carl, 227

Perry, Herman, 167
Peter Bent Brigham Hospital (Boston), 138, 139, 140, 141
Peters, Mary Jane, 77
Peters, Richard, 77
Pickens, Mrs. Staunton, 155
Piedmont Driving Club, 182
Piedmont Exposition (1887), 28
Piedmont Exposition (1889), 28
Piedmont Hospital, 138, 157–158, 160, 165, 170, 189, 207, 220, 221
Piedmont Sanatorium, 82
Pinckney, Charles, 13
Pine Center Garden Club, 167
Pinkston, John William "Bill," Jr., 180, 193, 201, 202, 208, 213, 220, 223, 225, 229, 233-235
Pittman, Louise Madeleine, 97
Pittman, Mrs. David, 97–98
Pittsburgh Courier, 177
Planned Parenthood, 256
Platt, Allan, 220
pneumonia, 121
Polk, James K., 5
Poole, George, 187
Powell, John, 160
Powell, Thomas S., 17, 18, 86
Presbyterian Hospital (Atlanta), 82, 98–99
Presbyterian Hospital (Philadelphia), 33
Princeton University, 63
Proctor, Henry Hugh, 81
Providence, R.I.
 hospital, 32
Provident Hospital (Chicago), 189
psychoanalytic institute (Atlanta), 165–166
psychoanalytic training, 165–166
public hospitals, 238
 economic rationale, 35, 50
 nature of, 9, 35, 50, 146, 222–223
Puckett, Clark, 57
Puerto Rico Anemia Commission, 74

Q

Quillian, Garnett, 94, 101–102

R

race violence, 1960s, 206
Race violence, 1906, 78–81, 180, 190, 191
radiology, 65, 140, 164
Radium Institute, 101
Ragsdale, I. N., 104
Rauber, Albert, 203
Reader's Digest, 222
Reagan, Ronald, 225

Reed, Thomas, 133
Reed, Walter, 61
Regenstein, Julius, 223
Regenstein, Mrs. Louis, 94
Regenstein, Robert, 212, 223, 226
Reinhardt College, 130
Renford, Edward, 237, 254, 262
Rhodes, Mrs. C. C., 11
Rice, John, 7
Richards, Dickinson W., Jr., 143
Richardson, Arthur, 151–153, 154, 156, 157, 162, 186, 192, 213
Rich, Mrs. Morris, 69
Rich's Department Store, 134, 183, 256
Rich, Walter, 94
Rivers, Eurith D., 125
Roberts, M. Hines, 180
Roberts, Stewart, 138
Robinson, Lyle, 132
Robinson, William, 57
Rockefeller Foundation, 91, 110, 117, 179
Rockefeller Institute Hospital, 141
Rockefeller, John D., 14, 15, 74
Rockefeller Sanitary Commission for the Eradication of Hookworm Disease, 74
Roentgen, Wilhelm, 65
Roe v. Wade, 233
Rogers, Revere, 187
Rolleston, Morton, Jr., 242–243
Rome Commercial, 24–25
Roosevelt, Franklin D., 124, 130, 133
Ross, Harold, 184
Rotary Club, 95
Russell, Herman J., 207, 208, 209, 210, 246, 292 n.30
Russell, Michael B., 265, 266
Russell, Richard B., 125, 166
Ryan White Comprehensive AIDS Resources Emergency Act, 198, 248

S

Sadler, John H., 202
Saint Bartholomew Hospital (London), 210
Salvation Army, 146
Savannah Poor House and Hospital Society, 3
Schrader, Mrs. R. F., 164
Schumann, Theo, 38
SCLC. *See* Southern Christian Leadership Conference
Scottish Rite Convalescent Hospital for Crippled Children, 99, 130, 173
Scottish Rite Medical Center, 251
Scott, Winfield, 23
Sexson, William R., 232
Shelton, Lee, 190, 191

Shepherd, Alana, 265
Shepherd Center (Atlanta), 265
Shepherd, William Clyde, Jr., 260
Shepperson, Gay B., 124
Sherman, William Tecumseh, 6, 8, 26, 134
Sherrill, A. F., 38
Shutze, Philip, 155
Sims, Walter, 108
Sisters of Mercy, 13–14
Skandalakis, Mitch, 242, 244, 254
Skellie, Bert, 266
Slater, Thomas, 114
Slaton, Jack, 69
Slavery By Another Name, 61
smallpox, 5, 9, 52, 56, 64, 72, 127
Smith, Alice Banks, 190
Smith, Claude, 61, 72–74
Smith, C. Miles, 185
Smith, Edwin, 190
Smith, Hoke, 78–79
Smith, J. R., 94
Smith, O. T., 120
Smith, Otis, 255
Smith, Relliford Stillmon, 114
Smith, Ruby Doris, 190
Smith, William Randolph, 119
SNCC. *See* Student Nonviolent Coordinating Committee
Snell, Donald, 262–263
Social Security Amendments of 1965, 193
Society of Catholic Medical Mission Sisters, 211
South Carolina State Hospital, 129
Southeastern Fire Insurance Company, 167
Southern Airways Flight 242, 216
Southern Baptist Convention, 105–106
Southern Bell Telephone and Telegraph Company, 167
Southern Christian Leadership Conference (SCLC), 188, 190
Southern Company, 130
Southern Dental College, 18, 72
Southern Homeopathic Medical Association, 27
Southern League, 28, 38
Southern Medical College, 13, 18, 42, 131
Southern Railway, 26, 139
Southern, Tom, 187
South View Cemetery Association, 167
Southwest Hospital and Medical Center, 221. *See also* Holy Family Hospital
Spalding, Hughes, 139, 151, 155, 162, 165, 171–173, 177, 212
Spalding, McDougald, and Sibley, 166
Spalding Pavilion. *See* Hughes Spalding Pavilion
Spalding, Robert D., 59, 71
Spanish-American War, 58, 59, 84

Spanish Flu Pandemic of 1918, 94
Spartanburg General Hospital, 129
Spelman College, 14–15, 30, 34, 84, 189, 191
Spelman Seminary. *See* Spelman College
Springfield, Ma.
   hospital in, 32, 33, 34
Spritzer, Lorraine Nelson, 172, 173
Standard Oil Company, 74
Stanley, O. J., 120
Stead, Eugene, Jr., 136, 138–141, 139, 142, 143, 145, 218
Steiner, Albert D., 99
Steiner Clinic, 99–101, 102, 125, 131, 154
Stetson, Eugene, 116
Stewart, William W., 189
Stiles, Charles Wardell, 73–74, 75
St. Joseph's Infirmary (Hospital), 12–13, 17, 49, 173, 166, 237
St. Luke's Episcopal Church (Atlanta), 15, 16
Stockton, F. O., 16
Stone, Harlan, 214, 216
St. Paul of the Cross (Atlanta), 212
Student Nonviolent Coordinating Committee (SNCC), 188, 191
sulfadiazide, 141
sulfanilamide, 120
sulfapyridine, 121
Sullivan, Louis, 214, 226, 227, 230
Summerall, Charles, 58
Summerall, William B., 52–54, 57, 66, 69, 86, 88
Sunday Telegram, 25
Sunshine, Harry, 167
SunTrust, 256, 265
Swift, Charles, 79
Swift, Lena, 79
S. W. Inman and Son, 63
Symbas, Peter, 217–218
syphilis, 67, 99, 182

T

Tait, C. Downing Jr., 164
Taliaferro and Noble Infirmary, 11
Talmadge, Eugene, 124–126, 125, 135
Talmadge, Herman, 166, 175
Task Force for Good Government, the, 242
taxation, 38
   Emory University and, 106–107
   fee-for-services model, 10, 50
   Grady hospital and, 38, 49, 50–51, 59, 85, 94, 105–106, 181, 206, 207, 222–225, 226, 235, 241–243
   hospitals and, 17
   property taxes, 207, 240, 245
   race and, 182
   special assessments, 10, 49–50

taxation (continued)
    tax revolt (1979), 224
    tax revolt (1991-1992), 240–242
The Atlanta Courier, 25
The Church of the Redeemer (Episcopal), 38
The Daily Herald, 25
The Hospital Survey and Construction Act (Hill-Burton Act), 170, 187
The Indian Removal Act, 23
The Interdenominational Ministerial Alliance, 185
The Johns Hopkins University, 33, 34, 67, 86
The Johns Hopkins University Hospital, 53
The Johns Hopkins University School of Medicine, 132
The Journal of the Medical Association of Georgia, 121
The Treaty of New Echota, 23
The White Company, 69
Third National Bank, 64
Thomas, Lillian, 84
Thompson, John Daniel "Dan," 164, 194–196
Thompson, Sumner, 250
Thomson, William D., 45
Thoreau, Henry David, 5
Thornwell College, 82
Thrash, Elmore C., 104, 109
Thymol, 74
Tibbs, Fannie, 67, 68
Time, 218
Todd, J. S., 16, 17
Truman, Harry S., 132, 170
Trust Company of Georgia, 116, 129, 130, 139, 166, 265
tuberculosis, 67, 72
Tucker, Cynthia, 229
Tucker, Henry Holcombe, 11, 19
Tucker, Mrs. Henry Holcombe, 11
Tulane University Medical Center, 86
Tuller, Mrs. William, 8
Turner, Fred J., 167, 168, 187
Tuskegee Institute (University), 208, 260
Tuskegee Veterans Administration Hospital, 175, 179, 189, 236
TWD, Inc., 265
Tygart, Algie, 67, 68
typhoid fever, 57

U

United Daughters of the Confederacy, 77
United Negro College Fund, 264
U.S. Commission on Civil Rights, 185, 187
U.S. Commission on Industrial Relations, 37
U. S. Department of Health, Education, and Welfare, 185, 194
U.S. Department of Public Health, 179
U.S. Public Health Service, 197
  Office of Malaria Control in War Areas, 148

U.S. Senate
    Commerce Committee, 192
United Textile Workers, 37
University of Alabama Medical School in Birmingham, 198
University of Chicago, 119, 175
University of Cincinnati, 138
University of Georgia, 11, 24, 44, 64, 77, 157, 165, 181, 237
University of Georgia Foundation, 166
University of Georgia Law School, 166
University of Iowa College of Medicine, 195
University of Maryland, 160
University of Michigan School of Medicine, 187
University of Mississippi, 197
University of North Carolina, 210
University of Oklahoma College of Medicine, 197
University of Pennsylvania, 131, 141
University of Pennsylvania Medical School, 210
University of Texas Medical School, 140
University of the South, 65
University of Toronto, 204
University of Virginia, 24
University of Washington, 142
Upton, Charles R., 13

V

Van Buren, Ebert, 191, 204
Vanderbilt University, 45
Vaughan, Virginia, 228
Veterans Administration Hospital (Atlanta), 152
Vidarabine, 198
Von Mering, Joseph, 204
Vroon, David H., 200–201

W

Walden, A. T., 190
Walker, Alex, 81
Walker, Charles, 256–257
Walker, Harry Leslie, 53
Wall, Bithel, 146
Ward, Horace T., 191
Ward, Richard S., 164
Ward, Sandy, 216
Warner, Clinton E., Jr., 184, 185, 186, 190, 221, 226
Warren, James, 139, 140, 142, 143
Warren, Roy D., 203
Watson, Tom, 78
Weens, Heinz, 140
Weiss, Soma, 138, 139, 141
Wellhouse, Henry, 100
Wenger, Nanette Kass, 218–219
WERD (radio station), 184

Wesley House, 37
Wesley Memorial Hospital, 66, 82, 112, 132. *See also* Emory University Hospital
Western & Atlantic Railroad, 4, 5
Western Electric Company, 234
West Georgia College, 157
West, Harry, 206
West Hunter Street Baptist Church (Atlanta), 188
Westmoreland, John, 4
Westmoreland, Willis F., 14, 16
Wheat Street Baptist Church (Atlanta), 183
White, Goodrich C., 136
White, John, 129
White, Louella, 137
White, Paul Dudley, 157
White, Walter, 107–108
Whitley, Richard J., 198
Wilkins, Roy, 185
Willard, Frances, 95
William A. Harris Hospital. *See* Harris Memorial Hospital
Williams, Dick, 242, 243
Williams, Sam, 265
Wilson, Bob, 228
Wilson, Charles, 11
Wilson, Frank, 146, 165, 166, 172, 180, 191, 192
Wilson, Frank L., Jr., 244
Winecoff Hotel, 146
Withorn, Abner Calhoun, 64
Wofford, Leon D., 129
Woman's Day, 218
Woman's Hospital (New York City), 64
Wooding, W. J., 57
Wood, J. W., 7
Wood, R. Hugh, 137, 149, 150, 152, 173, 174, 178, 179
Woodruff, Ernest, 116, 119, 130
Woodruff, Mrs. Robert W., 145
Woodruff, Robert W., 139, 143, 145, 146, 148, 149, 151, 166, 171
Woodward, A. J., 16
Woodward, C. Vann, 25
Woodward, James G., 51, 81
Works, George A., 119
World Health Organization (WHO), 197, 218
World War I, 58, 83, 84–85, 110, 166–167
World War II, 58, 135, 137, 140, 143, 148, 156, 234
Worley, Gwendolyn, 67, 68
Wright, Frank Lloyd, 53
Wright, Jackson, Brown, Williams & Stephens, Inc., 208
Wright, Louis T., 172
Wyatt, Clarice Marijetta, 184

Y

Yale University, 140, 142
Yancey, Asa, 175, 179, 187, 189, 191, 211, 221, 226, 236–237
Yates and Milton Drug Store, 167
Yates, Clayton R., 167, 177, 207, 212
yellow fever, 9
   Epidemic of 1878, 9–10, 11, 30
Young, Andrew, 196, 213, 228, 264

Z

Zeegen, Susie, 198
Ziegler, Peg, 216